Over Fifty-Five, Healthy and Alive

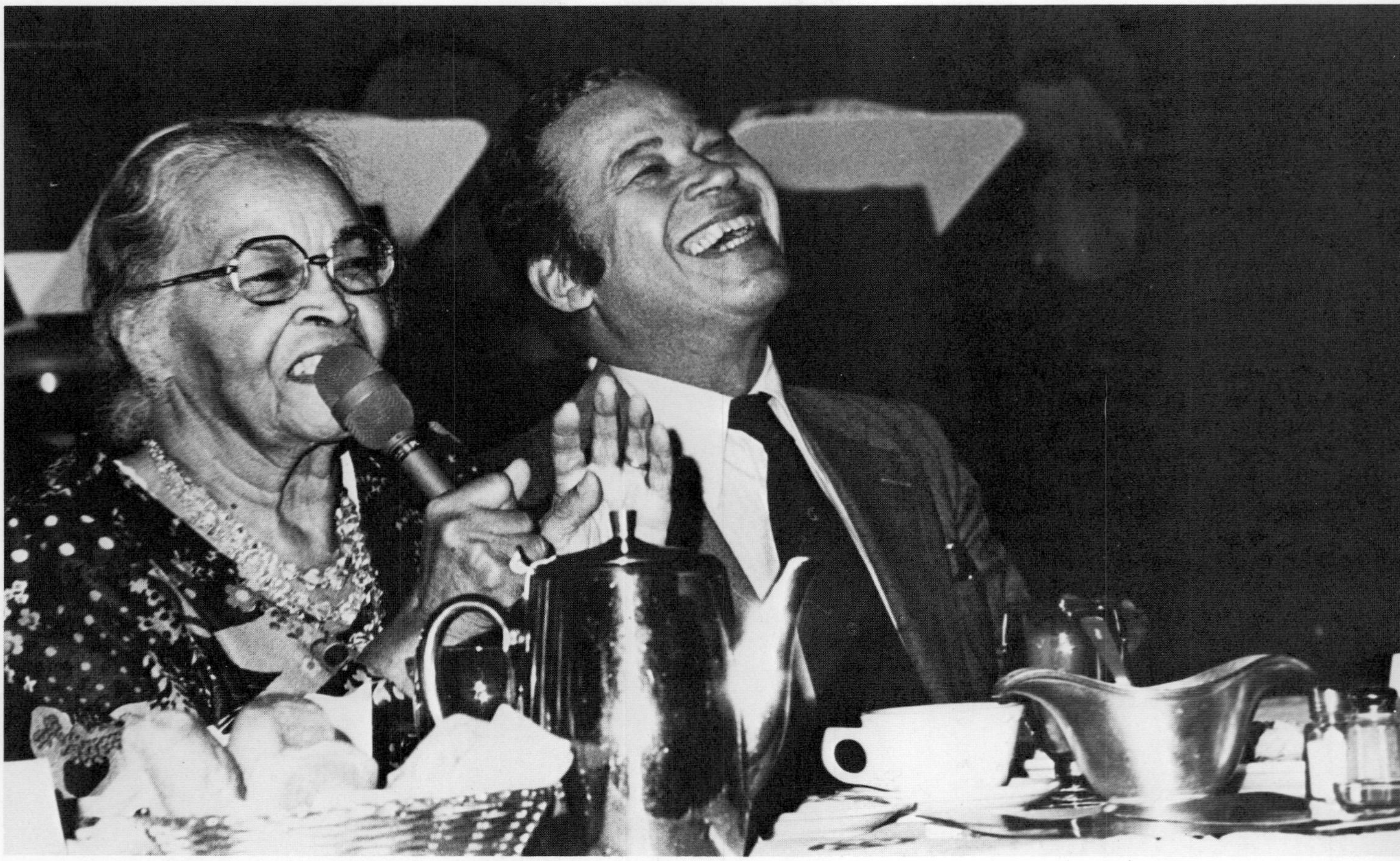

Over Fifty-Five, Healthy and Alive

A Health Resource For the Coming of Age

Hank Pizer, Editor

VAN NOSTRAND REINHOLD COMPANY
NEW YORK CINCINNATI TORONTO LONDON MELBOURNE

To the memory of my father, Harry Lewis Pizer

Library of Congress Catalog Card Number 82-2725

ISBN 0-442-27425-4 (cloth)
ISBN 0-442-27424-6 (paper)

Printed in the United States of America

Designed by Joyce Duffy

Photographs, unless otherwise noted: *Boston Seniority*, Betty Barry

Illustrations, unless otherwise noted: Peggy Clark

Published by Van Nostrand Reinhold Company Inc.
135 West 50th Street
New York, New York 10020

Fleet Publishers
1410 Birchmount Road
Scarborough, Ontario M1P 2E7, Canada

Van Nostrand Reinhold Australia Pty. Ltd.
480 Latrobe Street
Melbourne, Victoria 3000, Australia

Van Nostrand Reinhold Company Limited
Molly Millars Lane
Wokingham, Berkshire, England RG11 2PY

16 15 14 13 12 11 10 9 8 7 6 5 4 3 2 1

Library of Congress Cataloging in Publication Data
Main entry under title:

Over fifty-five, healthy and alive.

Includes index.
1. Middle age—Health and hygiene. 2. Aged—Care and hygiene. 3. Geriatrics. I. Pizer, Hank. [DNLM: 1. Geriatrics—Popular works. WT 100 096]
RA777.5.093 613′.0434 82-2725
ISBN 0-442-27425-4 AACR2
ISBN 0-442-27424-6 (pbk.)

Contents

Acknowledgments

My deepest appreciation to: Barbara Ravage, our editor, who worked extensively on the book; Alan Rinzler, who helped make the book possible; Stella Pizer, for her work in helping compile interviews; Dr. Carol Sawka, who worked on the neurology section; Dr. Michael Glenn, for helping read the manuscript; Dr. William Thomas, for his help with the section on death and dying; Julie Rubin at Massachusetts Eye and Ear; the Joslyn Diabetes Center; Sarah Bachrach, for helping with the nursing home interviews; The Age Page; Boston Seniority; The American Red Cross; The American Cancer Society; The American Heart Association; and Pat Knisely, RD, who helped with the nutrition section.

Foreword

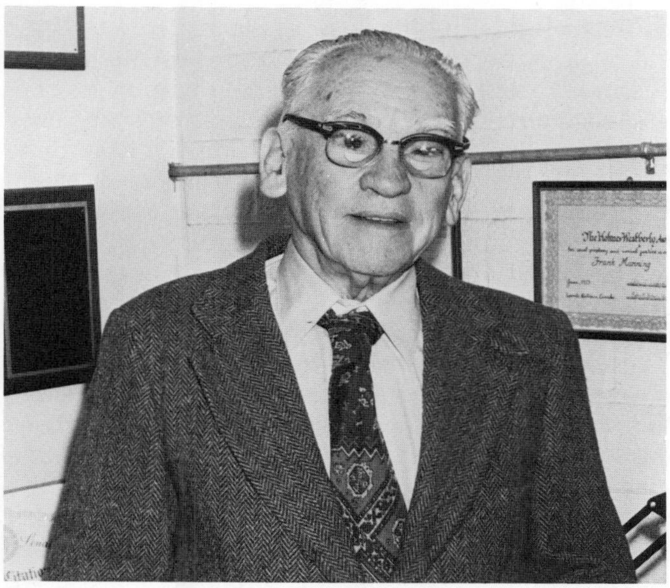

In the twentieth century, a rapid and unprecedented change occurred in America and other industrialized countries that profoundly affected the senior population. Mandatory retirement and the separation of many people from their communities and jobs created, for some, great hardships. This became an enormous challenge for all of us—young and old. We saw a need for the organization of older people to deal with this challenge.

The Massachusetts Association of Older Americans started in 1968 at a time when urban renewal was displacing thousands of elders without adequately providing alternate housing. It seemed to us that the creators of urban renewal were so obsessed with blueprints and demolition that they did not take the time to determine the impact on senior citizens. We began to deal with this change, as well as with problems like safety, health care, and nutrition. In short, we began to form a community life for all of us.

Americans first learned of the need to organize senior citizens during the Great Depression of the 1930s. Francis Townsend called for granting two hundred dollars a month to all seniors. The overwhelming response by thousands of people in favor of the measure did more to reveal the growth of the older population than any other single event that I can think of. Many people around the country were amazed: Americans had not realized that a crisis had developed because we, as elders, had been silent. Many of us, of course, have now broken that silence, but the need to advocate our desires remains.

The great social movements of the 1930s paved the way for Social Security, the forty-hour week, unemployment insurance, and bank savings insurance. Later the Older Americans Act, which set up nutrition, research, employment, transportation, health care, legal, and consumer programs for older people, became the Magna Carta for senior citizens. This has provided an open-ended call for social services and the widening of our access to quality health care.

This brings me to an extremely important issue: the future of health care for older Americans. Long-term care is the knottiest problem, since it is the most expensive, yet serves only 5 or 6 percent of us at any one time. We need to rearrange our priorities and allocate funds in a way that reflects the needs of all of us. This does not necessarily mean cuts in long-term care; it does mean finding ways to deliver this care. We need more services for people outside of institutional settings and a greater emphasis on preventive care.

There is also a shortage of nurses, physicians, and other medical practitioners skilled in geriatric care. The House Committee on Aging under Congressman Claude Pepper found that at least 80,000 nurses are needed and that very few doctors and nurses fully understand some of the symptoms and illnesses that affect seniors. I do not advocate a separate branch of medicine, but it is essential that better training in the subspecialty of geriatrics be provided in medical schools.

A problem of attitudes exists as well. Whenever a doctor tells me, "What do you expect at your age?" I tell him that I expect to get another doctor. A doctor who is a friend would not pose such a question. We need a more positive outlook from our medical care givers, so that all of our potential can be maximized as we age. Life for us should not be considered limited.

As the historian Arnold Toynbee pointed out, those societies that care for and consult with their elders are the most humane and most advanced. We must realize that older people cannot be separated from society. I am speaking now not only for the elderly, but for the young of today, who will one day become seniors. For this reason everything we do now touches upon the lives of all of us—young and old.

The quality of one's life depends to a great extent on what we know about our health and the efforts we make in taking good care of our bodies. Even with all of the advances in medical technique, the ultimate responsibility for good health lies within each of us. We should learn more about ourselves and our bodies, and we should make every effort to promote better health through the way in which we live. For this reason, a book such as this, designed to help us take better care of our bodies and be better consumers when we need health services, is an important step in a positive direction.

FRANK J. MANNING
President, Massachusetts Association of Older Americans

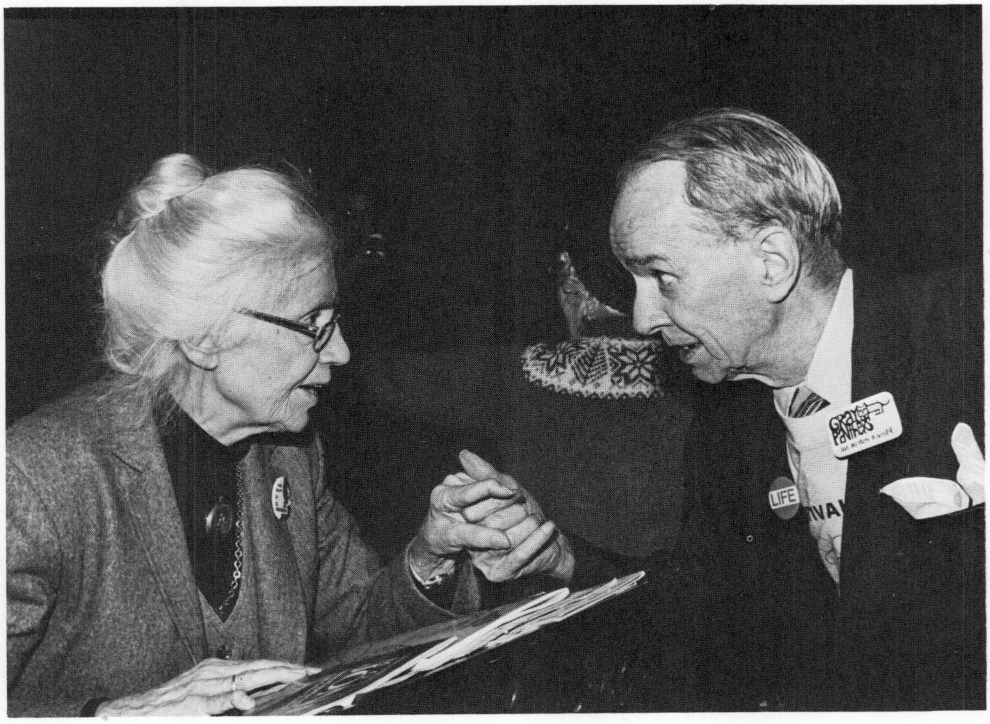

“I did not even think much about politics for most of my life. I was kind of a happy-go-lucky guy who was running around the country. I did not worry about who was president or governor. In fact, I did not vote until I was in Chicago. Mayor Daley, of course, was in charge then. I was a bartender. It behooved me to vote for Mr. Daley, as it behooved 'most anyone to vote for him, if you lived in Chicago. I voted, but I was still not interested in politics.

I became interested in politics when I could no longer work. I could not drive a cab or a truck, and I came to a nursing home. The first inkling I had of making any statements in public on political matters was when a gentleman told me he was starting an organization called LIFE—Living Is For The Elderly.

He wondered why we did not have any political organization in all of the nursing homes in the state. We had no way of influencing how we lived. There was no way of voicing our feelings about what was good and what was bad. I agreed, and we began to organize others.

I try to encourage others to take an active role in political life. I tell them that you have to get interested in something. You don't want to only eat and sleep and then go back to bed. Getting interested in something makes for a better life, and you won't feel sorry for yourself. I explain that it worked in my case and that I expect it will work in theirs.

As president of LIFE, I attend the meetings and find out what bills are going into the legislature that affect elderly people. Our politicians need our encouragement in order to be able to argue for us. They need to see a thousand letters in favor of a particular bill or to receive telephone calls.

All the politicians will say that they are for the elderly. I have never heard any say that they want to reduce benefits for seniors, but nevertheless, if we are going to vote, we should do it for someone we are sure of. That means meeting them and knowing their views before they get into office.

My political work has also helped me personally. It has given me something to have on my mind and has kept me mentally aware. Rather than just thinking about my troubles or physical ailments, I find that it keeps me happy and involved.”

—Roy Smith, 75

Introduction

The notion of what people over fifty-five can and should do is undergoing a monumental change in Western society. We are discarding the negative stereotypes that link aging with isolation, unhappiness, lack of productivity, and decline, and we are becoming aware of its true vitality. This is long overdue. Ageism, like racism, sexism, and other prejudices, disappears slowly and only through major efforts to change society.

Aging means changing on a personal level. Part I of this book speaks to these changes: how our bodies change; new ways of looking at marriage, family, and friends; sexuality; being a wise consumer; and looking at our own mortality.

Throughout this book, we have tried to formulate a new image for aging. In doing so we ran into the inevitable problem of having only old words to describe a new concept. Senior citizen, retiree, elder—all convey in some way the negative stereotype that we are trying to change.

After great deliberation I came up with the term *older*. But our editor was quick to point out that this is not grammatically correct. "You have to be older than someone or something," she said. And though I replied, "Over fifty-five," she was still not satisfied.

She is, of course, correct. So, throughout the book, when you see *older*, please forgive our grammatical error. Keep in mind that our language reflects our prejudices and we have yet to find a vibrant word to describe people over fifty-five. Perhaps we can think of one together.

Part I

Changing

From the time of conception until death, the body undergoes a normal aging process. It is unfortunate that this normal process is viewed negatively by our society. We focus on loss of vigor, rather than emphasizing experience. We look upon aging as unsightly and asexual, rather than as beautiful and romantic.

For instance, there is a commonly held prejudice that people lose their vitality as they grow older. Nothing is further from the truth. The United States Department of Commerce estimates that 47 percent of the men and 38 percent of the women over sixty-five (more than nine million people) exercise regularly. Most people in this age group have no limitation of their physical abilities, and the number who try vigorous activities is increasing steadily.

In addition, we have adopted the notion that older people are poor, socially withdrawn, and economically unproductive. This too is mistaken. The per capita income of people from fifty-five to sixty-four and of those over sixty-five rose faster in the last decade than for all other groups, except those in the forty-five to fifty-four range. Moreover, rather than withdrawing from society, people who have retired from successful careers are finding new careers at an unprecedented rate. And, only 5 percent of the people over sixty-five are in institutional living situations. Seventy-one percent live in their own homes, support their communities, and have no loss of mental function. In other words, they are active, independent people.

Since the turn of the century, the average life expectancy of Americans has increased by approximately twenty-six years. A similar increase is seen throughout the Western nations and, to a lesser extent, in other countries as well. It is estimated that more people over sixty-five are living today than have been on earth throughout the rest of history. Moreover, the growth of an older segment of the population will continue into the next century.

The upper limit of human life, however, apparently remains unchanged. In other words, the number of people living beyond age sixty-five has increased, but the number of people living past one hundred has not. If you are seventy-five now, you have about the same chance of living until seventy-six as you did a century ago.

The medical community is consequently shifting its emphasis from prolonging life to improving it for older people. The goal is to find ways to help people live better, without crippling disease, pain, or limitation. It is hoped that aging will not have to mean ailing.

Chapter 1
How We Change with Age

Hank Pizer, PA-C

Understanding the aging process throughout nature helps us to understand human aging. We should begin by realizing that, of all the mammals, humans live the longest. In this sense we have been the most successful in adapting to the stresses of nature. This adaptation has made us exceedingly complex in our biological makeup and our social organization.

Among mammals the Indian elephant comes closest to our life span, attaining about sixty years. The rhinoceros and horse can live perhaps forty years. Whales have even shorter spans. Only the great tortoises of the Pacific and some species of birds may outlive us, and they rarely do so in the wild. In nature even the smallest degree of slowing or loss of strength usually means death, as animals fall prey to their natural enemies.

We are different, however, in that we have designed an elaborate social structure to support us as we age. Society provides housing, sanitation, transportation, and medical devices like hearing aids, glasses, and dentures to help us live longer. Thus, human aging is a social process as well as a biological one. Other social factors may, on the other hand, detract from our fullest potential longevity. Eating and drinking to excess, environmental pollution, crime, overcrowding, and stress are all negative forces that contribute to premature death. The more we learn about the interaction of society and biology, the harder it is to separate the good from the bad or to be able to accurately quantify the effects of all the potential forces acting on us.

For instance, presbycusis is the medical term for the loss of hearing that often occurs with advancing years. Some loss is probably part of aging, yet we also know that noise pollution greatly aggravates hearing loss. This means loud noises at work, on the subway or bus, in our cars when we travel, in our daily lives in the city. It is hard to know where biology stops and environment takes over.

Longevity

Each living cell has a genetic clock programmed by its DNA that determines its ideal longevity. This clock differs for every species and explains in part why horses live longer than fish, fish live longer than butterflies, and so on. From the biologist's point of view, aging can be seen in the cell of every organism. Some scientists feel that certain essential chemicals within the cell are lost in the course of aging. Some cells, such as those in the muscles and the brain, contain very long-lived, but irreplaceable, chemicals. When these chemicals are lost or damaged, the cell dies, and it, in turn, cannot be replaced. Other researchers believe that cell death (and therefore aging) results from errors in the DNA that occur during cell division and reproduction. Whereas we do not yet know the precise biological mechanism of cell aging, it is clear that each of us has an internal clock that ticks off time from the moment of conception.

But longevity depends on more than just what happens to the cell or its DNA. Even if medicine cannot help us live beyond the upper limit of our cells' potential, our life-style can help or hinder our ability to approach that biological ideal. Right now considerable debate exists about what the upper limit is. Some scientists believe that it is over one hundred, whereas others contend that, for most of us, it is between eighty and ninety.

Medicine, however, still looks at death as the outcome of a specific illness. Dying of old age is not an acceptable cause on the death certificate and not part of the accepted curriculum of medical training. Yet the majority of us probably do die of old age. Someone who is eighty-five and dies of heart disease may actually have died of old age. The entire body was aging, but the heart was simply the first essential part to fail completely. In the near future, medicine will probably change its view of longevity, and death for people in their eighties and nineties may once again be considered the result of old age.

Throughout this book emphasis will be placed on ways in which all of us can control and improve the quality of our lives. Some of the insights come from studying other cultures, where people remain active and relatively free of limitation in later years. Other knowledge comes from our increasing understanding of what causes disease in our society. All of the contributors have tried to focus on the simple and practical things that you can do to improve your body and sense of well-being, independent of your chronological age. We have tried to avoid any expression, implicit or explicit, of the pat medical phrase, "What do you expect at your age?"

Clearly, exercise and nutrition are areas in which everyone over fifty-five can take positive steps. Studies of other cultures and of laboratory animals have demonstrated that *eating less,* maintaining a *lean* body and low weight, and getting some *regular* form of exercise are very important. Also essential are social factors like reducing stress levels and finding interesting and absorbing activities. People over fifty-five can remain active, even in the face of specific medical problems like arthritis, poor vision, or diabetes. With professional help and personal desire, you can find ways to adapt your life-style so that you can enjoy many kinds of activities. That is what is so special about human beings. We can adapt to many kinds of losses, both physical and emotional, and still find ways to create, change, and fulfill ourselves.

❝ Lillian and Charles are an example of a marriage that continues to work after thirty-five years. As she says, "It is no easy task." I think that anyone who has been in a long relationship knows that. It takes flexibility and a mutual commitment. Of the many interviews I did for this book, I was particularly struck by these qualities in Lillian and Charles's relationship. Moreover, their bonds seem to have gotten stronger over the years.

Making a marriage work means adapting to many stages of life together. They, for example, worked through the stresses of separation during World War II, building a business and a family, and now, retirement. Lillian stayed home raising the children for many years, although she says that she wished she could have worked. When the children were old enough, she returned to the business world. Charles accepted and respected that need.

As in all families, each child is different. Their son now lives with a young woman who has a child from a previous marriage. They accept this and are very loving to the youngster. Their daughter is a professional photographer who has an independent life-style. For awhile she lived in California, but despite the great distance they continued to have a close relationship with her. I think the movements and changes that their children have gone through have demanded great flexibility from Lillian and Charles. Families now must adjust to divorce, relocation, and relating to children from previous marriages. Lillian and Charles seem to have done this, and they maintain a warm, caring relationship with their children.

Lillian and Charles seem to enjoy each other and their retirement. They play tennis, bridge, and golf together and take classes to learn new things. They share a similar outlook on the world. After thirty-five years their relationship continues to grow.

LILLIAN: We're both retired now, and we really like being with each other. Retirement has given us more time to do things together, like play bridge; and we learned tennis and golf together.

CHARLES: I've always admired Lillian. She is a great cook, housekeeper, and entertainer. We take courses together and share the same political views. Over the years things have gotten better, especially now that there is more time to enjoy things. I have been lucky in that, at age sixty-six, my health is good.

LILLIAN: I'm sixty-three and pretty fit, except that I need a cataract operation. I miss many more balls when I play tennis, and I have to look at cards very closely to play bridge.

I am anxious to have the surgery over with and get back my normal eyesight. I found out I had this problem when my left eye started to hemorrhage. There wasn't any pain, but my vision all of a sudden got very shadowy and distorted. I was pretty scared, and it was important that I had Charlie to help me.

CHARLES: My life, I think, has been fairly typical of the men my age. I started to work when I was in junior high school, wrapping packages on Saturday in a shoe store. I also worked in a factory, where I made twelve dollars a week. Later I became a bookkeeper in a landscaping firm.

I graduated from high school in 1933. That was the Depression. I was in business selling newspapers, cigarettes, and soda. I did this until 1941, when I went back to the factory as an assistant foreman. They were making defense items for the war, and it was possible to make good money. Just before that I had tried operating a gas station for awhile, but gas was rationed so I couldn't stay with it.

We got married in 1942. I was supporting my parents, so I was classified 3A. My father had had an auto repair and radio shop from 1920 to 1938, but times had gotten tough, and he just couldn't make a living from it.

Then, in April, 1943, I was drafted and sent to China. I was there from November, 1943 to December, 1945. At the time I thought the army was terrible, but as it worked out, I didn't get to see much action. We were behind the Japanese lines for about six months, and I got amebic dysentery. It was awful. We had only sulfa pills for treatment, and they didn't work. I had been trained in artillery but was retrained in radio operations. Most of all I missed home and Lillian.

LILLIAN: I graduated from high school and got a job as a secretary. I earned eight dollars a week for a five-and-a-half-day week. To get to work, I had to walk from Mount Vernon to the subway in the Bronx. It was two-and-a-half miles each way. I remember that they took eight cents out of my pay for Social Security.

My brother was a brilliant student and went to City College. But he only lasted for six months because my father made him quit. He said that college was making him "talk radical." I did not like my father. He was cruel. He left the family one time. I loved my mother, who was a good person. In spite of my feelings, my father liked me.

When Charlie went into the army, I wrote him every night. Very often I had nothing to say, but I wrote anyway. Once I got a picture of Charlie in a Chinese guerrilla uniform.

CHARLES: Lillian's letters came all at once, when I could get mail. In the army you couldn't count on those things.

When I got back home we took an apartment. I tried to go back to school at N.Y.U., in engineering. Lillian had saved some money, and I had my back pay. It was a few thousand dollars.

LILLIAN: Our son was born in 1946, and we had a daughter in 1948. Our son was an easy child to raise, even though he had encephalitis. It was a mild case, and he turned out to be fine. Our daughter was more difficult to raise. She was her own mother. By that I mean that she was headstrong and always had her own way of doing things.

I was bored to death with the mother role. But I loved the children. I had wanted a family, and I'm basically a flexible person. So I accepted it and stayed home for fifteen years.

CHARLES: In 1949 I bought into a gas station. In 1957 I bought into a garage with a partner, and we got along very well. Business was good and I stayed on until I retired five years ago. There were many economic advantages to keeping the business, but at sixty-one I felt that I had had enough. I was anxious to retire and do other things.

LILLIAN: I went back to work after fifteen years at home. At first I got a temporary job, and then, when I got my speed back as a stenographer, I took a full-time job. I liked having my own money.

I retired at fifty-eight, when Charlie did. It was something we decided to do together. We take courses together and play together. I also feel like I want to take care of Charlie. I love my children and don't think that we will have any grandchildren. When my son's marriage broke up after six years, I felt very sad and hurt. But now he is with someone whom I like, and we love her child.

Sometimes I think of what it would be like if I were left alone. I feel that I would be able to be strong and independent, but that is not what I want to have happen.

CHARLES: Now I want to take care of Lillian. If I were left alone, I would feel a deep loss. I would be very lonely. After all, we have gone through so much of life together. But I try to think about the things to do now, and to have more to do with the time we have. ❞

Interview and comment
—Stella Young Pizer, 65

Aging in the Human Body

In recent years interest in the normal aging process has increased. Medical scientists want to better understand disease and to help devise ways of maximizing human potential. Individuals want to find strategies to cope with particular problems and to extend themselves in new directions.

A variety of coping strategies can be used to enhance our life-styles. We can wear glasses, use amplification for hearing, improve our control (rather than speed and strength) in sports, learn to lift and carry things with the correct posture, design our homes and workplaces for optimal safety and productivity. In this context the way we change in our bodies does not have to decrease our ability to produce and enjoy. Even with such difficult or restricting medical problems as cataracts, coping strategies can be developed.

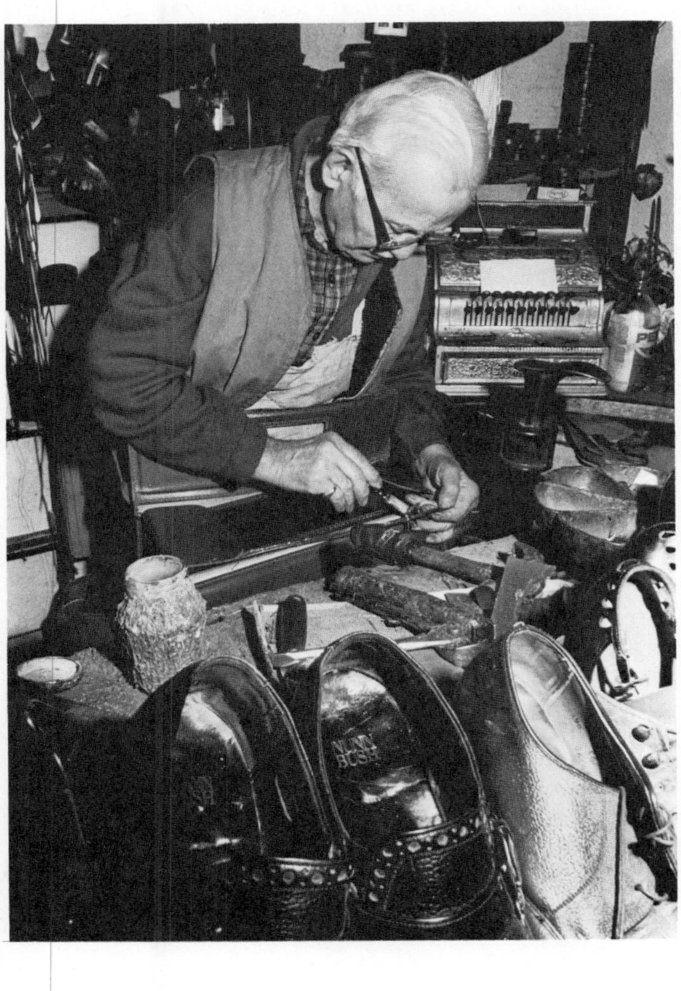

The Senses

Of all our senses, seeing is perhaps the most dear to us. Age brings changes in our vision, the most familiar of which is a stiffening of the lens of the eye, which results in difficulty seeing objects that are close. The lens also tends to cloud as we age, so that less light passes through the eye to the retina. Both of these changes are gradual processes that begin early in life, but we usually do not notice them until we are in our late forties or fifties. By age sixty most of us should wear glasses to help us see close objects and should provide ourselves with adequate illumination when we work and drive.

Along with the clouding of the lens comes a change in our color perception that most of us do not notice. Our ability to appreciate the "cool" colors of green and blue decreases because these wavelengths are filtered out to a degree by the dense lens. Because of this, the "warm" colors, the reds and yellows, tend to stand out in contrast.

Changes also take place in our hearing as we age. This too is a normal process, called presbycusis. Loudness is measured scientifically in decibels; approximately 20 to 30 percent of all people over sixty-five have a hearing loss of at least fifteen to twenty-five decibels. A loss of as many as thirty decibels is considered a very mild impairment, affecting only the ability to understand whispered speech or the rustling of leaves. But many may have a greater loss and experience difficulty hearing and understanding speech. You should be conscious of this; have your hearing checked if you find that you frequently turn up the television or think that people are mumbling. Normal hearing is critical for safety—to hear cars, people calling to us, and hundreds of other stimuli. Further discussion of hearing and hearing loss can be found in Chapter 11, *The Ears, Nose, and Throat.*

We do not know as much about the changes in our senses of touch, taste, and smell. These senses apparently remain fairly well intact for most people. Any change, therefore, should not be dismissed as normal. It may in fact be a sign of diabetes or some other medical problem that can be treated. These other senses are also important for our safety and well-being, so if you notice a change, you should seek medical advice.

The Heart and Lungs

Diseases of the heart, blood vessels, and lungs are still our number one killers. Scientists know a lot about the aging of these systems, yet it is still extremely difficult to separate normal aging from what we create by smoking, overeating, and living sedentary lives, from air pollution and other environmental factors. Moreover, basic assumptions within the medical profession are changing. For example, atherosclerosis (the depositing of fatty substances in the arteries) used to be considered a normal part of aging, but now that view is under question.

In the early 1960s, scientists began to study non-Western people in an effort to understand how they age. It was discovered that these people often had little evidence of atherosclerosis and coronary artery disease. The Masai of Africa, who eat a diet composed primarily of milk, meat, and blood, were found to maintain an incredibly high level of heart and lung function. In their later lives, they remained lean, did not have high blood pressure, and continued to be able to exercise to a degree generally unheard of in older Americans. Although many of them had parasitic infections, the older men could often perform treadmill tests with an endurance equal to that of a young Olympic athlete.

This kind of data revealed that exercise, smoking, air and water quality, and the type of work we do, as well as diet, are factors in how the heart and lungs age. No single factor or pattern can explain why we get heart disease, strokes, or other circulatory and respiratory problems. There are, however, identifiable *risk factors* such as high blood pressure, smoking, and obesity. We can minimize these negative influences by making positive changes in our life-style.

Most of the aging effects on the heart and lungs may be observed when we try to exercise strenuously. Our maximum heart rate declines and the overall ability of the heart to work up to maximum potential is decreased. For most of us, blood pressure also increases, which further increases the work that the heart must do to pump blood. All of this can be improved, *at any age,* with regular, vigorous exercise. If you have not exercised regularly for some time, you must begin slowly and gradually. But you can still work your way up to a strenuous program, whatever your age. Athletes over sixty-five often show heart and lung function comparable to, or better than, more sedentary people in their twenties and thirties.

People who exercise regularly have less coronary artery disease and lower blood pressure, and their hearts are better able to withstand stress. If they do get heart disease, it is usually less severe and occurs later in life. You will find a full discussion of what this means and how to start an exercise program in Part 2, *Body Maintenance.*

Other Organs

Changes in the kidneys, liver, muscles, intestine, and hormone systems have been documented by physiologists who study aging. Yet, in most cases, these systems function normally until we are in our eighties. The aging of these organs affects how we metabolize drugs; therefore these effects are important for doctors to understand when prescribing medicines. Older people often require less of a medication because the drugs they take stay in the body for longer periods of time.

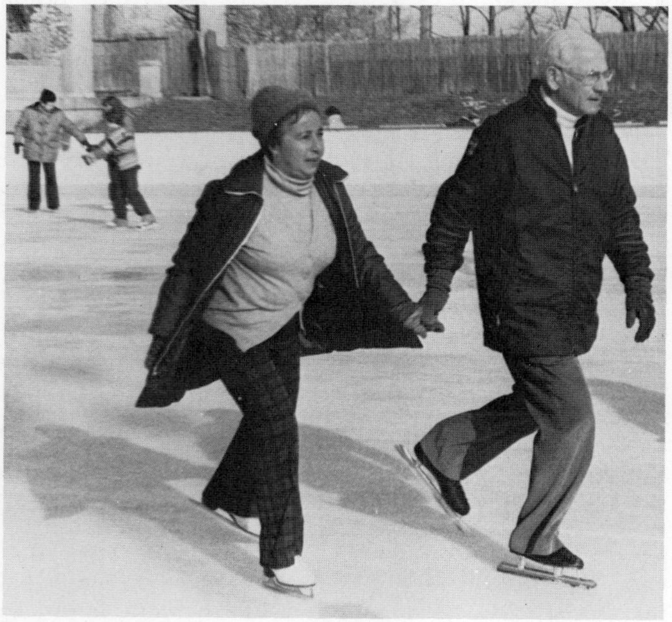

In most situations the changes associated with aging in these organs do not impair function. Constipation, for instance, is more likely to be related to poor diet and lack of exercise than to the aging of the intestine. Similarly, although we all lose some ability to metabolize sugar, diabetes is not a normal outcome of aging. The complications of eye and nerve degeneration that may accompany diabetes should not be considered normal aging either; they demand medical attention.

Mental Functioning

Normal aging does not mean that we lose our mental abilities. As a society, we tend to think of seniors as slow of mind or forgetful, and often condemn them for living in the past. These are perhaps the most devastating and unfair social stereotypes confronting older people. And, of course, none of them is true. Senility is a disease, an *abnormal* process, just like heart disease or arthritis.

Of numerous studies on mental functioning of older people, only those involving a timed test show a decline in mental ability with added years. Those tests draw an unfair and therefore inaccurate comparison, since younger people, closer to school experience, are more accustomed to taking tests. In addition, older people may be more conscious of being accurate on tests and try harder to work slowly and deliberately. Without illness, mental functioning does not decline with age.

Older workers generally have fewer accidents, demonstrate better attendance at work, make fewer mistakes, and usually have superior work records. The leaders of most industries and professions tend to be people over fifty-five. It is hoped that the practice of mandatory retirement at sixty-five, or at any age, will die out, like other antiquated notions about aging. People who want to retire should have that option, but healthy, vigorous, competent people should continue to work as long as they want. They are extremely productive for society and represent a lifetime of accumulated experience and wisdom.

Sexuality

Older people are also unjustly stereotyped as asexual or unattractive. Women usually go through menopause and become infertile between ages forty-five and fifty-five. Despite other physiological changes in the female genitalia, however, the clitoris is not affected by this physiological change and women continue to be capable of orgasm. A woman of eighty is as able to attain orgasm as a woman of twenty. In fact some women report increased sexual drive after menopause, possibly because they no longer need be concerned about birth control. Neither hysterectomy (surgical removal of the uterus) nor mastectomy (removal of the breast) prevent a woman from having an orgasm or enjoying sex.

Men do not undergo a physiological menopause, although age-related changes do occur in the male reproductive system. Men usually remain capable of producing children well into their seventies, and some men have produced children in their nineties. Men do tend to attain erections more slowly and to maintain them longer with advancing years. This does not mean that sexual relationships are not pleasurable. Impotence in an older man should not be considered a normal part of aging and deserves a complete medical investigation by a urologist.

One of the most devastating messages concerning aging is that older people are not physically attractive. This is particularly unfortunate for older women, who are rarely portrayed as beautiful by the media. This kind of negative image makes it more difficult for people to continue to have sexual feelings.

Moreover, it is still considered inappropriate for older men and women to be sexual. Adult children often send out the message that their parents either are, or should be, asexual. Open displays of affection are often thought to be embarrassing. And since many women outlive their spouses and we continue to have prohibitions about sex out of wedlock, older women are often unnecessarily forced into celibacy.

“ I am fifty-five years old, a young-looking and -feeling person. I am very energetic, involved in sports, politics and intellectual pursuits, as I have always been. As Satchel Paige said, "I don't know how old I would be if I didn't know how old I was."

My social life has remained active since my divorce in 1976. My friends have asked, "How come you are so busy? You're not a beautiful woman." I feel that I am only moderately attractive, but I get to meet people because I am sincerely interested in them. My male partners pick that up, I think, and find it attractive. I meet people by being out in the community, doing what I want to do. I have never gone to singles bars and go out only with people whom I want to go out with. I tend to go out most weekends, and that feels good.

I have not gotten into a permanent relationship since my divorce. But I have been meeting good people and had long and satisfying relationships. I am pleased that I have maintained friendships with the men I no longer date. That is what is important to me. I do not want to become permanently attached out of a compromise. I want to find someone whom I feel good enough about to say, "This is exactly where I want to be, no more new male relationships." Until that time, I will just assume that I will continue to have an active and diverse social life.

I guess in my world, conventions have not hampered the process of forming new relationships. I am a mixture of both unconventional and traditional values. I am not afraid of sex, and I am willing to take a risk and fail. Sexual demands have not been a problem, but I would just as soon participate in choosing to have the sexual relationship. I do not go to bed with anyone whom I do not want to do it with, but sometimes it is just like another part of a date. You just try it out.

I think that most women have not had good sexual relationships. That goes for women who are thirty as well as women who are sixty. They are still playing the game of having to please a man, so that he will like them and continue to ask them out. I think that some part of all of us thinks that it is a coupled world. We want to have a mate to go to the movies with, or to the museum, or to dinner. I have found that it is worthwhile to try to change that feeling, and I have not lost my old friends who are in couples because of it. I entertain as I did before.

I came out of my marriage, like many others, feeling somewhat insecure about new relationships. I was concerned with wanting to please, and I had some hit-and-miss sexual relations. It was not an overwhelming number either way. If I met someone and I was very attracted to him, that was great. But, if my interest waned or I was not taken with him, I discovered that I could not find satisfaction in the sexual relationship.

There is no relationship between the size of a man's penis, or his age, and my sexual feelings. I hope that men understand this and feel the same way about it. I have now gone out with men aged forty to over sixty, and the man whom I had the best sexual relationship with was sixty-two. Once you get to know each other, both men and women realize that we do not judge the quality of our sexual relationships on the basis of the number of orgasms the man has, or how many orgasms he thinks I have. Early in the relationship, my friend said, "Look, it may take you an hour to get ready for me, because this is new and we are just getting to know each other." I was always guilty about taking, feeling that someone else was working hard to give. And it did take half an hour at first. Now it only takes five or ten minutes. This is new to me, not only since my marriage, but just new.

Sometimes I find it hard to believe that I have gone through as many emotional changes as I have. For all of this, I feel more in control of myself and more fulfilled. It has been, in some ways, growth through pain, because it has not always been easy. I am living a rich life, certainly so since my divorce. If things stopped right now and I had to deal with something very negative, I would not forget all the good things that have happened. Being a single person has given me more self-confidence. Having what I feel to be a successful present has made me more optimistic about the future.

It is often hard for divorced women to find a career. I did not have any confidence initially, and I fell into a job working with adolescents. Perhaps they were replacing my grown children who had since moved away and set up their own lives. For me this job was naturally easy but not very challenging. I worked at it for four years. Three months ago I quit and took a vacation. Now I work in the political sphere. It has always been an interest of mine. I don't know how long it will last or how well I will do with it. But I love it. I enjoyed my three months off, but I felt that I had to get back to work. If nothing else, I needed the money. There is also no question in my mind that I want to work—to have new contacts with people and to continually refresh my life through my work.

One of the biggest problems has been the financial adjustment to being single. I was very comfortable during my marriage. It took me a year to stop signing Mrs. Dr. Davis on my charge accounts. No one sees me as a doctor's wife anymore. I would like to have more money. I know that I will probably not get into a relationship with someone who has no money, but on the other hand I will never marry for money. I expect to work.

There is no question in my mind that my life continues to get better. I think that I will take most of the responsibility for that. I will give my mother credit as well. She was widowed when she was fifty and had never worked a day in her life outside of the house before that. She went off to work and remained active in the community. She seemed to me to be a living example of the ability to make it. I have thought of her often and know that I can make it if she could. I am a coper, a survivor, and I love life. ❞

—Lois Davis, 55

There is more about sexuality in Dr. Alice Rothchild's discussion about menopause in Chapter 3 and in the section on genitourinary problems of men in Chapter 17. The basic point is that, in the absence of physical illness, sexual feelings and sexual relationships are normal throughout life.

Changing Ourselves and Our Society

The more we learn about normal human aging, the more it seems clear that we have been operating under some basic misconceptions. People do not necessarily have to wither and fade away. They can remain productive and integral to society until their death. There is no basis for considering senility or loss of vigor as normal.

Whereas medical scientists and gerontologists increasingly accept this view, society will inevitably adopt it more slowly. Older people need to emphasize their own vitality. As one geriatrician put it, "Run, don't rest." The human potential to improve, to grow, and to be fulfilled exists at any age.

We need to accept interlocking of mental, emotional, and physical abilities that almost always allows us to adapt to changes that occur in aging. In many of the personal stories that appear throughout the book, people emphasize how they have continued to be active in spite of physical changes. One man points out that he played basketball until he could no longer keep up with the younger players. He then switched to volleyball and squash. He did not stop exercising; he simply changed how he did it. We should remember that humans are incredibly adaptive. Beethoven wrote his Ninth Symphony when he was almost totally deaf. Milton wrote *Paradise Lost* after losing his sight. Betty Ford challenged the social stigma of breast cancer and remains a vigorous public figure. And Agnes DeMille fought the crippling effects of a major stroke and returned to the world of dance.

❝ My first wife had cirrhosis of the liver and, in her weakened condition, picked up meningitis. This resulted in the almost complete destruction of the inside of her brain. She lived for some fifteen months, most of the time in a condition called coma vigile, which meant that, while the electroencephalogram showed no cerebral waves above the brain stem level and she was in that respect dead, enough of the cells in the outer cover of the brain were alive so that her eyes were open. She would recognize someone coming into the room, stretch out her left hand (her right side being paralyzed), and lift up her face to be kissed. She was without speech and, of course, incapable of intelligible communication.

With around-the-clock nursing, she lived for fifteen months in that condition. During that time, I renewed acquaintance with a college sweetheart who had turned me down to marry a somewhat older man. He was, at that time, already established in a successful career, while I was still facing three years of law school. Becky and I began seeing each other while Marion was in her comatose state and had progressed so far that we were privately married in Cocoa Beach some ten days after Marion's ultimate death. Although Becky and I were both in our sixties, she being two years older than I, we had twelve happy years of marriage. Our temperaments were so suited to each other that I have no recollection of ever hearing an angry word from her or uttering one myself. Our physical bonds were very close and very happy until her heart failed on January 10 of this year. Her passing was apparently painless, without any outcry, and was quite unexpected, although she had had a heart attack some six months earlier.

I am now about to get married for the third time, to my secretary, who is beautiful, talented in music, and very temperamentally suited to me. This time my intended is twenty years younger than I, but the age difference does not so far seem to be a barrier to mutual adjustment or affection.

In my lifetime I have had a coronary, now old and well healed. I have had rheumatoid arthritis, numerous kidney stones, four skin cancers, and carcinoma of the prostate. I have had my appendix removed, my gall bladder removed, and I have had two hernia operations. Nevertheless, I am still active and go to the office every day. I refuse to retire from the practice of law until my partners ask me to do so. Many years ago, when I was fired from a position with a corporation, I made up my mind to spend the rest of my life doing something I enjoyed—trying lawsuits. I still enjoy trial work, and I do not want to quit until I feel I can no longer represent clients properly.

I have always regarded a desire to remarry after the death of a spouse as a compliment to the late marriage. The happier the marriage, the more one wants to remarry. I find that work is an anodyne to the loss one suffers from the death of a spouse. A few days after the death of my last wife, I went to Denver to try a lawsuit. The absorption into the trial, the thought and energy expended, almost succeeded for a while in blocking out the otherwise dreadful sense of loss and loneliness. ❞

—Stuart Ball, Sr., 76

As a society, we need to place greater emphasis on the role of experience that aging provides. If we push people out of our workplaces, families, and communities, we will lose a major national resource. As long as people *feel useful* to others, they will continue to be useful to society.

We also need to accept a notion of normal longevity. It is unlikely that medicine will find ways to promote longer living through greater technological advances. But as individuals, we can help ourselves live longer by changing our life-styles and the society around us. That means improving the quality of our housing, air, water, places of work, personal relationships, diets, and habits. We need to accept, on the one hand, that human life is finite and, on the other, that the potential for a long and full life exists at any age. There may be an upper limit to the number of years that we live, but there is no limit to the quality of life during those years.

Chapter 2
Coping with Change and Loss

Michael L. Glenn, MD

Change is the only constant in life. As the Greek philosopher Heraclitis remarked, "We do not step into the same stream twice." Situations shift, places are altered, and people we know (including ourselves) become different as they move through life's tortuous passageways.

When we are younger, we often find change invigorating. We may rush toward it, welcoming it as a source of growth and creativity. Sometimes we even embrace change for its own sake, eager to grow up, to leave old friends and family, to see new places, meet new people, and plunge ourselves into new adventures. Youth's impetuousness finds change tantalizing.

Yet much of this only *seems* so. Change for the young may be fun when it is a matter of choice, but when change is a necessity, imposed by life's events, it is usually a harsh challenge for anyone. Young people jilted in love can be just as unhappy as their elders when they experience divorce. Children thrust into dealing with a parent's death or with the frightening upheaval of parental divorce find the experience harrowing and overwhelming. There is nothing magical about the ability of young people to cope with change and loss; nor is there anything about aging that makes coping impossible. Each stage of life has its stresses; learning to cope is the task of living. Unfortunately, change *forced* upon us by the world and time may occur more often as we age.

Change and loss are two sides of the same coin. Every change involves a loss of some kind. And every loss dictates change.

The majority of life's major changes have to do with personal relationships. This should not be a surprise, since no man is an island unto himself. Each of us lives in a world peopled by others, and we are all intimately entwined. What happens to those close to us affects us, and what happens to us affects them.

When children grow up and leave the house, parents have to adjust to the empty nest—newly silent halls, vacant bedrooms, places not set at the dinner table. When a spouse grows ill or depressed, his or her mate must adjust. The loss of a loved one creates the greatest turmoil of all. When we leave a home whose rooms enclose memories of years gone by and of people no longer with us, we find the change of life's habits a devastating experience.

There is also the change we sense in our bodies. When we lose our capacity to move about quickly or experience weakness in an arm, infirmity in the heart, or notice our lungs no longer draw air as effortlessly as they once did, we have to find a new sense of our bodies' capacity.

The phenomenon is universal. All too often, though, with aging we have to deal with these changes from a weakened or more vulnerable position. Fortunately we may draw upon our experience and wisdom, which help pad the blow of a loss. This is perhaps the greatest gift of years and our most important resource.

How we experience change and loss depends on the delicate balance of negative and positive feelings within us. Feelings of failure versus feelings of adequacy, feelings of hope versus feelings of hopelessness create the basis upon which we meet the challenge. These feelings are not solely created in late adulthood. They have developed over a lifetime.

The ability to cope depends also on how many options we really have. The more resources of loved ones, money, and skills, the more capable we are to deal with loss. There is thus an interplay between forces affecting our lives and the feelings and attitudes we have about them. It is as complex as life itself; but we should not lose sight of the fact that loss also brings the potential for growth, not just sadness.

“ The surgeon who removed my malignant breast was examining the area where the surgery was performed. He looked at me with troubled eyes. "It appears I did not get all of the tumor. I can do no more for you."

"How long will I live?"

"About six months," he said.

I became an icicle encased in a void of anxiety. How could I tell my elderly parents and my only sister, a nurse?

The night was black, long, sleepless, but not depressing. For the first time in fourteen years, I was glad my husband was not living. I called aloud in the quiet of the night, declaring, "Somewhere out there someone can and will help me."

At sunrise I dozed off to sleep. The telephone awakened me at 7:30 A.M. with a heartening message from the surgeon. "Be at the hospital at eleven. A cancer specialist with a fine reputation will see you."

The doctor I saw that morning was a kind person, whom I related to at once. I felt encouraged when he suggested that deep radiation of the involved area would no doubt be a curative treatment.

"You will have to wait several weeks before there will be a hospital bed for you. The series of treatments every week will run into two or three months."

Two months later I was admitted to a four-patient ward. The three roommates opened my mind to a world I never knew existed. They were a prostitute, a drug addict, and an alcoholic. They talked, and I learned about another side of life.

Each day I received treatments. I was strapped into a chair in a closed compartment where rays were aimed at the infected area. A monitor outside timed and regulated the therapy. Meanwhile, I occupied my mind with healing thoughts of gratitude.

Metaphysical theory was a subject I had studied, and I could accept its logic.

Despite the fatigue that accompanies radiation treatments, I needed something to occupy my mind besides my roommates. Permission was granted for me to assist in the library. There I saw a book, *Someday You Will Write*. I started a book and have been writing ever since.

A year from the day the hospital released me cured, the cancer reappeared. A series of medications were prescribed. One by one they all became ineffective, or my body would not tolerate them. Finally, after fifteen years, radiation was again necessary as a last resort. There was a question whether added radiation was advisable, but we went ahead.

After fourteen treatments a blessed event took place. I was free of malignant tissue! I hope I am forever, as the radiologist predicts. I have an unending gratitude to the dedicated, patient, understanding physician who attended and advised my program of treatments for the past sixteen years, and who helped me to my current happy state of good health.

Several times during this period I decided to give up when the side effects of the medications made me miserable. Wouldn't it have been weak and stupid to have done so? I have learned that often the goal is around the corner, but it may be hard to see.

People divide themselves into two groups: those who hug trouble or illness close to themselves as they would a loved one, and those who take a positive view and cope, with courage.

When all of this started for me, I was sixty-four. I am eighty now. Many things were different then, but I remember that it wasn't until the fear and anxiety of having a malignant tumor gradually subsided that my mind began to function. Fortunately, I chose to cope, and I have had many rich experiences as a result. My mother once told me, "Nothing is bigger than you are. The choice is yours." That applies to us in both illness and good health. ❞

—Charlotie Harndon, 80

Many of us, as we grow older, become afraid of change. We live in constant anxiety and dread lest something go wrong. Feeling less capable of adapting to change, we become enmeshed in habit and routine, clinging to what is known and predictable, as if it were protection against the changes lurking ahead. Change, far from seeming the tantalizing fruit of youth, appears as a frightening monster. Closing one's eyes may be a way of saying that it does not exist. But no one can hold back the course of time; we can, however, change our attitude toward it.

Life's Stages

All years over fifty-five are not the same, nor are these years the same for all people. Some people become ill in their fifties; others remain healthy into their ninth decade. Some lose a mate early; others live as a vibrant couple beyond their golden anniversary.

For many the decade between fifty-five and sixty-five is a good period. The last ten years of one's job may be a time of fulfillment and deep satisfaction, of advancement and responsibility. For others, however, it may be a time of fatigue, of overwork and exhaustion, and of a sense of failure at one's lack of advancement. The growth of family offers rewards and enjoyments: grandchildren, family outings, a sense of

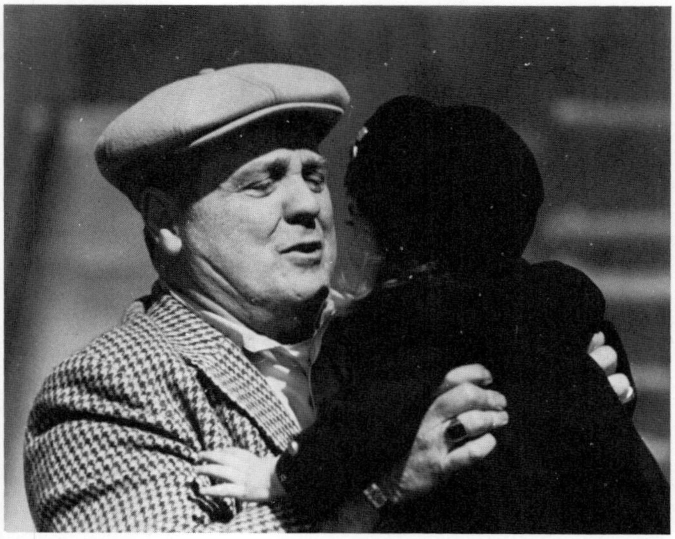

expanded personal contact and value. But those without families may feel empty. And those with sharp family conflict, bereft of warm contact with their children and close relatives, may feel a penetrating sense of loss bordering on despair.

These years are usually navigated without serious illness. With good health and an active exercise program, they can be a vigorous ten years. The mind remains sharp; the wit is quick.

The changes of menopause may affect how a woman enters this decade. The loss of the menstrual cycle does not signal the end of sexuality. Having understood this, many women enter the postmenopausal years with a deepened sense of themselves and their sexual identity.

The decade between sixty-five and seventy-five belongs to a different phase of life. For some it is a time of great happiness and a continuation of the good health and fulfillment of the previous decade. Retirement can bring new freedom, especially if one has a strong financial footing upon which to leap into new endeavors. With good health, energetic activity continues; and there is more time to enjoy interpersonal relationships.

For many, however, jarring insults may occur if change and loss rain down torrentially. We may experience the death of loved ones: wife or husband, brother or sister, close friends, and even children. Such losses are profoundly stressful events. A recent study has suggested, for instance, that 20 percent of men who lose their wives at this age will themselves die within twelve months.

Loss of a job or mate may also portend a sharp decline in one's standard of living. This may mean a change in housing, diet, and social activities. It is all too easy to become isolated from others if one cannot afford to go out or if one fears violence in the community. Inevitably this creates a loss of self-esteem. We feel helpless and hopeless—the future appears grim. We have lost our social usefulness because we no longer produce in the economic marketplace.

Facing such devastating losses, people often turn inward and act out the message of society that says they are senile or not useful. They may hesitate to involve themselves actively in social functions, parties, family events, and discussions. This is a tragic loss, not only for them, but for society as a whole. Their experience is lost forever for all of society.

The decade between seventy-five and eighty-five may be filled with further loss. The marriage surviving this far is lucky indeed. More people have developed chronic illness or disabilities and have to endure changed living arrangements. Elderly grandparents may find themselves shuttled between their children's homes, subject to the persistent anxiety of feeling in the way. Some people are even abused, much as small children may be abused, scapegoats of society's wear and tear on the entire family.

But not everyone goes through a decline after age seventy-five. Many continue to work or remain active in social and political endeavors. Every physician who treats seniors knows of people who remain incredibly active in spite of chronic illnesses like arthritis, hypertension, or diabetes. Many excellent stories deal with this period, such as Willa Cather's *The Professor's House* and Tillie Olsen's "Tell Me a Riddle."

This last stage of life presents challenges that dwarf all previous tasks and call upon reserves of understanding, patience, and acceptance to keep us moving ahead.

Even death can vary in its meaning. Two of my patients, both women in their seventies, developed terminal cancer of the colon at the same time. The first lived alone, bitter and isolated, timid and fearful. She lived her last months in an atmosphere of dejection, not really accepting her illness, but instead being occupied by a dozen different petty annoyances of life all at once—the light bill, the neighbors who made noise, and so on. Her final days were lonely and must have been an extreme hardship for her.

The other woman was quite poor, but she had a close male friend and she was loved warmly by a family of nieces. Although she went through the same stages of anger at her cancer, hope that its spread might be arrested through chemotherapy, and finally despair at her progressive decline, her last months were not empty. Instead they were filled with the support and solace of her friend and family, support she eagerly accepted and appreciated.

Strategies

Coping with any problem begins with being honest about it. It is no myth that advancing age can bring sickness and sorrow, as well as growth and enjoyment. So, let us start with the truth.

As we age, our bodies do weaken. Our organs undergo wear and tear. Hearts become less efficient. Lungs become less resilient. Our bones may thin and become more fragile. Our ability to regulate body temperature is impaired. Serious illness may affect any part of the body. And our minds may weaken, making us forgetful, less able to control emotions, more subject to worry.

Our social networks may also dissolve. We lose important people and with them parts of ourselves. We may lose our access to meaningful places—homes and towns—and to things we treasure.

Finally, we may lose certain hopes, goals, or ambitions. Ideals that had gripped us for years may suddenly appear forever beyond our grasp. We may perceive ourselves as less worthy, less valuable, less lovable.

These are profound losses, difficult to integrate and still continue with an optimistic, yea-saying attitude on life. Perhaps we should be asking how so many people manage to keep going, to keep their spirits up. What is their secret?

The answer is that the human spirit has tremendous strength and resiliency. Losses can be dealt with, and most people manage to move past them and on to other things. They come to accept what has happened and to create new goals, new relationships. Just as surely as loss occurs, people manage to endure. To be sure, no one emerges unscathed from the cauldron of loss. We are all changed, transformed by each experience. But these changes create room for growth. Touched deeply by loss and tragedy, we have the capacity to adapt and integrate our lives onto another level.

I have often heard it said that life is what you make of it. Young people are constantly telling older people to "just get more active in things" or "stop feeling sorry for yourself." I am not talking about this kind of Pollyanna attitude, which often denies the reality of people's feelings. I am talking about a challenge to all of us not to be thrown by sickness or loss, a challenge to go on with our lives, seeking meaning at each instant.

This is a matter of attitude. It has two parts: first, not to succumb to anxiety about what *might* happen; and, second, to deal honestly with whatever changes *do* take place, and to try to move ahead.

One of my patients is eighty-four. She attends a Golden Age group every day. She has many friends whom she speaks to intimately, consoles, advises, and, in general, relates to warmly. She exercises. She bowls. She plays the piano for her friends, as she has done ever since she was ten. She constantly gives of herself. She is a woman whose attitude belies the losses she has endured—that of a husband and a very close aunt with whom she lived for many years, as well as serious heart and lung disease. Without a doubt she is a model to all who know her.

Not everyone can be as outgoing, cheerful, and open as this woman. Part of the reason stems from the social

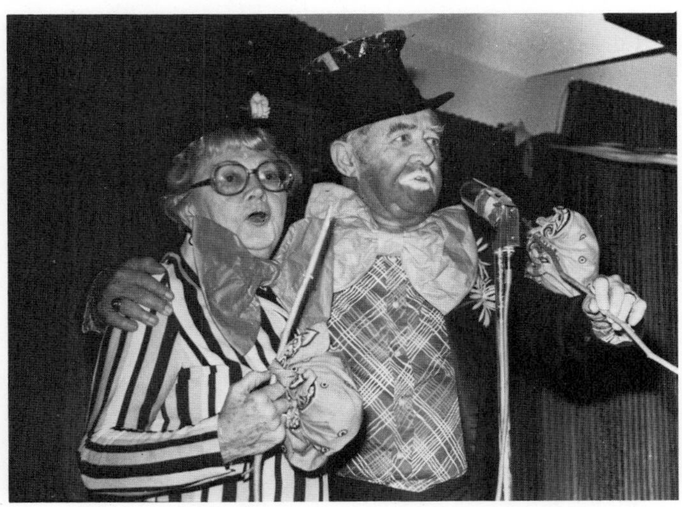

attitudes all of us grow up with. We are conditioned to fear getting older. We are afraid of dying, and we are afraid of everything that seems to bring us one step closer to death. Thus, we are uneasy around wrinkled skin, false teeth, hearing aids, wheelchairs, artificial limbs, and canes.

One way we handle fear is by denying it. This can come up as glibness regarding real misfortune, falling back on half-hearted admonitions to try harder or keep a stiff upper lip. These usually signal our own inability to deal with the problem. Denial is also the basis for free-floating anxiety. By not being clear about what we in fact have to cope with, we can create a living hell of each day—worrying about what might happen, restricting activities, giving up when we could go on. Getting past denial means beginning with the facts of one's own situation. This is the key to coping with change and loss.

Coping rests, therefore, on an honest appraisal of things. What problem has brought about the change? What options do I have for dealing with it? We can assess our strengths for dealing with adversity, as well as focusing on our weaknesses. Good health, a sense of humor, or a successful prior experience in dealing with a similar problem may be assets we can draw upon.

We can assess the support available from others. Are there family, friends, a close physician, or a minister who will help? There is no need to keep that stiff upper lip. Turn to others.

Lastly, we must look within ourselves for reasons to continue moving forward. What values do we give to life that can help combat both real and vague anxiety, as well as the depression that comes from loss?

At this point we often encounter the paradoxical answers that religion or poetry provide. Those who have lost often appear to have found much through their acceptance of life's process and an understanding of human experience. They express this in their writing, painting, music. Those who might be expected to fall apart often create a new sense of themselves through these outlets or from the appreciation of the work of others who have also suffered loss.

It is an attitude one cannot assume superficially. It has to be earned through hard struggle against adversity.

One of my patients, a woman of sixty-four, had an extremely protective husband. She was about one hundred pounds overweight and was supposed to be very fragile emotionally, having suffered two breakdowns earlier in life. She was said to be schizophrenic.

When her husband fell ill, he begged me to keep it a secret from her, lest she worry. As his illness progressed, he also pleaded with the other physicians to keep the truth from her. He had developed a cancer of the lung, and its course was rapid and fatal. Deep down, he understood what was happening to him, but his main concern was protecting his wife from that knowledge and its consequences.

I was filled with fear and uncertainty. How would this woman cope with her husband's rapid decline? How could she stand to lose him? I readied myself for her imminent collapse.

But she understood quite well what her husband was going through. She understood how important it was for him to think he was concealing the pain and hurt from her, thus protecting her as he had tried to do for so many years.

As he lay dying, his breath rattling in the grip of thick cords of mucus, she spoke to me in the visitor's lounge.

"Tell me the truth, doctor," she said. "Is he going? Is there any hope for him at all?"

"What do you think?" I countered, afraid to answer her directly.

"I think he looks bad. Very bad." Her tone possessed such honest openness that I was drawn to look at her more directly. She met my gaze.

"I think you're right," I said. "I think he's failing. We're trying all we can, but I'm afraid he hasn't more than a day or two to go."

Suddenly she moved to console *me*. "I know you're doing all you can, doctor," she said. "You've been doing your best."

"Have you anyone to help you with all you'll have to do?"

"My brother."

"You should probably be starting to make arrangements then."

"Yes." She looked at me, nodding. "Yes, I should, shouldn't I."

Her husband died that evening. She took charge of the necessary rituals, the burial, the ceremony. Not once, it seemed, did she flinch. There was not even a hint of a breakdown.

About three months afterwards, she visited me in my office, requesting "some of those shots" that she occasionally took to tide her over tough periods. The shots were vitamin B_{12} and homeopathic doses of female hormones. As important to her as getting the shots, I understood, was a chance to chat, obliquely and informally, to talk about her fears and sadness.

She confided how afraid she had been when her husband died. She had experienced his death as a great loss but also as a great challenge for her to overcome. She felt he would have been proud of her for not collapsing. That thought was her consolation.

"I think he would have been proud," she said. "I know I wasn't sure myself if I had it in me. But I knew I had to do it, for his sake."

She did not collapse, as many might have predicted. Instead she found strength that she, and her husband, did not know she had. Her grieving process was lengthy and appropriate. Several other times, at two- or three-month intervals, she would appear in my office, requesting the shots. During that time I would talk with her, and I found that she continued to find ways to cope with life without him.

After this experience, I resolved never again to prejudge anyone's capacity to deal with adversity.

Chapter 3
Menopause and After

Alice Rothchild, MD

Menopause has been a taboo topic for far too long. Often it has been a subject that we as women are ashamed of and do not discuss publicly. We may feel awkward about mentioning a hot flash or one of the other symptoms associated with menopause. Women are now beginning to talk about menopause more openly among themselves, and physicians are reevaluating and rethinking some long-standing assumptions about menopause.

Unfortunately, our culture generally looks upon menopause as a disease. You may have heard it associated with insanity, obesity, the decline of one's life, cancer, and a vast array of other completely unrelated maladies. The trouble is that no one speaks of it in a positive way. Nor do they understand it in the *normal* context of aging. This is a serious problem, because about half the population are women, for whom this normal physiological process is inevitable.

If you have already undergone menopause, you may be tempted to skip over this chapter. I urge you to read on for several reasons. You may have had some unpleasant, upsetting, or confusing experiences during menopause, and their emotional and physical effects may continue into your present life and attitudes. I would like to dispel some of the myths about menopause in the hope of countering those effects. Furthermore, you may be among the many women who are being treated with estrogen, tranquilizers, or other medications for "menopausal symptoms," and I would like to put forward some of the arguments against such treatments and suggest some alternatives to them. I will explain what menopause is, the changes that result, and the misconceptions, so that you can understand what happens physically when body estrogen levels fall.

Physical Changes

Menopause is a normal part of life. It is not a sudden event, but a period of gradual decline in the frequency and regularity of the menstrual cycle. Just as the menstrual cycle is regulated during the fertile years by the brain and the body's sex hormones, so is the series of metabolic and hormonal changes that comprise menopause regulated by hormonal chemicals in the brain. Women do not use up their reservoir of potential eggs, and the brain, not the ovaries, controls the menopausal process.

It is a common misconception that after menopause women no longer produce any sex hormones. In fact, the ovaries continue to produce estrogen and progesterone; the adrenal glands and fat cells also produce estrogen. What does happen during the *climacteric* (the time during which the functioning of the ovary gradually declines or slows down) is that the ovaries become unresponsive to signals from the brain and ovulation occurs less frequently. Menopause is, strictly speaking, the last menstrual period. The process of declining responsiveness of the ovary is, however, a gradual one. During this entire period and thereafter, the body still has estrogen.

The time in her life at which a woman goes through menopause is affected by many factors besides her chronological age. Climate, emotional factors, heredity, nutrition, socioeconomic status, and general health have an effect. Furthermore, for some women the climacteric may occur over months, for others, over years. In other words, although most women go through menopause between the ages of forty and fifty-four (average age is fifty), there is no single normal age for menopause. Interestingly, recent studies have shown that women are experiencing menopause at a somewhat later age than in the past, possibly because of the effects of better nutrition in adulthood.

Many physical changes occur after the last menstrual period. The ovaries become smaller, and the vagina may also become slightly smaller and narrower. These changes are often represented to women as the end of femininity and beauty. Sexuality and femininity do not, however, depend on the size and texture of the sex organs.

Atrophic vaginitis is the term that is used to describe a group of changes that occurs in the vagina when estrogen levels decrease. It is an unfortunate term because it sounds like a dreaded disease. It is not, and regarding or treating it like one is part of the sexist thinking about menopause. Moreover, these changes do not happen to everyone, nor are they a serious problem for the majority of women to whom they do. Atrophic vaginitis occurs because of a thinning of the tissue that lines the vagina when estrogen production decreases. During intercourse the vagina may feel dry or irritated. *Senile urethritis* (another unfortunate term), or thinning of the tissue around the opening to the bladder, may also occur for the same reason. Urination may be more frequent. This is because the urethral tissue loses some of its tone and cannot maintain itself in the face of pressure from a full bladder.

Another common symptom of menopause is the hot flush, or hot flash. Referred to in medical terminology as *vasomotor disturbances,* hot flushes are sensations of heat rushing through the body. They are most commonly felt in the upper portion of the chest and face and may last from a few seconds to a few minutes. Sometimes these feelings are accompanied by chills or sweats. We do not know exactly why they occur.

Emotional Changes

It may surprise you to learn that many of the emotional changes that frequently accompany the physical changes of menopause are not caused by physiological factors and need not necessarily be a part of the menopausal experience. Rather, they often come about because of negative attitudes and expectations toward older women that prevail in our society.

The language of menopause reflects these attitudes. You may have heard that menopause is the time in which women outlive their ovaries, or the time of living decay. One of the most offensive advertisements in a medical journal I have ever seen is for a medication to eliminate "the menopausal symptoms that bother *him* most." None of these prejudices is true.

Some women do complain of increased nervousness, insomnia, headaches, or irritability during menopause. It is unclear whether these symptoms are more closely related to the decrease in body estrogen or to social pressures that place stress on menopausal women. We do know that hormones have an emotional effect during the time that women have menstrual periods, so there may be an effect when the level of these hormones is reduced.

The range of this emotional impact is probably not as great as is reported in the medical literature; assessments of women's emotional changes are often fraught with sexist attitudes. Treating a woman with an estrogen pill will not cure the stresses related to children leaving home, changes in marriage, entry or reentry into the job market, or fear of aging. It is clear to me as a gynecologist that teenagers and new mothers have a higher incidence of irritability and depression than do menopausal women, and yet no one rushes to balance their hormone levels with pills.

“ Looking back on it from the vantage point of "over fifty-five," I would have to say that it was the time that marked the Rubicon crossing in my life. It was not actually as simple as crossing a river; it was an entire coming together of a lot of currents in my life that had to be rechanneled, dammed up, or dealt with in a new way. Perhaps more than a Rubicon, it was a watershed.

My six children were practically all grown. Rearing them had kept a structure in my life that I both liked and needed. My oldest and youngest are sixteen years apart, so I have had over thirty years of childraising.

At the same time, my husband was facing drastic and traumatic career changes. His work had structured his life in much the same way that raising six children had structured mine. We turned to each other for comfort and found it difficult to understand each other's situation. This was going on not only for us, but also for many of our friends. There were new challenges to face and a new context to view them in.

What I felt was a totally personal experience, which also came as a complete surprise. I had *not* dreaded turning fifty, nor for that matter any of the other decades that marked my life. But suddenly I felt that I had discovered the secret of old age, and that in our society there is very little market for it. It seemed that overnight I began to feel saggy, wrinkled, creaky, and achey in all of my joints. I had been a person who had enjoyed good health all of her life.

What I understand now is that many of my feelings were really parts of the "empty nest" syndrome. I had come late to this problem because my last child was born when I was forty. What ailed me, of course, was depression. It had not come overnight, nor did I lick it overnight.

After a series of medical tests, which ruled out any physical problems other than the normal wear and tear of aging, we looked for professional help from a psychiatrist. I found a competent therapist and began looking more closely at myself. With plenty of moral and financial support from my husband, I also began to look for something to do outside the home. After a brief try at real estate, for which I was totally unsuited, I took courses at a special education center that trains people to become remedial or supportive tutors. I began teaching youngsters with learning disabilities. It has been a career that is rewarding and stimulating, and one that utilizes all the skills that I had acquired raising six children.

Menopause? I guess that there was a time when all this would have been blamed on that. If *menopause* is taken to mean over-the-hill, no-longer-needed, what-am-I-going-to-do-with-the-rest-of-my-life, nothing-I-can-contribute-out-there kinds of feelings, then I guess it was a factor. But men seem to suffer the same doubts and fears, so we should come up with a new word.

My advice is to find something to do in the world that really interests you. Take care of yourself. In fact, be good to your body. Eat and drink right, but also enjoy a little overindulgence now and then. Try some form of regular exercise. I am addicted to an exercise class at our Y that meets at six in the morning, five days a week. Also stay friends with young people. The exchange between generations is stimulating and rewarding.

Do not apologize for your age. You do not have to engrave it on your forehead, but on the other hand, you do not have to lie about it. ”

—Ellen Garfink, 58

Sex after Menopause

Sexual feelings after menopause depend to a large extent on our surrounding social relationships. This means that women are deeply affected by the feelings and attitudes of the loved ones around them. Some women feel pressured not to have sexual feelings. This may be because others feel that sexual activity should be associated with childbearing, or because they feel that older women should not be sexually active. We should remember that the function of the ovaries has very little to do with sexuality in humans. The sexual response to menopause has more to do with one's attitudes about sex than with the levels of hormones that are being produced. In other animal species, the female is usually sexually active and capable of reproduction until death. Humans are unique in having a period of infertility at the end of the life cycle. There is, however, no requirement that this period be less sexual than before menopause, nor is there any evidence that having a full sexual life after menopause is abnormal. Some women, in fact, feel more sexually interested because they no longer have to worry about birth control.

Estrogen Replacement

The decision whether or not to take estrogen replacement medications for menopausal symptoms is an important one that a woman should make in concert with her physician. These replacements are not entirely

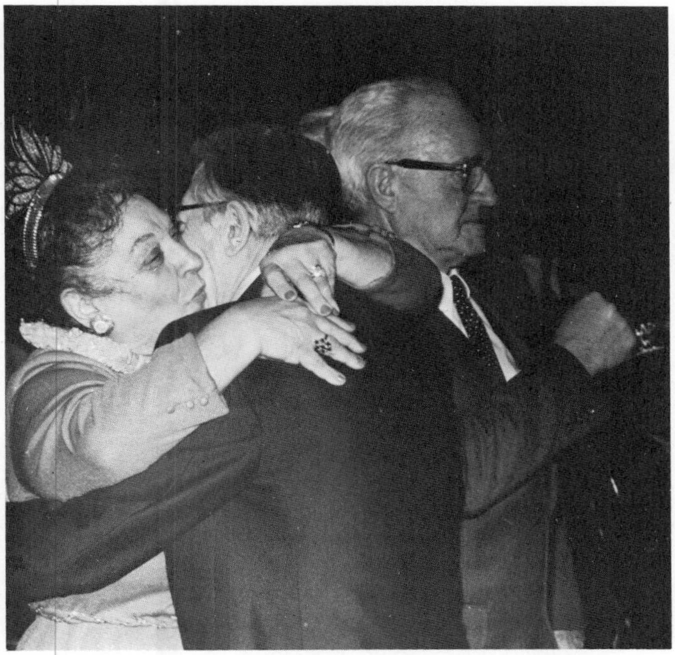

benign; in fact, a large body of data links them with an increased risk of cancer of the lining of the uterus (*endometrium*). This risk increases with the length of time and the amount of estrogen taken. The risk persists, even if estrogen use is discontinued, probably for at least one year. Overall, it is estimated that a woman who takes estrogen replacement, such as Premarin, has a 7½ times greater risk of developing endometrial cancer than does a woman who has never taken it.

Some other side effects of estrogen replacement should also be considered. Estrogen replacement probably increases the risk of forming blood clots (*thrombophlebitis*) and high blood pressure. Contrary to some popularly held beliefs, it does not prevent arteriosclerosis, also known as hardening of the arteries. Fibroids of both the uterus and breast are more common in women on estrogen replacement therapy. Other side effects include bloating (feeling gassy and distended), weight gain, fluid retention, and irregular vaginal bleeding.

It is now recommended that estrogens be taken cyclically; for instance, three weeks on and then one week off. In other words these medications should probably not be taken each day of the month. A book called *Feminine Forever* that came out a few years ago advocated taking estrogens as an anti-aging measure. There is no evidence that estrogens retard aging in any way, and they should be taken only for a specific medical problem related to reduced estrogen production.

Other Strategies

What are some of the strategies for dealing with bothersome menopausal symptoms? Dryness in the vagina may be successfully treated with an estrogen cream. This reduces the amount of estrogen that the entire body is exposed to, although some estrogen is absorbed from the vagina. A nonestrogenic cream lubricant can be substituted for an estrogen cream. K-Y Jelly is a bland lubricating cream that can be purchased in the drugstore without a prescription. Almost any kind of lightly scented emollient cream will do. For women who have not had intercourse for some time and who feel that the vagina has narrowed, a lubricant and a dilator used for a few weeks prior to intercourse may be all that is needed. The dilator may be obtained at a drugstore, and a gynecologist should be able to explain its use. In addition, more foreplay prior to intercourse and some lubricant spread on the lips of the vagina (*labia*) or penis may solve the problem.

For many women psychotherapy and discussion groups with other women may be more beneficial than estrogen replacement, especially for insomnia, depression, and irritability. Local women's groups may be able to provide information about these services; if not, gynecologists or internists may be helpful. Some doctors may prescribe tranquilizers, but again, I urge caution. All too often tranquilizers are given without an adequate understanding of the nature of the problem. They may help cover up the issues rather than resolve them. As you can see, I favor using medications as a last resort. I regard menopause as a normal part of aging, and as such see estrogen replacement or tranquilizers as an intervention only when other strategies for adjustment fail.

Osteoporosis, sometimes called thinning of the bones, has also been linked with menopause (see Chapter 18, *The Skeleton*). It is not known whether estrogen replacement is beneficial for osteoporosis. Good nutrition and active physical exercise routines may be more helpful than taking estrogen. Again, I recommend trying nonmedical strategies first, before going to estrogen replacement.

Many of the feelings that women have during menopause are directly related to the stress of aging and of being a woman in a society that is going through dynamic changes in both these areas. I urge you to find a medical provider who understands these social issues, as well as the medical ones, so that rational decisions can be made. Taking drugs, especially those that have some serious element of risk associated with their use, should not be a substitute for dealing with the important issues that you face at this stage of your life.

Chapter 4
Coping with Death in the Family

Hank Pizer, PA-C

Most of us face dying without any experience to draw upon. It usually comes about suddenly. Even for cancer victims, death usually occurs within a few months to a year, and families are taken by surprise. It is normal to feel overcome by the suddenness of the events. Our loved ones are literally with us at one moment and then gone forever. This suddenness is, above all, awesome.

My father's illness came upon us in this way. It was around the Labor Day holiday that he fell on the floor while trying to reach the bathroom. He was taken immediately to the hospital, where he spent some time undergoing tests, treatments, and observation. He remained out of the hospital but received treatments as an outpatient throughout the autumn months. By the beginning of December, he was completely bedridden, emaciated, unable to feed himself or control his bowels and bladder. Although this was not a particularly unusual or rapid course, it seemed so to us.

Unhappily we felt that we could no longer take care of him at home. We had not been prepared for this possibility and had not made alternative arrangements. I think that we expected he would be able to return to the treatment hospital where he had originally been hospitalized. Unfortunately, acute-care hospitals, where people are initially taken for treatment, are not set up for the terminally ill. They do not receive insurance payments for this kind of care. The combination of the speed of the events and our lack of knowledge about the system left us unprepared for dealing with this problem.

We should have been better prepared for all of this by the medical staff. They should have told us of the possibility of his rapid decline and of the importance of making arrangements for the future if this should occur. Fortunately, hospice programs throughout the country have been established for this purpose. They are discussed in Chapter 5, *Hospice,* by Dr. Paula McBrine. Hospice provides skilled people who are both sympathetic and experienced in dealing with the psychological and physical problems of dying. In many ways treatment hospitals are least qualified for this job, whereas hospice centers specialize in it.

> “I had been married for thirty-five years. Had my husband lived, I would now be married for forty-five years. In this kind of long, sometimes checkered relationship, there were many ups and downs. But most of the days and years fell somewhere in the middle.
>
> I had my own career and my own friends. I had created my own momentum, with reference to my own achievements, which included for me my work, education, political activity, and social life. All this I did while raising a family. Some of my pursuits were seriously directed, while others were quite frivolous. I loved to play cards, for instance. I was never a heavy gambler, but I liked pitting my intelligence against chance. Above all, I think my life had a high level of activity, some of it exhausting, some stimulating.
>
> On the outside I suppose we had the trappings of suburban, middle-class life. Yet there was an inner restlessness and many dreams about unrealized ambitions and experiences.
>
> In looking back, the onset of my husband's illness was barely noticeable. One day while he was driving, I noticed, sitting next to him, that he was coming perilously close to cars parked on the right. Was it my misperception, or his? Ever taciturn, he did not complain, except that occasionally he had headaches.
>
> Shortly afterwards he fell onto the bathroom floor. I had to help him up, and we got medical attention. The neurologist said that he might have had a seizure. I asked if it was petit mal, and the neurologist said that, at his age of sixty, it would be a grand mal. He gave my husband some medication, and I took over the driving. He went back to work, and we resumed our lives.
>
> However, things got worse. By early December my husband was back in the hospital. I visited each afternoon. One day he said, "I'm not getting any better." I was well aware of this but told him I thought there was some improvement. I told friends I thought he was terminally ill, but I never told him.
>
> He died on December 31. He had been comatose for about five days. I told no one that day. Friends had a right to celebrate a traditional New Year's Eve.
>
> About two weeks before he died, the social service unit at the hospital asked me to find what they called a long-term nursing facility for him. He was in a treatment hospital, and he was no longer a treatable patient. The facilities that were suggested presented enormous obstacles to me. How was I to visit, since they were far away from my home and work? I had heard about the capricious state of patient care in these facilities and did not feel comfortable with them. In a sense his death relieved him and me of a possibly more degrading and ignoble experience.
>
> My son left home about five days after my husband's death. He had made previous plans to relocate. I was left alone with my loneliness and depression. For months I thought I heard my husband's key at the front door at 6:00 in the evening, when he usually returned from work. When spring came, I imagined I saw him picking weeds out of the lawn. I had my work, my friends, my card games, my political and social interests. These were extremely important. They helped alleviate the terrible sense of loss.

Sometimes I felt I was going into a depression. Because I had these resources, I did not succumb; but I know that the partner left behind suffers a great wrenching. You feel that you are drifting, buffeted about, and aware of and frightened by oblivion. One of my friends told me sometime later, when she had lost her husband, that she wanted to go into the bedroom closet and never come out.

Guilt seems to be the overriding legacy of the living partner. It occurs with the death of a parent as well. All the should-have, could-have, would-haves haunt us with an unremitting frequency. What we do not stress enough for the living partner or remaining relative is the pleasure, support, and well-being that the one left behind offered in the relationship.

Since we cannot arrange a simultaneous demise with our mates, we all have to think about a time when we will have to live in a single fashion. We must develop resources along the way which can be called upon at some time in the future. ❞

—Stella Young Pizer, 65

Often treatment-oriented and well-meaning medical providers do not tell the patient or the family the complete prognosis. They remain overly optimistic, in part because this helps them adjust to the stress of treating seriously ill patients. This approach, however, does a disservice to families. In our situation my father's initial medical assessment included a seizure, a stroke, or brain cancer. Our physicians tended to emphasize stroke or seizure at first. In looking back from the vantage point of having worked in cancer care, I know that the signs weighed heavily toward cancer. The staff was trying to be helpful, but it served only to divide our family and give us false hopes. My mother sensed that it was a tumor, yet my sister and I clung to the more optimistic possibility. This made us feel that our mother was being overly pessimistic.

In dealing with the medical system, all of us need to understand how physicians and nurses often approach death and dying. They paint a portrait of optimism, but we should learn to see through it. Ask your care givers to spell out exactly what they think the likely future will be and to explain the possible adverse situations. Plan for the serious illness as well as for the possibility of recovery. Because it helps them cope, medical people share some element of denial in their own way of dealing with dying. As a patient, or as part of the family of a patient, however, you will need to know the good and the bad in order to make decisions for the future.

Families bring to the dying situation all of the problems they had prior to the illness. In stressful moments these long-held feelings come out with great intensity. In my family, my mother and sister revived many of their differences, as did my mother and her sister. I felt separated from these problems, and this renewed my commitment to leave home as soon as the illness was resolved. My father and I had not been particularly close, and we both found it hard to talk about his illness, family problems, or necessary arrangements.

This is a reason for families to seek the help of a social worker, hospice worker, psychologist, clergyman, or medical care giver, who can help resolve some of the inevitable personal problems that arise. This person should be someone trained and experienced in working with families who have a loved one who is seriously ill or dying. Friends and neighbors can be supportive, but they should not be relied on for dealing with intense family issues. This takes training and a professional distance. Seek out the guidance of a skilled person early, before the issues become too heated and serious misunderstandings result. If you feel that your medical care giver cannot provide this service, try the hospice program.

Both the patient and the family go through emotional stages after learning of impending death. These were first characterized by Dr. Elisabeth Kübler-Ross. First, there is denial, in which the ill person and the loved ones cannot talk openly about the problem. Next there is anger, when we feel cheated; then bargaining, when we look for a cure or a miracle. That is followed by depression, when the reality sets in and overwhelms us. Finally, there is acceptance.

It is normal for each person in the family to go through all of these stages. In fact, they occur with many kinds of loss, among them the dissolution of a marriage, the loss of a job, or moving. Death, of course, brings them out with maximum intensity. Moreover, it is common to feel more than one of these at the same time. In other words part of us may be bargaining for a cure while another part is feeling denial, anger, or depression. Feelings have no clear-cut lines, and they tend to come in uncontrollable waves. There are big swings up and even bigger swings down.

Be aware that dying breaks down the usual social conventions. People tend to act in extreme ways, and unless we understand this, there may be terrible guilt about things that are said and done. A friend recently experienced the sudden death by drowning of her husband. She told me that one of the most comforting things she was told was that whatever she felt was okay. In my family we needed someone to say this very simple thing to us, so that we could have our feelings without recrimination or guilt. This kind of service can be provided by a person who is experienced in counseling the terminally ill and their families.

❝ We were married before I went into the service, more than thirty-five years in all. She died of a kind of cancer called multiple myeloma.

It first started with something like rheumatism in her legs. She carried a cane for a short time, but it was cancer all that time and it did not get better. She was sixty-six when she died, and she had been sick for only two years. I said to her once, "Don't you ever get sick before you are sixty-five." We were fooling. By God, about three or four months after sixty-five, she started to get the pains and aches that we thought were arthritis.

One time she asked me if she was going to die. I said that they were doing their best to try to keep her alive, but eventually it would affect her whole body. She lost so much weight that she seemed to weigh nothing. At the end she was on dialysis, but she got steadily worse.

I knew that she wasn't going to make it. She would look at me as if she knew the end was coming. I kept putting my doubts aside, hoping that she would get better. I would get her weight up six or seven pounds, and then in one day she would go for dialysis and all the weight would be gone. It was all fluid.

I felt that she was in terrible pain most of the time, and life for her had become useless. She would say, "I pray to God to take me." I didn't feel that, but I hoped something would happen because she was getting no better. She was suffering and hardly eating. At the end she did not have enough strength to eat a piece of bread.

Both my children were married by then, so I had to take care of her myself. I miss my wife quite a bit. I still think of her as a person. I talk to her. Everyone does that when someone dies. I ask her, "What do you think about this?" or "How do you think this will be?" knowing that she is dead and gone. You talk like that and keep up a conversation, though you know deep in your heart and mind that she is dead. She is still with me. I can still think of various places that we have been and the fun that we had together. ❞

—Joseph Lawlor, 76

Dr. William Thomas is a psychiatrist with whom I worked in cancer care. He points out that, whereas all of the stages that Dr. Kübler-Ross describes are normal phases in the dying process, the real difficulty lies in getting stuck in any one of them. For instance, in my family we could not get past the stage of denial. None of us could talk with my father about what was going to happen. That included our emotions as well as certain mundane issues like the disposition of his business and property. Fortunately, my mother had experience in attending to the family's financial affairs. This is an important fact of life that many people are unprepared for, however, and here again trained counselors can help.

Being stuck in the bargaining stage is very much like becoming fixed in denial. It becomes difficult to say the things that really need to be said because no one wants to admit the truth. It also makes people prey to charlatans who promise miracle cures. Having a relationship with a medical care giver whom you can trust is therefore extremely important. If you understand the extent of the illness, it aids in resolving the bargaining stage.

The anger stage is particularly devastating for everyone. The anger divides the family. In the hospital seemingly endless anger, on the part of the patient or family, compromises medical care. The staff tends to avoid the patient and the family. Relieving this anger depends on being able to acknowledge and release one's feelings. Sometimes the anger results from the illness; at other times it comes from deepseated feelings. Whatever the cause, it is normal to feel angry and to express it, but there are limits beyond which the anger is destructive. Exceeding that limit is a signal to get immediate help from your physician or a counselor.

Becoming mired in depression makes it impossible to enjoy the final months and days of life. Depression makes one immobile and also tends to isolate the depressed person from others. Ideally the final moments should be shared with loved ones. This includes children and grandchildren, who are particularly important in family life. It was a tragedy that in our situation the hospital did not want my young nephew to visit his grandfather. Families should work out children's visitation privileges before a loved one enters the hospital.

Inevitably the issue of dying at home versus dying in the hospital must be settled. There is no right or wrong in this. We were not able to cope with the daily care that my father needed. Unfortunately, the hospital staff was not helpful in finding aides who might have come into our home, and no hospice program was available to us at that time. Having a family member die at home can be very stressful, and you should not try to take on this responsibility alone. Hospitals have twenty-four-hour nursing and medical staffing for the enormous task of caring for the seriously ill. You should not take this on without aid from others. The burden will stress everyone more than the difficulties encountered with dying in a hospital. You will need occasional visits from a nurse, possibly a doctor, aides, and perhaps volunteers who can help move, feed, and spend time with the ill person. Again, the hospice program in your area should be a resource for organizing all the necessary supports.

It is not realistic to expect that the medical care givers can solve all of the problems that dying and death bring up in families. Certainly no one could have eliminated my need to move away and establish my own life, nor change the fact that my mother was losing her companion of a lifetime. But trained, sensitive professionals can be helpful. It is best to seek them out and to avoid taking on the entire stress without help. The isolation, loneliness, and incredible needs of a dying person can be overwhelming. No one should have to shoulder all of the emotional and physical burdens alone.

Most of us need others to validate our feelings. Just knowing that what you feel is normal—no matter how sad, frightening, angry, or embarrassing—helps. If there is one central message that I have to share it is that, during stressful moments, it is best to be able to share one's feelings. This is the essence of family. If you cannot do this on your own, ask a counselor or your medical care giver to help you talk through the issues in a family meeting. The greatest tragedy is, perhaps, not the dying, but going through it alone.

Chapter 5
Hospice

Paula McBrine, MD

Hospice is a term for palliative care for people with terminal cancer. The word is an old one, and it means shelter for weary travelers on long and difficult journeys. This is an accurate metaphor for the individual with a terminal disease who has lived a long life and is now at the end of his or her journey.

The hospice program involves caring for the family as well as the dying person, with a total support system that includes medical, psychological, and spiritual help. It is palliative care. The goal is caring, not curing. It originated at St. Bartholomew's and St. Christopher's hospitals in England. The first hospice in the United States was started at Yale University in 1974. Since then many hospice programs have been established throughout the United States.

Above all, the hospice attempts to alleviate the panic of the dying person and his or her family. Few of us come to the death of a loved one knowing what to expect and what to do. It is the job of the hospice staff to help guide the family and to aid them in making the sort of medical decisions that often place unbearable demands on the patient and family.

In contrast to conventional acute-care hospitals, hospice accepts that the person is dying. Treatment is directed at alleviating the unpleasant and painful symptoms of the disease. In the acute-care hospital, attempts may be made to keep the patient alive for as long as possible. In the hospice program, the concern is with the quality of life prior to death, not in extending life. The effort is to remove the stressful symptoms with the expectation that what remains of a person's life may be used to its utmost—in fact, enjoyed. Dr. Cicely Saunders, who has been instrumental in establishing the basic principles of the hospice program at St. Christopher's Hospital, outside of London, has said, "The aim is to enable the patient to go on living through this part of his life as himself, and not as an uncomplaining residue."

Hospice involves volunteer services, often performed by others who have cancer; specially trained nurses, homemakers, and aides; and physicians who are dedicated to the hospice concept. The focus is on relief of physical and emotional pain and improving the quality of life before it ends. As a physician in such a program, many of my skills are directed at treating pain in a way that provides continuous relief without altering mental functioning. We want people to be able to function as actively as possible, as if they did not have pain and did not take medication. I also try to reduce anxiety and to control the nausea that often accompanies terminal care.

Unfortunately, dying people frequently feel abandoned by the people that they need most because of the taboos that we share about dying. We are all afraid of pain and death, but we do not communicate openly about our fears because we too are afraid of dying. Dying impresses upon us our own mortality and vulnerability, as well as the fear of loss and loneliness. In hospice we do not blame each other for these feelings, but understand that they have been around us for quite some time. We help the dying person and the family to talk about these things so that they can enjoy their last moments together to the greatest extent possible.

When an individual comes to us for hospice care, we assess his or her physical, emotional, and spiritual needs and those of the family. We try to plan a comprehensive approach that brings the family together and provides support on a twenty-four-hour basis. This has been very important to the program. Often the most critical moments come at night, when the physician may not be available. For this reason the support system of volunteers plays an important role.

I am often asked if people need a special place to die. I think that the answer is no. The issue is not where people die, but the supports that are provided to help them with their feelings and physical needs. It is not the flowers in the vases or beautiful music playing that helps, but the love and understanding of others. This can be provided in a hospital, home, or hospice.

There have been many problems to overcome in establishing hospice in America. Funding has been difficult, and often insurance carriers will not pay for hospice services. It has also been difficult to change attitudes among the general public and within the medical community concerning what the care of the dying person should be. In our present system, we can accommodate acute care and nursing homes but little in between. Often cancer patients do not fit into either of these spaces. They may not be receiving active medical treatment because their cancer is too widespread, but they may be too ill to enter a nursing home. Hospice is the logical alternative. It is hoped that we will see the growth of the hospice movement and its extension into the care of those with terminal illnesses other than cancer. Beds should be allocated in hospitals for this purpose, and insurance carriers should reimburse for this service. In addition, more physicians, nurses, and other care givers should be trained in hospice skills.

Hospice Programs

To find a hospice program in your area, consult first with your physician. If you are still uncertain about how to find a hospice, call the nearest hospital or medical college with a department of oncology. (This is the medical specialty that treats cancer patients.)

Further information, along with a listing of hospice programs in your region, may be obtained from:

The Association of Community Cancer Centers
4733 Bethesda Avenue
Washington, DC 20014

The National Hospice Organization
765 Prospect Street
New Haven, CT 06511.

If you are interested in organizing public support for the hospice concept, contact:

Hospice Action
P.O. Box 32331
Washington, DC 20007

Cancer patients are often in need of financial assistance. Information concerning available help may be obtained from:

The American Cancer Society
777 Third Avenue
New York, NY 10017

Cancer Care, Inc.
One Park Avenue
New York, NY 10016

United Way
801 North Fairfax
Alexandria, VA 22314

Additional organizations and government agencies that can provide information and assistance to cancer patients are listed in the back of *Breast Cancer Digest,* which can be obtained from the United States Department of Health and Human Services, National Institutes of Health, Bethesda, MD 20205. Ask for Publication No. 80-1691.

Chapter 6
Avoiding Consumer Fraud

Jerilou Hammett

People over fifty-five have some special difficulties in being good consumers, particularly with respect to health care. To begin with, they rely on these services more often and hence are more vulnerable to fraud. For instance, you are 100 percent more likely to get an electrocardiogram (EKG) at age sixty-five than you were at age forty. Sales of eyeglasses, hearing aids, and other medical appliances almost tripled in dollar expenditures from 1950 to 1977. Nursing homes have grown from a $1-billion-a-year industry in 1950 to a $24-billion one today. Sales of drugs and health related sundries have risen fivefold during the same period. People over fifty-five are the principal consumers of these items and services.

❝ All of us over fifty-fivers should raise our aging, spotted, arthritic hands in a salute to Madison Avenue. They have discovered us. After all these years of being the heroic generation who fought World War II, we have become the new market. We knew we were there all the time, but why did it take so long for them to find us?

As a friend of mine put it wistfully, "You know, when we were kids, adults were in style. Now that we are adults, kids are in style." But that was a few years ago, and things are being remedied. Now *U.S. News and World Report* featured us on the front cover of its September 1, 1980, issue and announced that a new era is in the making.

It seems that the hucksters have latched onto some statistics that say we have an annual income of $350 billion. I guess it struck those little rascals that there was a lot of "going for the gusto" potential in us after all . . . at least with our credit cards, checkbooks, and charge accounts.

The aforementioned magazine went on to say that the trends are unmistakable. Commercials are already featuring "older" models. So far they are still fixating on losing one's complexion around age thirty-one or swigging Geritol at thirty-five, but it is a look at the future. Patience—our day is coming.

Can you imagine the possibilities? Helena Rubenstein already has, and is coming up with a special line of cosmetics. Maybe their ads will run something like: "Why should you look young at thirty-two? Want to do something about that smooth, youthful complexion? Try Instawrinkle Creme-Eternal 57. Do Grays have more fun?" Women will say, "I am really forty-two, but I put sixty-one down on my employment application. I did not want to be turned down because of my youth."

All of this makes my head reel and my blood pressure rise. But you have not heard it all. Levi Strauss is going to do a new line of jeans just for us older "girls." What label will we be reading on elderly behinds? Will they go for the vulgar—"Old Wives' Tails"—or will it be French designer chic: *"Le Dernier/Derriére Cri"* (roughly translated: The Last Hurrah)? I can't wait . . . well, yes, I can.

I do have a plan for salvaging some good from all of this. Once this trend is fully established and fifty-five and over is indeed where it is all at—when no one can be too thin, too rich, or too old, when Ted Kennedy is too young to run for president—we can raise our collective voice (there are more than forty-five million of us) and yell: "So listen up, you rotten kids, and listen good! We are in charge here now, and we don't trust *anyone* under forty. So put that in your pipe (along with all the other stuff) and smoke it!" ❞

—Ellen Garfink, 58

Older women are commonly disadvantaged as consumers because of the constraints of traditional sex roles. As many women become widowed, their vulnerability is increased. Difficulty reading fine print on contracts, insurance policies, and medical consent forms may pose additional difficulties for both men and women.

Lack of mobility often restricts access to information, as well as the opportunity to compare prices. For example, shopping around for a walker or prescription drug is more difficult for many older people. Convenience and closeness may become important factors when choosing a pharmacy. In a community of seniors, the pharmacy may not be as competitive as one in a more mixed neighborhood. Lack of mobility also may mean relying on television or other media for information about health-related products. Not all of this information is accurate or helpful.

Health problems also make people vulnerable to promises of miracle cures and other questionable medical schemes. Fear of aging and loneliness tend to increase susceptibility to products that offer youth and beauty.

Consumer Tips

Despite all this, it is possible to be a more aware consumer. Following are some tips for protection against fraud:

1. Be suspicious of door-to-door sales, especially of people who come to the door without having been called. Require identification of all salespeople.
2. Do not feel pressure to sign a contract. Before signing, ask the advice of a lawyer, trusted friend, or knowledgeable family member.
3. Know the exact cost of any planned purchase, including charges for finance, handling, installation, and service and maintenance.
4. Do not make a large down payment before the work or service is performed; do not make final payment until fully satisfied.
5. If uncertain about a product, consult an independent, reliable source. This can be the attorney general's office in your state, Better Business Bureau, newspaper, television, radio, police, consumer agency.
6. Do not rush into any purchase. Shop around.

There are some particular areas to be wary of in regard to health care. Older people spend $4 billion on unnecessary health insurance or additional benefits that are of little value. They purchase coverage for items already included in Medicare or a pension plan insurance policy. I am aware of a woman in her seventies who purchased a plan that included coverage for pregnancy. Your state insurance commission or state agency on aging should be able to answer questions about purchasing health insurance.

Sometimes seniors receive fewer services than they should because they are covered by Medicare or Medicaid. The physician or other provider bills for services that were not performed, and since the billing is direct to the carrier (not seen by the patient), the patient has little control over the situation. You can monitor this by getting a full list of all services and charges and having them reviewed by your insurance commission or another medical provider.

Drugs are the largest out-of-pocket medical expense for most people. Laws differ from state to state, but in general you can ask your medical provider or pharmacist to substitute a generic equivalent for a brand name medication that will be less costly. You can also ask if a less expensive type of medication can be prescribed that will offer similar results. This is especially true for antibiotics. In many cases combination medications are prescribed that are considerably more expensive than single-agent medicines, but which offer little additional benefit. An example of this are pain killers and cold preparations that add aspirin to other ingredients. Often you can purchase just the single ingredient for a far lower price and take a generic aspirin that can be purchased reasonably in your pharmacy or supermarket. It is always a good idea to remind your medical provider to choose the most cost-effective alternative.

Medical charlatans often appeal to older people, especially in areas where conventional medical services are difficult to obtain, expensive, or not very helpful. Cures for arthritis, wrinkles, balding, cancer, or obesity are examples. No magical creams or vitamins will increase potency or reverse the effects of normal aging. Do not buy dental plates from mail-order catalogs or newspaper advertisements. They will not fit properly. Similarly, hearing aids and eyeglasses must be fitted to meet particular needs, and that should be done by a trained person.

Any item priced at twenty-five dollars or more that is purchased in your home or outside of the seller's usual place of business is subject to the three-day Cooling-Off Rule of the Federal Trade Commission. The rule allows three business days to reconsider the purchase and to return the item or cancel the sale. The salesman is obligated to explain this cancellation right, and it must also be included in the contract. The contract must be dated and include the name and address of the seller. You do not have to give a reason for canceling the sale.

Funerals are a large expense for many families, and the decision on the size and type of funeral are not always made with a full understanding of the costs and alternatives. In 1979 the average cost of a complete funeral was $2,500, and funerals costing $5,000 were not uncommon.

Two brochures may help in planning a funeral: *Where There Is A Will* (two dollars) and *Smoothing The Way* (twenty-five cents). They provide information regarding both wills and funeral plans. They should be obtained before there is a death, so that sensible decisions can be planned. They are available from the Continental Association of Funeral and Memorial Societies, Inc., 1828 L Street NW, Suite 1100, Washington, DC 20036.

Redress

In 1978 Congress passed the Older Americans Act. It mandated services for older Americans in diverse areas such as nutrition, research projects, employment, transportation, health care, the legal system, and consumer affairs. The act prohibits discrimination against older Americans, and governmental agencies are empowered to enforce the law and aid individuals in seeking redress.

Consumer Resource List

If you have a question or complaint regarding the purchase of an item, a service, or medical care, a number of agencies and groups can be contacted for help. A complaint about medical practice should be referred to your state's board of medicine, insurance commission, state or county medical society, or attorney general. Other sources of information and/or avenues of redress are listed below.

Particular Medical Need

Administration on Aging
Office of Human Development Services
U.S. Department of Health and Human Services
200 Independence Avenue SW
Washington, DC 20201

Alexander Graham Bell Association for the Deaf
3417 Volta Place NW
Washington, DC 20007

Allergy Foundation of America
19 West 44th Street
New York, NY 10036

American Academy of Dermatology
820 Davis Street
Evanston, IL 60201

American Cancer Society
777 Third Avenue
New York, NY 10017

American Dental Association
211 East Chicago Avenue
Chicago, IL 60611

American Diabetes Association, Inc.
Two Park Avenue
New York, NY 10016

American Dietetic Association
430 North Michigan Avenue
Chicago, IL 60611

(continued)

American Foundation for the Blind
15 West 16th Street
New York, NY 10011

American Geriatrics Society
10 Columbus Circle
New York, NY 10019

American Health Care Association
1200 15th Street NW
Washington, DC 20005

American Heart Association
7320 Greenville Avenue
Dallas, TX 75231

American Lung Association
1740 Broadway
New York, NY 10019

American Parkinson Disease Association
116 John Street, Suite 417
New York, NY 10038

American Printing House for the Blind, Inc.
1839 Frankfort Avenue
Louisville, KY 40206

American Red Cross
17th and D Street, NW
Washington, DC 20006

American Speech-Language-Hearing Association
10801 Rockville Pike
Rockville, MD 20852

The Arthritis Foundation
3400 Peachtree Road NE
Atlanta, GA 30326

Concern for Dying
250 West 57th Street
New York, NY 10017

Division for the Blind and Physically Handicapped
Library of Congress
Washington, DC 20542

Epilepsy Foundation of America
Suite 406
1828 L Street NW
Washington, DC 20036

Gerontological Society of America
Suite 305
1835 K Street NW
Washington, DC 20006

Goodwill Industries of America, Inc.
9200 Wisconsin Avenue
Washington, DC 20014

Institute of Rehabilitation Medicine
400 East 34th Street
New York, NY 10016

International Association of Laryngectomees
c/o American Cancer Society
777 Third Avenue
New York, NY 10017

Leukemia Society of America, Inc.
800 Second Avenue
New York, NY 10017

Myasthenia Gravis Foundation, Inc.
15 East 26th Street
New York, NY 10010

National Association of the Deaf
814 Thayer Avenue
Silver Spring, MD 20910

National Cancer Institute
Information Office
Bethesda, MD 20014

National Council on the Aging
600 Maryland Avenue SW, West Wing 100
Washington, DC 20024

National Heart, Lung, and Blood Institute
National Institutes of Health
9600 Rockville Pike
Building 31, Room 5A52
Bethesda, MD 20014

National Institute of Arthritis, Metabolism and Digestive Diseases
c/o Dr. George Brooks
Westwood Building, Room 637
Bethesda, MD 20014

National Kidney Foundation
Two Park Avenue
New York, NY 10016

National Multiple Sclerosis Society
205 East 42nd Street
New York, NY 10017

National Parkinson Foundation, Inc.
1501 NW Ninth Avenue
Miami, FL 33136

National Rehabilitation Association
633 South Washington Street
Alexandria, VA 22314

National Society to Prevent Blindness
79 Madison Avenue
New York, NY 10016

National Spinal Cord Injury Foundation
369 Elliot Street
Newton Upper Falls, MA 02164

Parkinson's Disease Foundation
William Black Medical Research Building
Columbia Presbyterean Medical Center
640 West 168th Street
New York, NY 10032

Recording for the Blind, Inc.
215 East 58th Street
New York, NY 10022

Rehabilitation International
432 Park Avenue South
New York, NY 10016

Rehabilitation Services Administration
Department of Education
330 C Street SW
Washington, DC 20201

Sister Kenny Institute (rehabilitation)
Chicago Avenue at 27th Avenue
Minneapolis, MN 55407

(continued)

Consumer Resource List (*continued*)

United Ostomy Association
2001 West Beverly Boulevard
Los Angeles, CA 90057

Appliance Repair

If your appliance needs repair and the dealer does not provide this service, contact the manufacturer at its headquarters. If they do not help, write:

Major Appliance Consumer Action Panel (MACAP)
20 North Wacker Drive
Chicago, IL 60606

Include the type of appliance, brand, model serial number, and dealer's name and address.

Consumer Information

You can obtain a catalog that lists over 200 federal publications of consumer interest by writing to:

Consumer Information Center
Pueblo, CO 81009

Debt Collection Information

Fair Debt Collection Practices Project
Federal Trade Commission
Washington, DC 20580

Energy Questions

Department of Energy
Tel: 1-800-424-9245

Questions of Fraud

Director, Bureau of Consumer Protection
Federal Trade Commission
Washington, DC 20580
Tel: 202-523-3727

Housing

Department of Housing and Urban Development
Division of Consumer Complaints
Washington, DC 20410
Tel: 202-755-5353

Junk Mail

You can have your name removed from junk mail lists by requesting a "name removal order blank" from:

Mail Preference Service
Direct Mail/Marketing Association
Five East 43rd Street
New York, NY 10017

Lending or Financial Affairs

Housing and Credit Section
Civil Rights Division
Justice Department
Washington, DC 20530
Tel: 202-739-4123

Medicaid/Medicare

Health Care Financing Administration
Department of Health and Human Services
Washington, DC 20201
Tel: 202-245-0312

Product Safety

Consumer Product Safety Commission
Consumer Services Branch
Washington, DC 20207
Tel: 1-800-638-2666
(In Maryland: 1-800-492-2937)

Social Security

Check your local telephone directory under US Government. If there is no office, check your local post office for a time when social security representatives visit your area. Or write:

Division of Public Inquiries
Social Security Administration
6401 Security Boulevard
Baltimore, MD 21235
Tel: 301-594-7707

Tax Information

The Internal Revenue Service (IRS) has a toll-free number listed in your tax package or telephone directory. If you wish to write, address correspondence to: IRS District Director, Problem Resolution Program, for your district.

Veteran's Information

Veterans Administration
810 Vermont Avenue, NW
Washington, DC 20420

Other Problems or Information

American Association of Retired Persons
1909 K Street NW
Washington, DC 20049
202-872-4700

National Council of Senior Citizens
1511 K Street NW
Washington, DC 20005
202-347-8800

National Association of Area Agencies on Aging
1828 L Street NW
Washington, DC 20036
202-223-5010

Legal Services for the Elderly
132 West 43rd Street, 3rd Floor
New York, NY 10036
212-595-1340

National Caucus and Center on Black Aged
1424 K Street NW
Suite 500
Washington, DC 20005
202-637-8400

National Indian Council on Aging
PO Box 2088
Albuquerque, NM 87103
505-766-2276

National Pacific-Asian Resource Center on Aging
618 Second Avenue
Suite 243
Seattle, WA 98104
206-622-5124

A number of avenues are open for investigation into age discrimination. Discrimination in federally assisted programs should be investigated through the particular agency or the Office of the General Counsel, U.S. Department of Health and Human Services, 200 Independence Avenue SW, Washington, DC 20201. The American Civil Liberties Union has a handbook called *The Rights of Older Persons,* which can be purchased from Avon Books, 250 East 55th Street, New York, NY 10019, for $2.50.

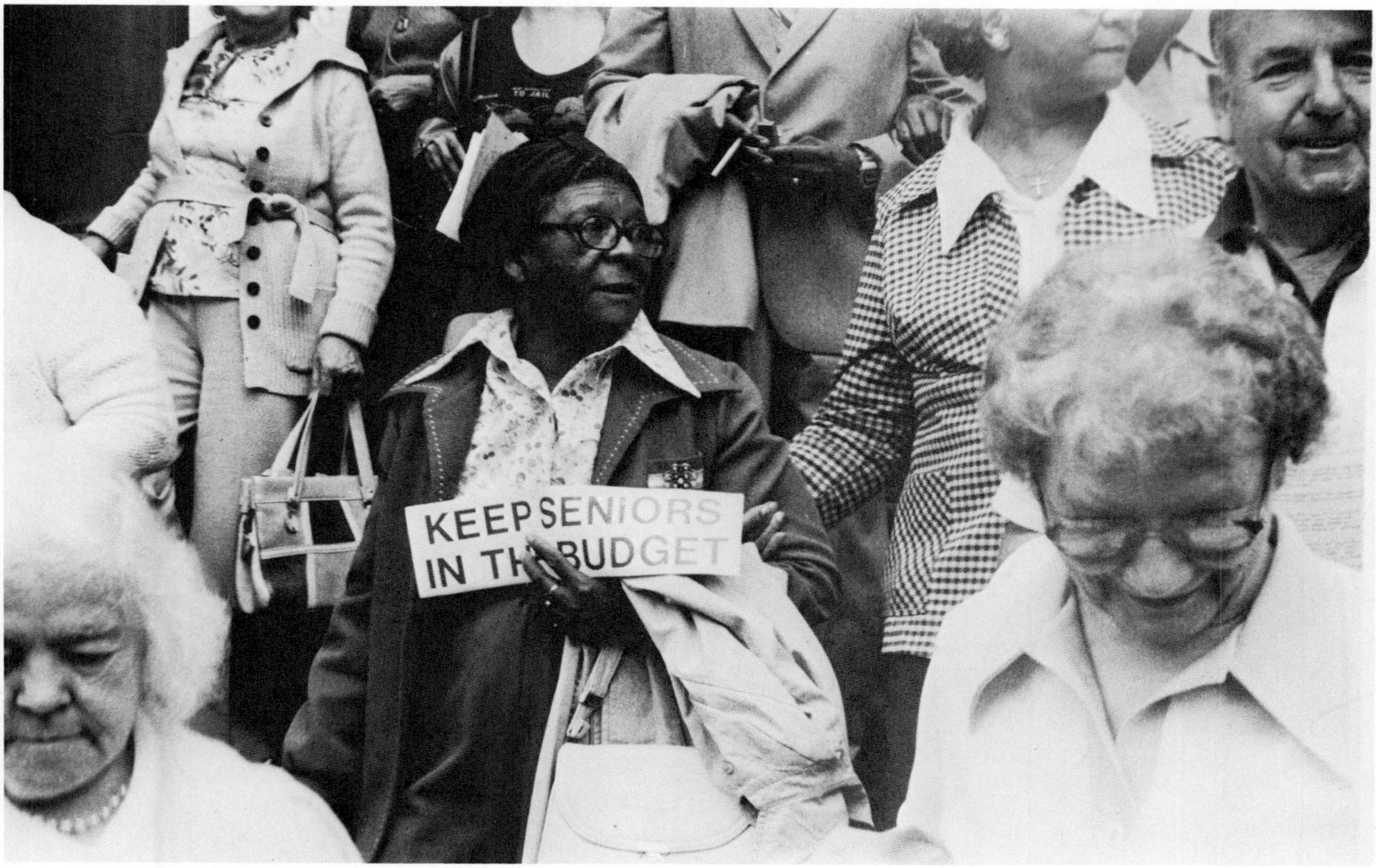

Part II

Body Maintenance

Most public health experts agree that good health is affected more by what we do for ourselves than by what our doctors can do for us. By that I mean by changing our daily patterns of living we can institute health practices that may promote longevity, increase the quality of life, and prevent illness. The two most relevant areas in which we can make these changes are eating and exercise.

It does not matter whether you have never exercised, are overweight, have a physical impairment, or consider yourself nonathletic. You can begin a program of regular exercise that will improve your physical fitness and is tailored to your individual needs.

Similarly, whether you like so-called health foods or not should not affect whether you can eat a balanced, healthy diet. You can eat well even if you travel for a living, have a limited food budget, or do not like to cook.

These are health choices that we all can make, regardless of age, sex, race, income, or ethnic origin. I think that you will quickly find that you feel better, look better, have increased energy, and a more positive outlook on life if you improve your diet and physical fitness. Good nutrition and regular exercise are, perhaps, the most important measures we can initiate for ourselves and do not become any less important with increasing years. In fact, they probably become more important for living an active, healthy, and vibrant life.

Chapter 7
Physical Fitness

Patti Marcus, RPT

Even if you have never exercised, are completely out of shape, have had a heart attack, have arthritis, or have difficulty seeing or hearing, some kind of exercise program can be designed to improve your health. Studies with both laboratory animals and humans have shown again and again that regular physical activity improves longevity and overall health. Just as important, it improves one's general sense of well-being. If you maintain your proper weight and continue a regular form of physical exercise, you will reduce the chances of having many common medical problems, including heart disease, diabetes, stroke, osteoporosis, and lung disease.

Begin with a form of exercise that you enjoy. No specific exercise routine will be presented in this chapter, because there is such a wide range of exercises and sports from which to choose. It does not matter what you pick as long as it is something you like, because that will encourage you to do it regularly. Once you find out what you like to do, you can join a Y, health club, swimming pool, or gym, or do it on your own or with friends.

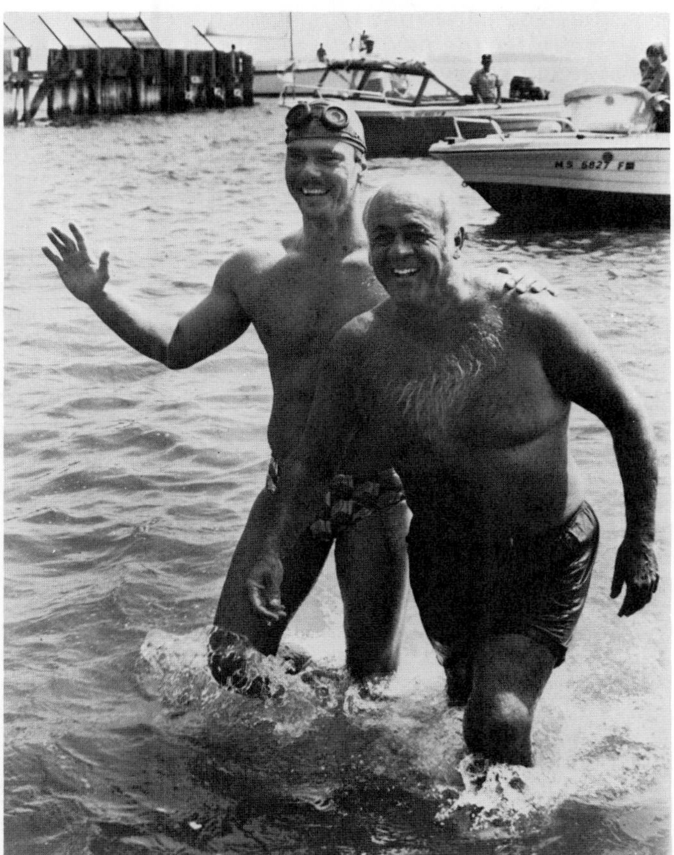

If you have physical limitations, you should pick a form of exercise that is compatible with your problem. For instance, if you have problems with your sight, swimming in a pool is a safe and easy way to exercise, because it does not require hand-eye coordination. You can work this out with your physician (if he or she is interested in physical exercise), the group that you join (many clubs and Ys have staff that can counsel you), or a sports medicine clinic. You can find a sports medicine clinic through the department of orthopedic surgery in most city hospitals, the Yellow Pages (under clinics, hospitals, or orthopedic physicians), or your country or state medical society.

Designing an Exercise Program

An exercise program should improve strength, flexibility, and the function of the heart and lungs. For most people this begins with increasing suppleness and proceeds to cardiovascular conditioning and finally muscular strength. If you set realistic goals and choose a form of exercise that you enjoy, you are likely to find that exercise becomes integral to your daily living.

“ I am seventy years old, and I have been active my entire life. I have been a member of the YMCA for at least fifty years, and I go regularly to work out. I have enjoyed many kinds of exercise. When I was younger, I was an amateur boxer, and I won the National Junior Championships one year.

I never married. Perhaps it was that I had the Y in my blood. But I have stayed close with my family. I have brothers and sisters who have children, and I spent years taking my nieces and nephews down to the Y to have fun and to exercise.

I stopped boxing during the Depression, in 1936. At that time I was working in the liquor business, and I continued to do that for about thirty-five years. Then I moved to a factory and supervised the quality of the parts that were being manufactured.

I finally retired at age sixty-six. Retiring was not so different, except maybe that I did not have to get up early in the morning if I did not want to. I guess I just did not want to be under the clock anymore. I still go down to the Y all the time, at least four or five days a week. There are a bunch of us guys who have been going down there since I can remember. We are in that age bracket in which we all say we are sixty-five, but some of us are a good bit older, going on to seventy-five and seventy-eight. We are all still going down there and exercising, having fun, working out, staying in shape. I have known many of these men for over fifty years.

When I stopped boxing, I took up handball and swimming. Then it was volleyball. I was too short for that, though. I could set up, but I really couldn't block the taller fellows. Over the years we did practically everything, including jogging. We started a one-hundred-mile club here that is still going.

After the fellows got too tall for me to play volleyball, I took up squash. That was about twenty years ago. I have been playing squash ever since. Sometimes I break that up with jogging.

I have learned that it is best for me is to vary things. When I was a kid it was ballparks, playing baseball, then boxing, volleyball, running, and now squash. I don't know why I do it, probably it has become a habit. I get so much pleasure out of it. It is my way of keeping out of being still and stagnant. That stagnant business, you can have it.

I try to win of course, but it is all in fun. It's not to win at all costs, like it used to be, when you were young. You have to be smarter than that. I have had a few accidents on the squash court—stitches over my eye. That was in the last few years, and I have learned to change my pace a little.

But most of all we get pleasure out of it. There is nothing like exercise and physical fitness—the way it feels and what it does for your circulation. I have never had any real medical problems, although I do take blood pressure pills. I am supposed to take two hydrochlorothiazides a day, and I get regular checkups. So far my blood pressure has remained normal. I told the doctor that sometimes I take only one pill, or not even that, and he said that it was okay.

I think that the big thing is that I feel good and my weight is down. About twenty years ago I got heavy for awhile. I was over 150 pounds, and now I am about 135. I remember that one day I got on the scale, and I couldn't believe the weight that I had put on. So I stopped eating so much and started exercising more. That was when we were running. And I have been feeling good ever since. If I have to go someplace, let's say it is two or three miles, I will walk rather than taking the car. Exercise has become a way of life. My advice is that we should all keep active at different things. Find different kinds of exercise so that you stay interested in it, and it keeps on being fun. ❞

—Joe Ricci, 70

Aerobic Conditioning

Aerobic exercise is any form of physical activity that improves the function of your heart and lungs. In the course of such activity, your body increases its ability to use oxygen, and therefore, your endurance increases. Running, swimming, calisthenics, cycling, and competitive sports in which your heart pumps *forcefully* and you breathe *deeply* and *rapidly* are aerobic. In general, weight lifting, yoga, and stationary exercises improve strength and flexibility but are not aerobic.

A simple formula for estimating whether you are exercising to get an aerobic effect is:

$$(220 - \text{age}) \times .75 = \text{aerobic heart rate.}$$

If you attain this heart rate while exercising, you are probably getting an aerobic effect. For example, if you are sixty years old:

$$\begin{aligned}(220 - 60) \times .75 &= 160 \times .75\\ &= 120 \text{ beats per minute.}\end{aligned}$$

Most people over fifty-five who are out of shape should not begin with an aerobic program. Work up to it gradually with vigorous walking, moderate calisthenics, or stationary cycling that do not increase your heart rate to an aerobic level. Also, get a thorough medical checkup before starting to work out vigorously.

Your age does not prevent you from starting an aerobic exercise program. It just may take you a little longer to prepare for it. If you want to read more about aerobics, try *The New Aerobics,* by Dr. Kenneth Cooper (Bantam Books).

Flexibility

The first consideration for anyone beginning an exercise program is total body flexibility. The majority of adults who are injured while exercising are those who have led sedentary lives and then began to exercise too vigorously. If you work behind a desk, nine to five, Monday through Friday, or have not exercised in many years, you are not ready to go the first weekend out.

Begin by considering your own body. Are there particular areas of tightness that often ache when you lift things or exert yourself? If so, these are areas that deserve special attention while warming up and cooling down. The tight areas for most people are: lower back, heel cords (Achilles tendon), and hamstrings (muscles from the buttocks to the back of the knee). For people with arthritis, the hands, shoulders, and neck may also be stiff areas.

I suggest that you perform the flexibility exercises shown on the following pages daily. In other words, even if you are not going to work out that day, you should still do some stretching. This takes only a few minutes, is invigorating, and will keep your muscles supple. If you cannot do this daily, try to do it at least four days a week. Even if you cannot do it that often, you still will benefit by any number of times that you can. Some activity, especially stretching, is better than none at all.

These flexibility exercises should be performed for five to ten minutes both before and after your exercise routine. The particular type of exercise that you pick does not alter the flexibility routine. If you are taking a dance class, yoga, or some other exercise class, your instructor may have a special warm-up, cool-down routine for stretching. Stick to that program. In any case, find some form of stretching that you enjoy, and work at it.

Planning Your Exercise

Once the flexibility exercises are part of your regular routine, you can begin an exercise program to improve strength and endurance. An efficient program should include three or four workouts a week of at least thirty to forty-five minutes. This will improve both your flexibility and cardiovascular (heart) and respiratory (lung) functioning. If you cannot exercise at this minimum, you should still do whatever you can. You should be particularly conscious not to overdo, however, so that you do not injure yourself.

It is up to you to find the kind of exercise that is most enjoyable and rewarding. No single kind of exercise is best for the average person.

Three basic rules should be followed while exercising.

1. Take your pulse at regular intervals. This can be done easily at two places on your body: the radial artery and carotid artery. The carotid artery is at the angle of the jaw (near your ear); the radial artery is on the wrist.

When taking your pulse, begin by feeling for it with the index, middle, and ring fingers; feel by gently placing the finger tips in the carotid or radial areas (see

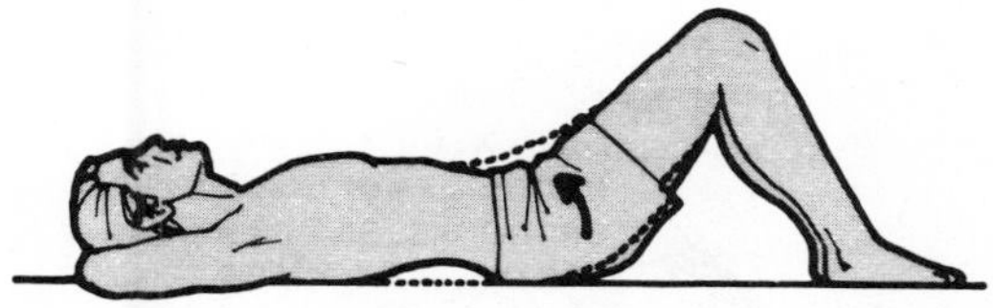

1.

Lie on your back with knees bent and hands clasped behind neck. Feet flat on the floor. Take a deep breath and relax. Press the small of your back against the floor and tighten your stomach and buttock muscles. This should cause the lower end of the pelvis to rotate forward and flatten your back against the floor. Hold for five seconds. Relax.

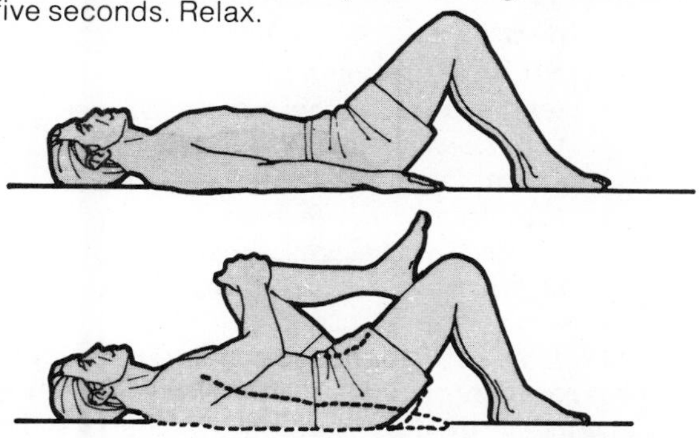

2.

Lie on your back with knees bent. Feet flat on the floor. Take a deep breath and relax. Grasp one knee with both hands and pull as close to your chest as possible. Return to starting position. Straighten leg. Return to starting position. Repeat with alternate leg.

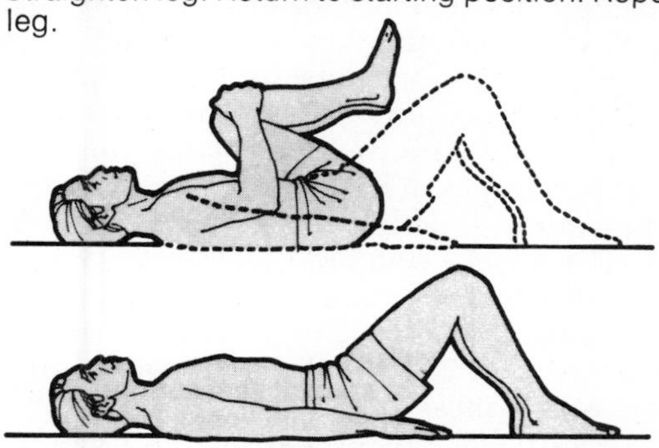

3.

Lie on your back with knees bent. Feet on the floor. Take a deep breath and relax. Grasp *both* knees and pull them as close to your chest as possible. Hold for three seconds, then return to starting position. Straighten legs and relax.

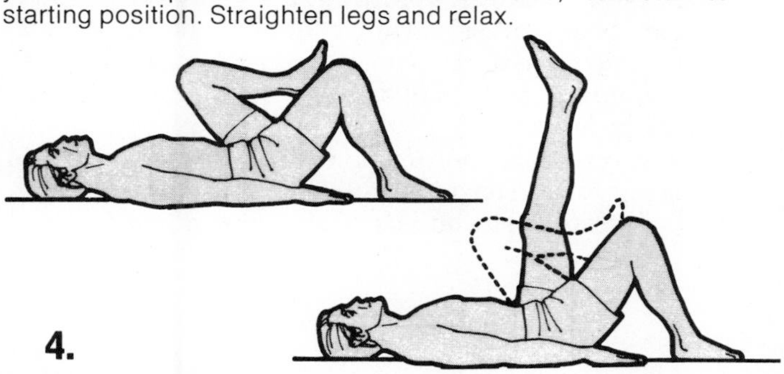

4.

Lie on your back with knees bent. Feet flat on the floor. Take a deep breath and relax. Draw one knee to chest. Then point leg upward as far as possible. Return to starting position. Relax. Repeat with alternate leg.

NOTE: This exercise is useful in stretching tight hamstring muscles, but is not recommended for patients with sciatic pain associated with a herniated disc.

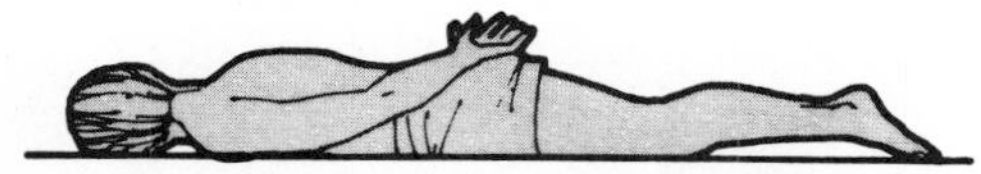

5.

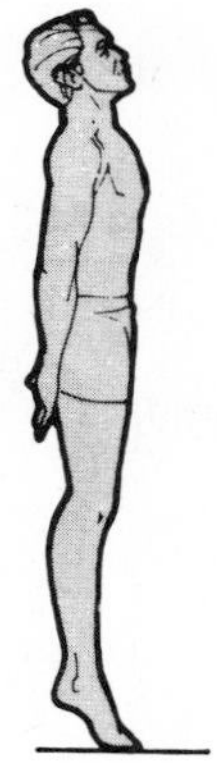

a. Lie on your stomach with hands clasped behind back. Pull shoulders back and down by pushing hands downward towards feet, pinching shoulder blades together, and lift head from floor. Take a deep breath. Hold for two seconds. Relax.

b. Stand erect. With one hand grasp the thumb of other hand behind the back, then pull downwards toward the floor; stand on toes and look at the ceiling while exerting the downward pull. Hold momentarily, then relax. Repeat 10 times at intervals of two hours during the working day. Take an exercise break instead of a coffee break!

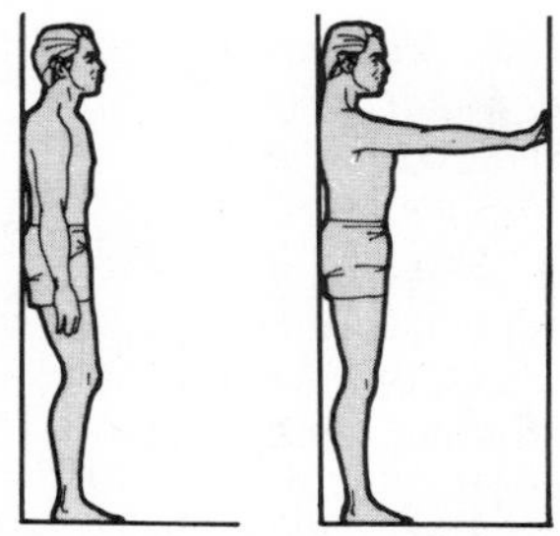

6. Stand with your back against doorway. Place heels four inches away from frame. Take a deep breath and relax. Press the small of your back against doorway. Tighten your stomach and buttock muscles, allowing your knees to bend slightly. This should cause the lower end of the pelvis to rotate forward (as in Exercise 1). Press your neck up against doorway. Press both hands against opposite side of doorway and straighten both knees. Hold for two seconds. Relax.

The following exercises (7, 8, 9) should not be started until you are free of pain and the other exercises have been done for several weeks.

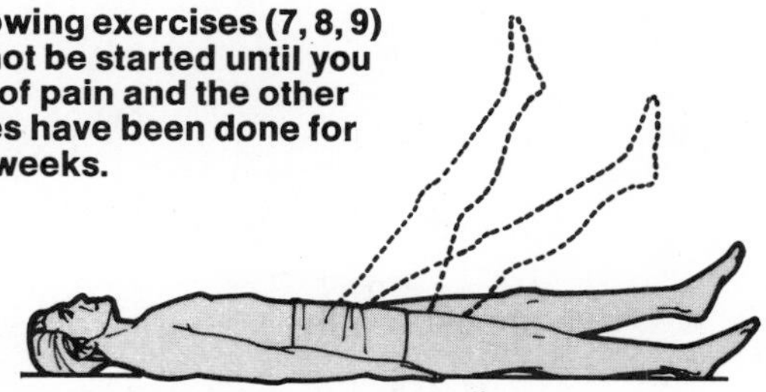

7.

Lie on your back with your legs straight out, knees unbent and arms at your sides. Take a deep breath and relax. Raise legs one at a time as high as is comfortable and lower to floor as slowly as possible. Repeat five times for each leg.

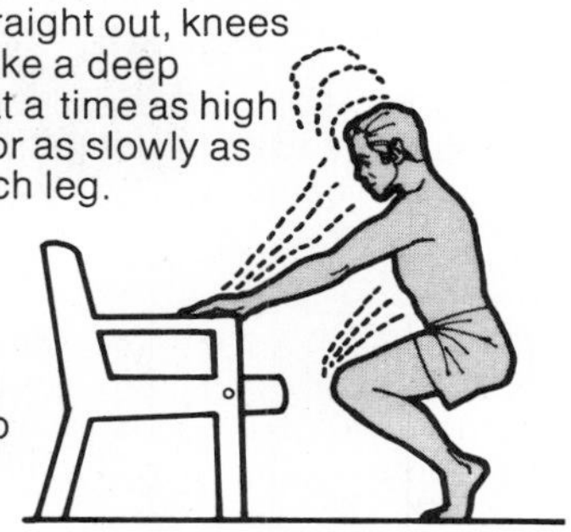

8.

May be done holding onto a chair or table. After squatting, flex head forward, bounce up and down two or three times, then assume erect position.

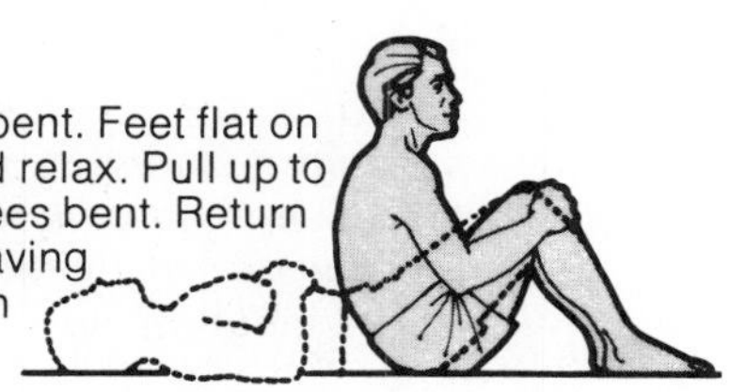

9.

Lie on your back with knees bent. Feet flat on floor. Take a deep breath and relax. Pull up to a sitting position keeping knees bent. Return to starting position. Relax. Having someone hold your feet down facilitates this exercise.

Exercise Set #1: The Back

These are standard back exercises that should be followed in sequence. They are called Williams back exercises *and are also used for people with back pain. They maintain flexibility of the back muscles while strengthening the abdominal muscles. Each step should be repeated five times. (Reprinted with permission: Riker Laboratories, Northridge, CA.)*

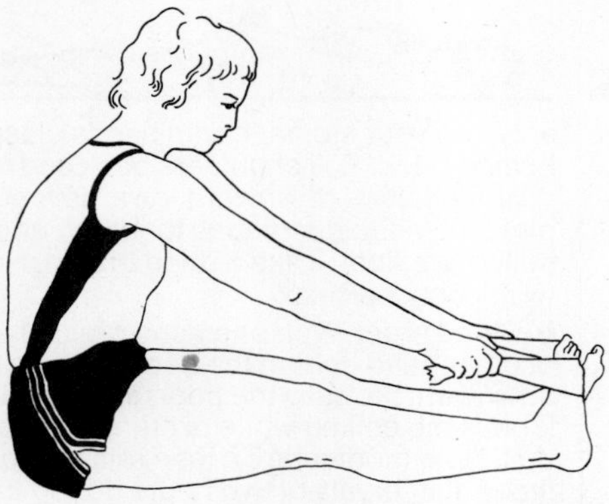

Exercise Set #2: The Heel Cords (Achilles Tendon)
Sit on the floor with your legs extended and toes pointing toward the ceiling. Place a medium-sized towel (dish size) around the upper third of one foot. Holding both ends of the towel, pull your foot toward you. Be sure to keep your heel on the floor. Do only one leg at a time. Hold the stretch to a slow count of four. Repeat, for each leg, five times.

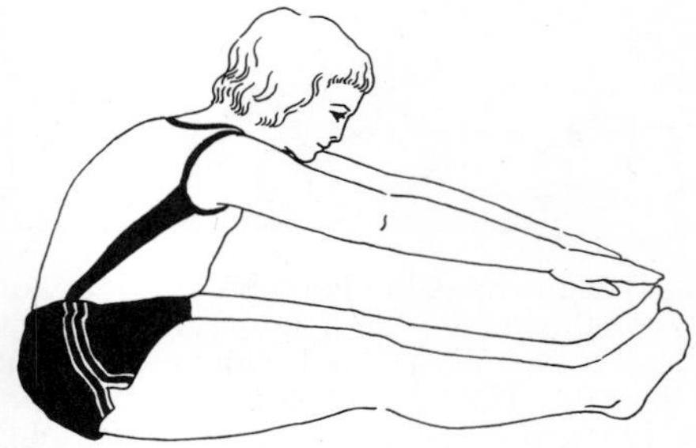

Exercise Set #3: The Hamstrings
Sit on the floor with your legs extended and toes pointing to the ceiling. Lower your torso toward your knees. Do not stretch your feet. Feel the stretch in the muscles of your buttocks and thighs. Hold to a count of four. Repeat five times.

page 34). Do not use your thumb. Take your resting pulse by counting the beats and timing with a watch. You can take your pulse for thirty seconds and multiply by two. Then take your pulse at regular intervals (for instance, after fifteen minutes of exercise) to monitor your body function.

Take your pulse more often during the first few weeks of working out. Avoid exercising to the point of a forceful, bounding pulse or chest pain. As a general rule, exercise only until your pulse is thirty to forty beats per minute above your normal resting pulse. For example, if your normal resting pulse is 80 beats per minute, do not exceed 110 to 120 beats per minute. For people who are unaccustomed to vigorous exercise, 110 to 120 beats per minute should be considered a safe upper limit regardless of what the resting pulse is. You can increase this gradually, as you improve your fitness.

2. Be aware of signs of distress. In other words, be sensitive to the signals that your body is sending out. Any unusual pain, shortness of breath, nausea, lightheadedness, dizziness, vomiting, uneven pulse, bounding heart beats, muscle cramps, or chest pain are signs to *stop* and *rest*. If you continue to exercise, do so at a less vigorous pace. Report these symptoms to your medical provider.

3. Always do a *cool-down* routine of walking and stretching for at least three to five minutes after vigorous exercise. Let your body slow down *gradually*.

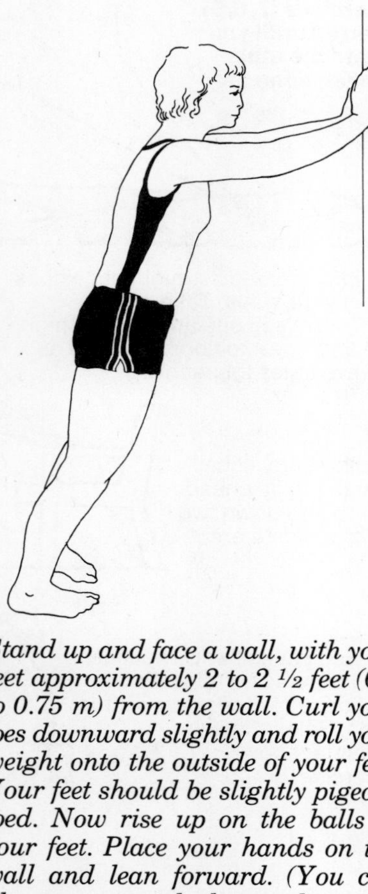

Stand up and face a wall, with your feet approximately 2 to 2 1/2 feet (0.6 to 0.75 m) from the wall. Curl your toes downward slightly and roll your weight onto the outside of your feet. Your feet should be slightly pigeon-toed. Now rise up on the balls of your feet. Place your hands on the wall and lean forward. (You can also use a car, telephone pole, or tall chair for support instead of a wall.) You should feel the stretch in your calves. Hold to a slow count of four. Repeat five times.

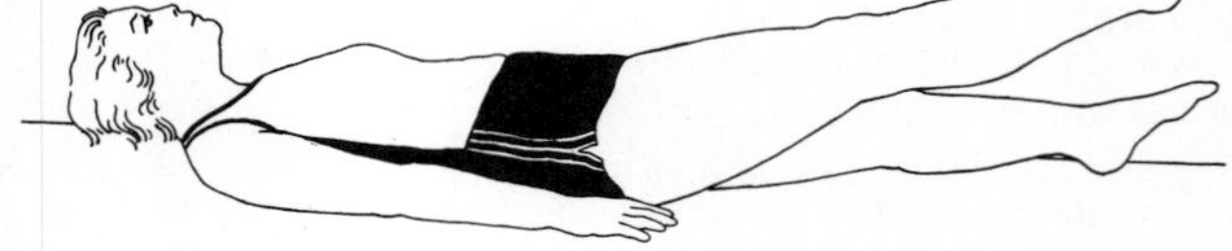

Lie flat on your back. Raise one leg toward the ceiling. Keep your leg straight while you lift it. Raise only one leg at a time to prevent back strain. Hold to a count of four. Repeat five times.

Exercises:

Stand under a hot shower for five to ten minutes and perform the following exercises, twice daily if possible.

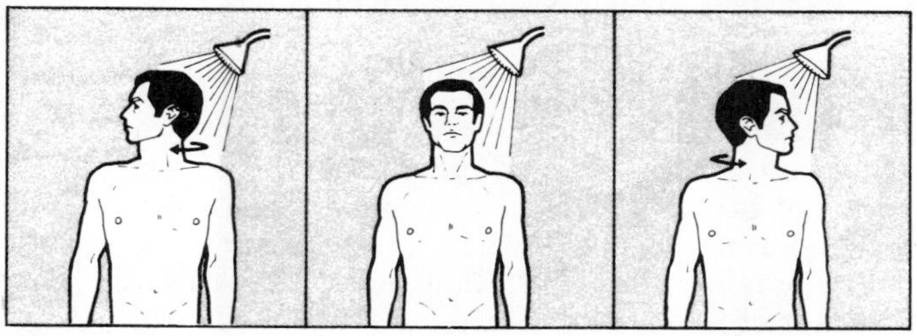

1. Stand erect. Turn head slowly as far as possible to the right. Return to normal center position and relax. Turn head slowly as far as possible to the left. Return to normal center position and relax.

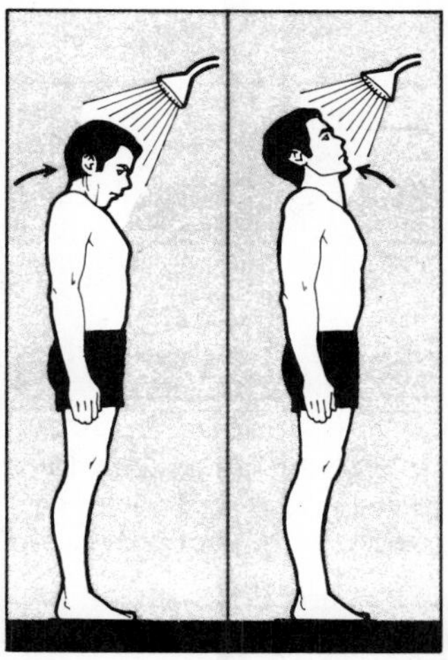

2. Stand erect. Try to touch your chin to your chest, slowly. Raise head backwards, looking up at ceiling, slowly.

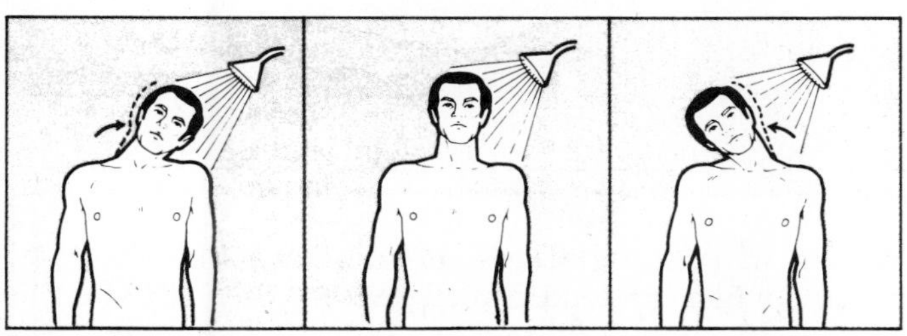

3. Stand erect. Try to touch left ear to the left shoulder. Return to normal center position and relax. Try to touch right ear to the right shoulder. Return to normal center position and relax.

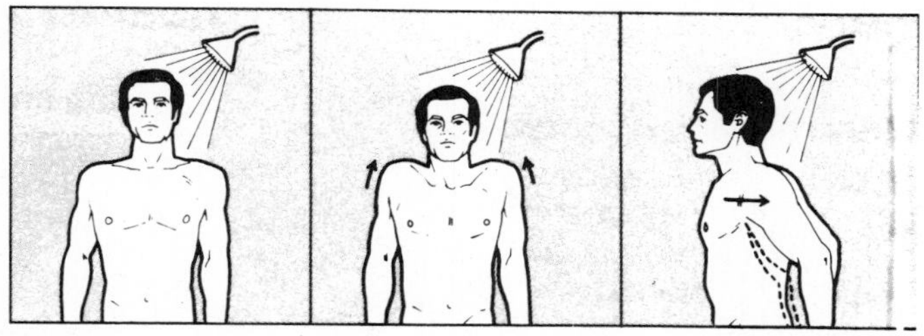

4. Stand erect. Raise both shoulders as close to the ears as possible and hold as you count to five. Relax. Stretch your shoulders backward as far as possible and hold, then relax.

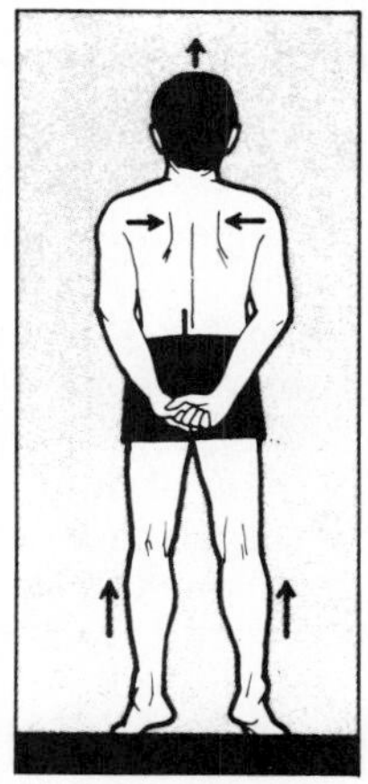

5. Stand erect. With one hand, grasp the thumb of the other hand behind the back, then pull downward towards the floor. Take a deep breath, stand on toes, and look at the ceiling while exerting the downward pull. Hold momentarily, then exhale slowly and relax. Repeat ten times.

Perform these exercises twice daily, preferably after a hot shower.

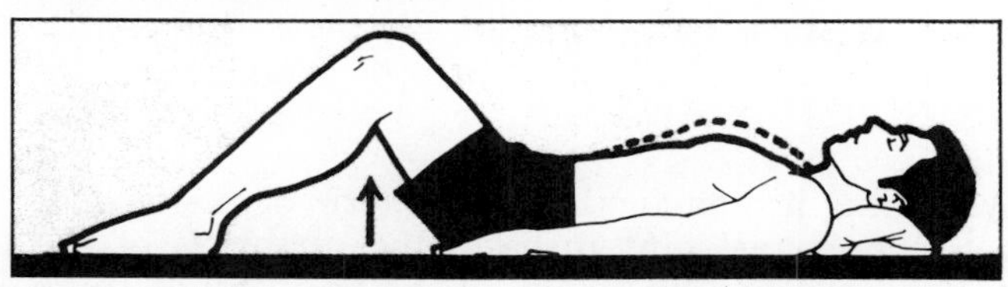

6. Lie on back, knees flexed, with a small pillow under your neck. Take a deep breath slowly, fully expanding chest, then exhale slowly. Repeat ten times.

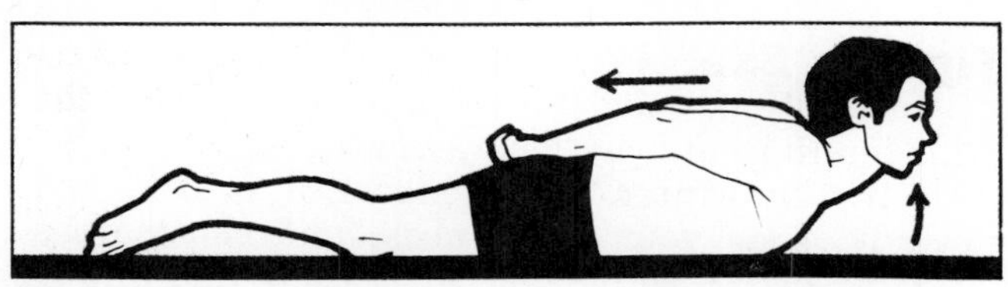

7. Lie on your stomach with hands clasped behind back. Pull shoulders back and down by pushing your hands toward your feet, pinching shoulder blades together, and lift head from floor. Take a deep breath. Hold for two seconds. Relax.

Exercise Set #4: The Neck and Shoulders

Stand erect while performing these stretches. If you are particularly stiff, you may want to perform them in the shower, as shown. This is not necessary, however, if you do not find the exercises painful or difficult. (Reprinted with permission: Riker Laboratories, Northridge, CA.)

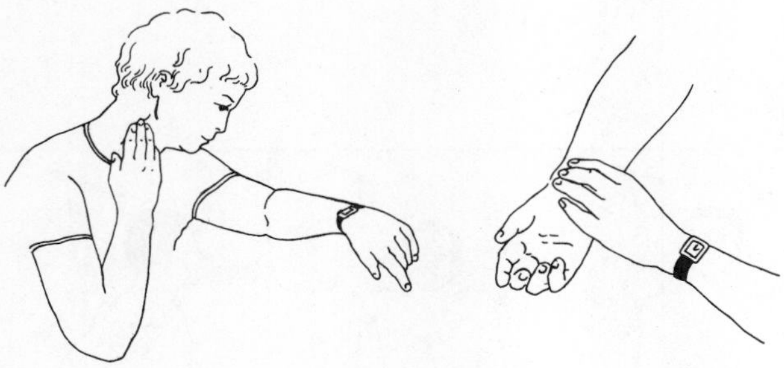

Taking the carotid (left) *and radial* (right) *pulse.*

Picking Your Form of Exercise

The following information can help you decide what form of exercise to start with. Remember that the most important quality of any exercise is that you *enjoy* it, so that you will want to do it on a regular basis.

Walking

Natural limitations on the speed of walking make it safe for almost everyone, and it is especially suited to people with heart disease. It also provides an opportunity to get out into your neighborhood or into the countryside. You get a chance to meet people and see new sights, and there is little risk of strains or sprains.

If you have had a heart attack, you should be able to walk at least one-half mile by the sixth week after leaving the hospital. By the eighth week, you should be able to cover a mile without difficulty. (See Exercising after a Heart Attack, pages 36–38).

Swimming

In the proper environment, swimming is a wonderful aerobic exercise that strengthens the upper extremities as well as the legs and abdomen. Unless you were a good swimmer earlier in life, however, this can be a very strenuous beginning form of exercise. Try to find a "buddy" to swim with or go to a pool that has a lifeguard.

Swimming is a particularly good form of exercise for people who have joint disease (like arthritis of the knee) or have had an injury to the back. Since these joints do not bear your body weight when you swim, there is less pain or chance of injury.

Until your endurance and strength are built up, avoid the overarm crawl. Instead, swim the breaststroke, backstroke, sidestroke, or dog paddle. Avoid cold water, as it can lower your body temperature dangerously fast.

Bicycling

Bicycling is another good aerobic type of exercise that does not strain the joints, because your body weight is supported by the bicycle. A stationary bicycle in your home or office will allow you to work out in poor weather or in a crowded city. In good weather bicycling is a great way to get out into the fresh air.

Adjust the bicycle so that your legs move freely. If you have back problems, avoid a ten-speed bike in favor of a one- or three-speed bike that allows you to peddle upright, with your back straight. Adjust the handlebars so that you do not have to bend over. Avoid excessively tight gripping of the hand grips, as this is an isometric exercise that can stress your heart.

Rope Jumping

Ten minutes of jumping rope equals thirty minutes of jogging! It is a very strenuous form of exercise and may not be safe if you have heart disease. Also, it may be difficult to learn if you are not experienced from earlier in life. If you get the knack, however, it is a good way to exercise in your office or home when the weather is bad.

When jumping rope, place one foot down at a time and alternate stepping your feet through the rope (this is often called skipping rope), rather than jumping with both legs at once. Skipping rope will guard against jarring the hip and knee joints.

Dance

Any form of dance can improve your fitness, but not all forms are aerobic. Vigorous dancing, as in a square dance or polka, may produce an aerobic effect that will benefit your heart and lungs. The most important consideration is to increase your heart rate to 75 percent of its maximum. This need not occur on your first attempt but, as with other athletic activities, comes with practice.

Tips on Exercise

- Pollution is *bad* for everyone. Consider the air quality outdoors before venturing out.
- In the winter, or whenever it is cold and windy, keep your head, neck, and chest areas warm with clothing that fits loosely and allows your skin to breathe.
- Be careful when exercising in hot or humid conditions, which are potentially more dangerous than the cold. Drink ample quantities of fluids like Gatorade, orange juice, lemonade, and other liquids that supply salt, sugar, and water. These nutrients are depleted during strenuous exercise. People on salt- or sugar-restricted diets should consult their physicians. E.R.G. is a powdered drink with the necessary salts that can be purchased in running stores. Reduce your exercise routine when the temperature exceeds 80°F (27°C) and/or 75 percent humidity. Wear a hat when exercising in the sun.
- Avoid heavy meals up to two hours before and one hour after exercising.
- Avoid hot showers, saunas, and steambaths immediately after strenuous exercise. The shock of the heat may direct blood to your skin and away from your heart.
- Rest when ill.
- If you are used to wearing shoes with heels, find an athletic shoe that has an elevated heel.
- It is usually better to increase the time and distance you exercise, rather than emphasizing speed.

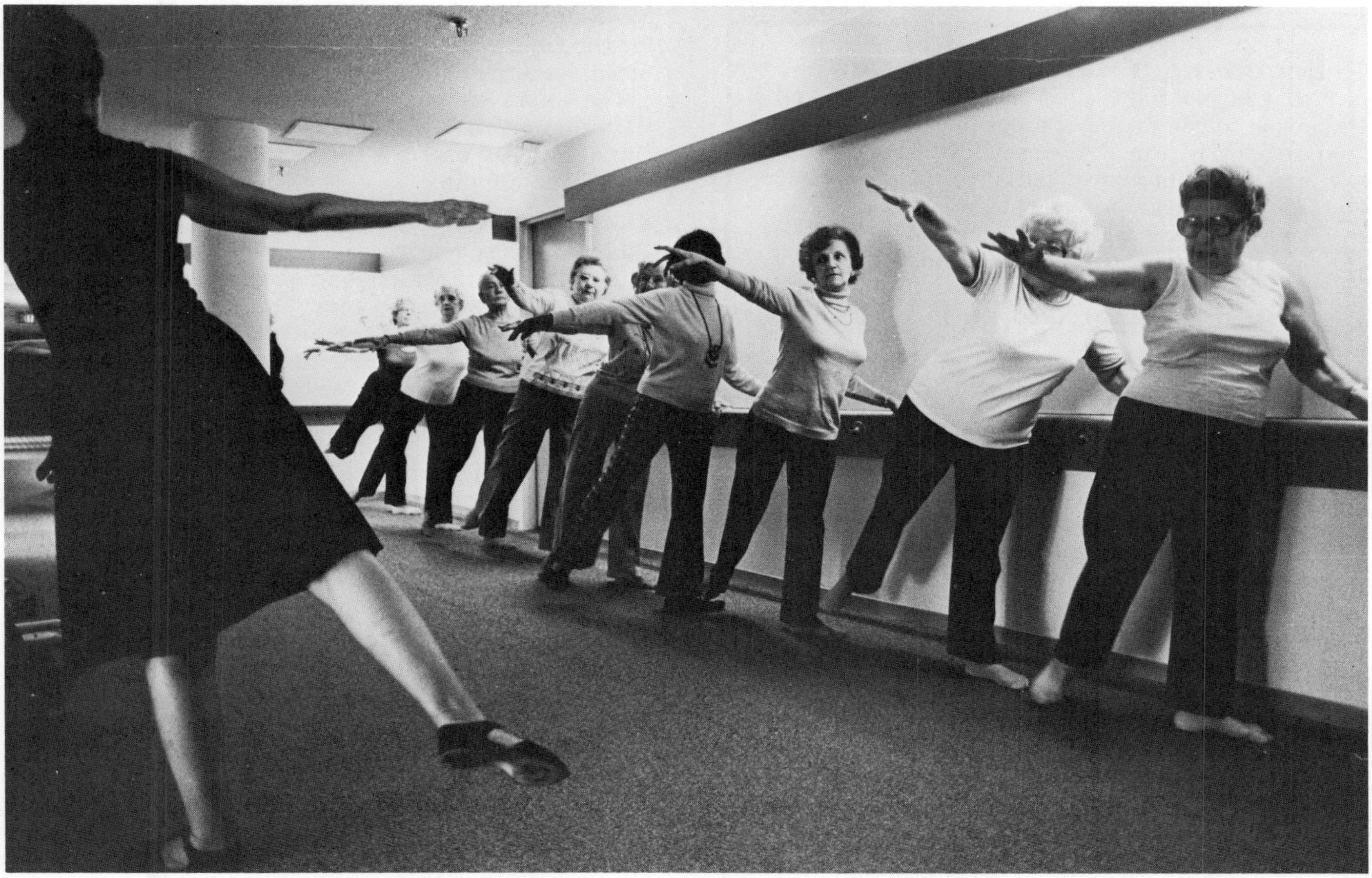

A recent popular means of achieving and maintaining fitness is aerobic dance or Jazzercise. Not really a dance in the traditional sense, aerobic dance consists of vigorous movement performed with lively music to achieve an aerobic effect, as well as improve muscle strength and endurance.

Many clubs, exercise spas, and Ys offer traditional dance and aerobic dance classes, often for a modest fee. The benefits are aesthetic as well as physical, as you learn to move more gracefully and to appreciate the increased suppleness of your body. The dance can be performed in a leotard or in loose-fitting clothing. If you perform barefoot, do so cautiously to avoid blisters or other foot injury.

Yoga

People who are unfamiliar with the many positions of yoga too often dismiss it as a form of exercise because they know only the lotus position or headstand. The ancient art of hatha yoga in actuality consists of a wide variety of breathing, stretching, and loosening exercises that range from the very simple to the extremely complex. These exercises increase your flexibility, improve your ability to concentrate on and control your muscles, and relax your body and spirit. Although it is not an aerobic form of exercise, yoga is enormously beneficial because it reduces tension and improves muscle tone.

Yoga classes are taught in exercise clubs, Ys, in private lessons, and in many community centers. Although there are a number of different types of hatha yoga, there is probably no single form that is best for the average person.

Yoga can be performed by many people who cannot, for one reason or another, participate in vigorous sports. It is safe, can be practiced daily in the privacy of your home, alone or with others, and involves no expensive equipment. Once you become familiar with a yoga routine, you may find that it becomes an integral part of your daily life and a useful way of relaxing your mind, body, and spirit.

Running

If you are not used to running or have not exercised for some time, you should begin a running program very gradually. It is also advisable to see your medical provider for a physical examination before you begin. Chapter 13, *The Heart,* contains more information in this regard.

Most people should begin with walking and then graduate to a routine of vigorous walking alternated with jogging. From the walk-jog cycle, you can increase your routine to a jogging only and then to a more strenuous run. The chart on page 36 gives a sample routine for beginning. You can progress at your own speed and tailor each week's activity level to your needs. Remember, before you begin to run in the run/walk routine, try vigorous walking. Monitor your breathing and pulse as was previously described. Do

Beginning a Running Program

If you are not accustomed to running and wish to begin such a program, the following routine is a model from which to start. Remember that you should have clearance from your medical provider before engaging in any new physical activity and that the routine should begin with a warm-up period of stretching and end with a cool-down period of stretching and reduced activity as described in the text.

The number of sets refers to repetitions of the run-walk cycle of steps. A set is *one* run-and-walk combination. This schedule is based on three workouts per week.

Days	Run (number of steps)	Walk (number of steps)	Number of Sets*
1–6	50	50	5 . . . 10
7–12	50	40	5 . . . 10
13–18	50	30	5 . . . 10
19–24	50	20	5 . . . 10
25–30	50	10	5 . . . 10
31–36	75	10	5 . . . 10
37–42	100	10	5 . . . 10
43–48	125	10	5 . . . 10
49–54	150	10	5 . . . 10
55–60	175	10	5 . . . 10
61–66	200	10	5 . . . 10
67 . . .	individualized program		

* Increase number of sets by one each day at each level of exercise. Stop and rest if signs of distress appear.

(Reprinted with permission of Hubert deVries, PhD, from "Tips on Prescribing Exercise Regimens for Your Older Patient," *Geriatrics,* April, 1979.)

not advance to jogging if you have any of the danger signs that were mentioned.

Special Considerations

For the most part, physical limitations, time constraints, modest finances, or being away from the gymnasium should not prevent one from exercising. These are special considerations that require some mental and physical adaptation but are usually not insurmountable. Continuing with an exercise program in the face of these conditions will help you maintain a healthy body and a positive outlook.

Exercises for Home, Office or Traveling

Sometimes you may not be able to get out to run or you may not have time for a trip to the gym. At other times you may be traveling on business or for pleasure and be unable to find a place to work out. You can still do some basic exercises in your home, office, or hotel room that will help you keep loose and fit.

As before, always begin with your warm-up stretching and finish with a period of cooling-down stretches. Your active routine should be thirty minutes or more. Even if you do not do the active part of the warm-up, however, try to do the stretches. You will stay flexible for the time when you get home and can resume your normal exercise routine.

The chart on page 37 provides a sample routine that emphasizes abdominals, leg, back, and arm muscles. The only exercise aid not normally available is a rope for jumping.

Exercising with Arthritis

When most people think of arthritis, they think of osteoarthritis, in which joints become stiff and painful from general wear and tear. The joints that are most often affected are the hands, knees, hips, neck, and lower back. The directions that follow are directed at people with this kind of arthritis. If you have rheumatoid or gouty arthritis (see Chapter 18, *The Skeleton*), you may have some special needs to consider before beginning an exercise program. You should work this out with your medical provider before beginning.

The objective of the exercise program is to maintain normal range of motion and muscular strength. Exercise should be started before function is lost. If some motion and strength has been lost, however, they can be improved—or at least not further lost—with a regular program. For the most part, exercise should not be performed during periods of pain and inflammation.

There are two types of exercises: *active* and *resistive.* Active exercises maintain range of motion through movement. Resistive exercises increase strength by working against a weight or force that opposes the movement. Weight lifting, for instance, is resistive because the weights impede motion.

In general, arthritic sufferers should begin with active exercises and progress to resistive exercises only if they do not have pain. An active exercise can be converted to a resistive exercise by adding a weight or by having another person manually resist the movements.

Heat is of potential benefit for arthritis. It relaxes the muscles and reduces irritation in the joints. Applying heat before exercise may make movement less painful and exercise easier and more pleasurable. Moist heat can be applied with a warm towel, hot shower, or steam bath. Melted paraffin and mineral oil baths can also be used for hands, feet, or elbows. A special setup and instruction from a trained medical person are necessary for this. Without proper instruction, burns may result. For most people warm towels and showers are an easy, inexpensive, and satisfactory alternative.

The chart on page 38 provides a sample exercise routine for joints that are commonly painful and stiffened with osteoarthritis. Use this guideline along with the advice of a medical provider.

Exercising after a Heart Attack

In the last decade or so, physicians have come to feel that exercise is important after a heart attack. It not only promotes health and avoids invalidism, but it creates a more positive self-image. After a heart attack, it is extremely important to work out an exercise routine with a cardiologist.

Exercise of some kind usually begins within a few days of admission to the hospital. This may mean sitting up in bed, with gradual progression of activity to

Exercises for Home, Office or Travel

Warm-up: Stretch for 5 minutes (minimum)
Dynamic period:

1. Jump rope, or
Hop in place with both feet together, or
Step up onto a stool that is eight to sixteen inches (20 to 40 cm) high, then step down. Alternate feet.
PERFORM any one of these exercises for ONE minute.
REST for THIRTY SECONDS.
REPEAT activity-rest cycle THREE times or more.

2. Single leg lifts (front)
Lie on your back and lift right leg about six inches (15 cm) off ground. Let it fall to the floor. Repeat with left leg.
PERFORM lifts FIVE to FIFTEEN times with each leg.
(Lift only one leg at a time to prevent back strain.)

3. Single leg lifts (back)
Lie on your stomach and lift right leg about three to five inches (7.5 to 12.5 cm) off ground. Let it fall to the floor. Repeat with left leg.
PERFORM lifts FIVE to FIFTEEN TIMES with each leg.
(Lift only one leg at a time.)

4. Jumping jacks
Stand with legs apart at shoulder width, and hands at your sides. Jump and spread your legs to the sides and simultaneously raise your arms above your head and clap them together. Return to standing position with feet together and arms at sides.
REPEAT jumping jacks FIVE to TWENTY times.

5. Hop-kick
Stand with feet at shoulder's width. Hop on left leg and swing right leg to the side. Simultaneously swing right arm to the side. Try to touch your right leg to your right hand. Repeat with left leg.
PERFORM on each side FIVE to FIFTEEN times.

6. Push-ups
Place both hands on a chair, bed frame, stool, or other solid object. Stretch your body out so that your back is straight and your feet are about six inches (15 cm) apart. Lower your chest, and then push up with your arms. (The lower the object, the more difficult the push-up. When accustomed to push-ups, place your hands on the floor.)
PERFORM push-ups FIVE to FIFTEEN times.

7. Sit-ups
Lie on your back with legs bent so that your heels are twelve to eighteen inches (36 to 48 cm) from your buttocks. Clasp your hands behind your head. Pull your chest up and forward and touch your right elbow to your left knee. Return to the floor. Repeat, touching left elbow to right knee. (The farther your heels are from your buttocks, the more difficult the sit-up.)
DO each side FIVE to FIFTEEN times.

Cool-down: Stretch at least three to five minutes

Total time: Thirty to forty-five minutes, depending on the number of repetitions in each exercise and the rest period in between.

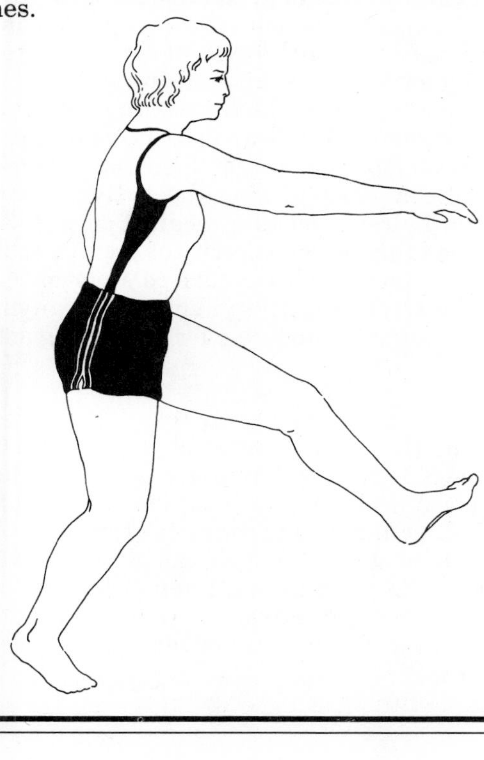

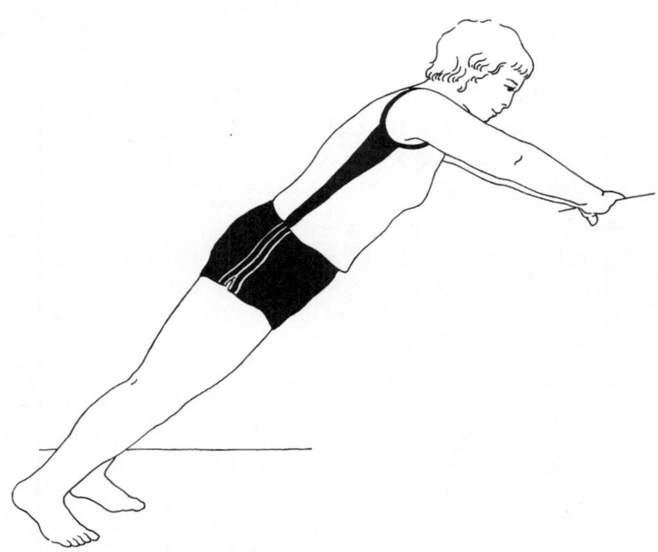

Exercises for Arthritis

The Wrist

1. Close all fingers and thumb to a tight fist, then open to full extension of fingers.
2. Turn a door knob (resistance can be provided by someone holding other side of knob).
3. Shake wrist.
4. Wring out assorted sizes of wet cloth.

The Fingers

1. With palm flat on table, raise and lower fingers one by one.
2. Make an O by touching thumb to fingertips one at a time.
3. Crumble a sheet of newspaper into a small ball with one hand.
4. Squeeze a small rubber ball or sponge.
5. Pick up coins or buttons of assorted sizes.

Neck and Shoulders

See exercise set #4, page 33. Exercise may be performed in or out of the shower.

The Hips

1. Lie on back; raise and lower leg slowly (a) with knee straight; (b) with knee bent. Perform on each side.
2. Lie on back, with legs straight. Slide legs wide apart to the side and return.
3. Lie on back, with legs flat on bed. Stretch first one leg then the other downward, then shrug each hip upward.
4. Stand between two chairs, grasping backs for support. Swing leg back and forth. Alternate legs.

The Knees

1. Sitting or lying on back, with knee bent, tighten muscles of entire leg, then straighten the knee.
2. Sitting on floor, keeping leg straight, lift knee off floor.
3. Sitting, gradually bend leg over edge of a table high enough to allow leg to dangle. Bend and straighten the knee. (Sandbags of gradually increasing weight can be hung over the ankle as the leg strengthens. You can make them by filling socks with beans or purchase them in a hospital supply outlet or athletic shop.)

The Ankles

1. Bend foot up and down slowly.
2. Turn foot in and out slowly.
3. Sitting, rotate the foot in a cranking or circular motion.

Perform as many exercises in each category, for as many repetitions, as are comfortable.

Exercising after a Heart Attack

Remember:

- begin only after medical clearance
- stop at any sign of distress
- avoid all burst activity and isometric exercise

First Twelve Weeks

Very light and light activity. Increase heart rate no more than thirty to forty beats per minute above normal resting heart rate.

Weeks Twelve to Twenty

Increase activity level gradually in consultation with a doctor. Avoid snow shoveling, heaving, lifting, and other exercises that cause strain (isometrics).

Weeks Twenty-one and after

Continue to gradually increase activity, as a doctor directs. Gradually increase length of exercise routine, e.g., from three times per week to four to five times; from thirty minutes to forty-five minutes. Avoid sudden bursts of activity, such as sprinting and heavy lifting, in favor of slowly increasing endurance. Watch for signs of distress.

walking and taking care of washing, dressing, eating, and going to the bathroom.

Once home, it is important to get clearance from a medical provider to gradually increase activities. This usually means light housekeeping, personal care, and visiting friends. All *bursts* of activity, like lifting, carrying heavy objects, and straining should be restricted at first. This form of exercise imposes a large demand on the heart. Nausea, light-headedness, chest pain, and sweating are signs of distress. These symptoms indicate a need to stop the activity and rest. They should be reported to a medical care giver.

Depending on the severity of the illness, heart attack victims can probably return to a normal life-style and regular physical activity. The accompanying chart provides a sample timetable for increasing activity levels.

✽

Almost everyone is capable of finding an exercise routine that will improve physical fitness and mental outlook. It does not really matter whether you have a weight problem, a modest income, are mostly housebound, or have some physical limitation. With effort and some direction, you can find a program that is tailored to your needs. Even if you do only a small amount of regular exercise, you will find that you will feel better about yourself and improve your overall health.

Chapter 8
Nutrition

Gerry Marcus, RD

Good nutrition is something that all of us can provide for ourselves to feel better, look more attractive, and probably live longer. Research data increasingly demonstrates the importance of diet in preventing and controlling many of the major health problems of society: high blood pressure, diabetes, heart disease, ulcers, hemorrhoids, diverticulosis. It is now thought that many forms of cancer may be linked to diet. By eating better we can improve our health and prevent many medical problems.

With eighty million overweight people in the United States, overeating is one of our most alarming problems. Obesity is related to our food preferences, which are established in childhood and reinforced by the media, the fast-food industry, and a fast-paced lifestyle. We consume far too many fatty foods (such as large quantities of red meats), refined carbohydrates (table sugar and white flour products), processed foods high in salt and chemical additives, and snack foods (chips, cookies, and candy) that add calories without providing nutrition.

Instead of these foods, we should be cooking more for ourselves and emphasizing whole grains, fruits, vegetables, fish, and poultry. These foods supply basic nutritional needs without unnecessary calories. Studies of cultures where people live longer than the average American show that these people eat about half the daily calories that we do. Not only do we eat the wrong foods, but most of us eat too much.

Losing Weight

The concept of appropriate weight is one of great controversy. Yet most people over fifty-five are extremely weight conscious. If you are concerned about your weight, ask your medical provider whether you should begin a reducing program. If you then feel that you should lose weight, you should be aware of some important facts.

Reducing the total number of calories consumed daily should be a goal for most of us. Rather than starving ourselves with quick and easy weight-loss diets, we should change our basic eating habits. Carbohydrates are not the primary cause of obesity; fat is a greater problem, simply because it is a much more concentrated source of calories. We get this fat from excessive intake of meats and dairy products. For example, a five-ounce steak has 500 calories, 8 percent of which comes from fat. A five-ounce potato has only 110 calories, only a few of which are from fat. At Michigan State University a study was performed in which two groups were given an equal daily allotment of calories. One group ate twelve slices of whole wheat, high-fiber bread. Although both groups ate the same number calories, the group that ate the high-fiber bread lost more weight. We do not know exactly why this should have been so, but it now appears that a whole-grain, whole-food diet can be more useful in promoting weight loss than a diet of equal calories made up of refined carbohydrates and fats.

People over fifty-five lose weight just as younger people do, with one important difference. As we age, most of us require fewer daily calories to keep our body weight constant, probably because of the diminution of two factors: basal metabolic rate and activity level. For instance, the average person between fifty-one and seventy-five seems to require 10 percent fewer calories than a person of equal size who is younger. After seventy-five the basic daily caloric requirement usually drops another 10 percent.

One way to lose weight more easily, and to do so without feeling starved, is to exercise regularly. Studies have shown that exercise not only burns added calories for the time you are exercising, but also increases your basal metabolic rate for up to fifteen hours after your period of activity. That means that you burn additional calories because your body stays "revved up" for a period of time after your exercise routine. Furthermore, some people claim that they feel less like eating so much when they are involved in a regular exercise program.

Adding fiber to the diet also probably helps with weight reduction. Fiber, like that found in bran, is not digestible; hence, it does not add calories. It is therefore filling without adding to your weight. You can eat more bulk, which digests slowly, yet you do not add calories. Fiber also increases the regularity and frequency of bowel movements, so that fewer calories may be absorbed as the food passes through the digestive system.

Contrary to popular belief, advertising, and the media, no miracle diet will make you lose weight. To reduce, you have to take in fewer calories than you

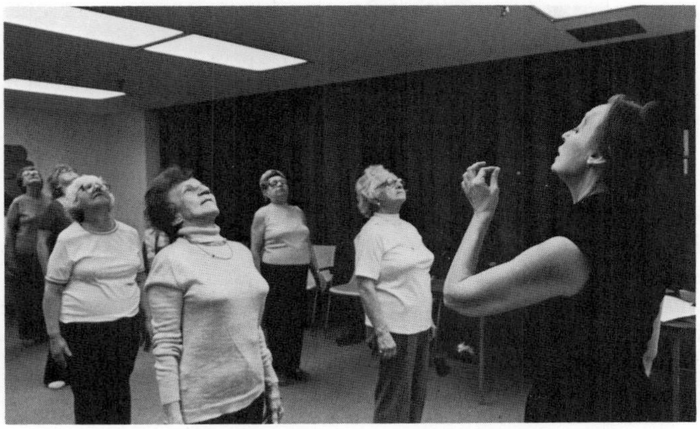

need to maintain your body weight. There is no magical way around this fact.

As a general rule, one pound (0.45 kg) of body weight equals 3,500 calories. Therefore, if you eat 500 calories less than you need to maintain your body weight each day, you should expect to lose one pound (0.45 kg) a week (500 calories times seven days equals 3,500 calories, or one pound).

For example, a sixty-year-old woman who is five feet four inches tall needs about 1,800 calories each day to maintain her current body weight. By eating 1,300 calories each day for a week, she can expect to lose a pound (0.45 kg) per week. If she is fifteen pounds (6.75 kg) overweight, it will take three or four months to lose the weight. (To find out the amount of calories you need for your height, weight, and age, consult a medical practitioner or registered dietician.) A regular exercise program will help her lose this weight somewhat faster, as well as making her body look more trim. Exercise will also increase her ability to burn off calories more rapidly in the future, because she will be replacing fat with muscle. Fat does not burn calories, whereas muscle does.

Weight loss should be gradual. Crash diets not only do not work, but they are dangerous. They do not work because people fail to change their regular eating patterns. Hence, crash dieters tend to gain the weight back after the diet ends. Dieting effectively means learning new eating patterns that help keep one's weight constant at the desired reduced level.

Some hints may help when dieting. Overweight people often claim that they skip meals, do not eat breakfast or lunch, and yet still seem to gain weight. Studies have shown that eating a large, highly caloric meal at night is more likely to put on pounds than three or more smaller meals spaced throughout the day. Still, many of us follow the pattern of starving all day and gorging at night. We may go out to a show and then go out to dinner, and then go to sleep. Or we eat with friends, beginning our meal at nine or ten at night, and then retire to bed. This means that we are consuming the bulk of our calories at a time when we are sedentary and cannot metabolize them efficiently. You can still dine late, but try to enjoy a small meal along with your socializing.

Eating large amounts of proteins to produce ketones will not suppress your appetite and make you lose weight. In one study one group of rats was fed a high-protein diet while the other received a diet with a normal mix of carbohydrates and protein and the same number of calories. The latter group gained less weight.

Part of a weight reduction program involves learning to cook and enjoy a different kind of diet. If you are used to having large portions of red meat, you should be aware that this will make dieting more difficult than if grains, vegetables, and fruits are your mainstays. This is because meat contains large quantities of fat. You can still eat meat, but you should find ways of emphasizing other kinds of foods as well. For instance, you can stir-fry Oriental-style dishes that have small pieces of meat mixed in with vegetables. You can also begin to eat more poultry and fish. These foods have a lower fat content than beef, pork, and lamb.

Dieting means *relearning* patterns of cooking and eating that are built up over a lifetime. This is a profound process. You should see dieting as a change in life-style, rather than merely a program of weight reduction. Weight should come off gradually, accompanied by increasing daily exercise and one's personal awareness of eating habits. In that way the weight will tend to stay off, rather than fluctuating up and down according to whether you are dieting or binging.

Keeping a Food Diary

Often people are unaware of how many needless and useless calories they consume each day. One way to be more aware of what you are eating and to make changes in your basic dietary patterns is to keep a food diary. The diary is designed to make you aware of the unnecessary calories you consume each day, such as that extra brownie or the three spoons of sugar you add to your morning coffee.

To do this, you must keep the diary, along with a basic calorie-counting guide, with you at all times—during work, when socializing, even when traveling. Keep your record in a small notebook that you can carry with you easily. You should mark down the time, the food, and the approximate amount of everything you eat and drink at the time you do it. Try not to rely on your memory so that you will not omit snacks, alcoholic drinks, and desserts. The accompanying chart is a sample page from a food diary.

At the end of two weeks, add up your calories and get an idea of how many unnecessary calories you consume, and in what form. Some may eat too many fatty meats; others may drink unnecessary alcoholic beverages. Others find that they snack far more than they had realized. The food diary will give you clues

Time/Date	Food	Amount	Calories	Salt
Monday				
8 A.M. breakfast	coffee/milk	1 cup	30	7 mg.
	buttered toast	2 slices	245	10 mg.
	grapefruit	1/2	45	
10 A.M. snack	coffee/milk	1 cup	30	7 mg.
	muffin	1	140	5 mg.
12:30 P.M lunch	sliced chicken	3 ounces	115	15 mg.
	bread	1 slice	70	
	coffee/milk	1 cup	30	7 mg.
6 P.M. dinner	lamb chop	1 (3 ounce)	360	20 mg.
	white rice	1 cup, cooked	60	10 mg
	green salad/vinegar dress	medium	140	20 mg
	beer	1 glass (8 oz.)	110	

as to where you can cut your daily calories without curtailing the intake of essential nutritional needs.

Eating and Aging

Unless you have special medical problems that require dietary treatment, good nutrition does not differ significantly after age fifty-five. Despite the 10 percent reduction in calories previously mentioned, we have the same basic needs for protein, minerals, vitamins, and other nutrients as we age. That means it is worthwhile to make extra efforts to avoid foods with empty calories, because there is just a little less leeway for eating highly caloric foods that are not very nutritious.

Some older people have dentures that slip or fit poorly and make eating difficult. If your dental work does not fit properly, go back to your dentist and have it realigned. Dentures should not make eating a normal diet impossible.

Women after menopause may find eating foods rich in vitamin D and calcium worthwhile. Osteoporosis occurs most commonly in women after menopause (see also Chapter 18, *The Skeleton*) and may also be seen in older men. It may be aggravated, or even caused, by poor dietary intake of calcium and vitamin D. Therefore, older men and women should be conscious of taking in adequate amounts of these substances. You do not necessarily need vitamin or mineral supplements; rather, you can assure adequate calcium and vitamin D with a diet of dairy products (use those made with skim milk to minimize your intake of fat), dark leafy vegetables (like kale, collards, and mustard greens), and turnips. In addition, vitamin D is made on our skin by sunlight.

The debate over the need for and use of vitamin supplements is highly controversial. In general, most nutritionists do not feel that people need vitamin supplements if they eat a normal diet. Unless you have a medical problem for which they are prescribed, you probably do not need them. They should not be used to make up for a diet based primarily on junk foods, processed foods, or snacks.

Furthermore, some of the nutritional supplements may be dangerous. For instance, a recent report cited dolomite, often taken to replace calcium and magnesium, as containing lead, arsenic, mercury, and aluminum—all potentially dangerous substances. Large doses of vitamins A, D, E, and K are also potentially harmful because excess amounts of these vitamins are stored in fat cells rather than excreted by the body as some other vitamins are. If you think you need vitamins, consult your medical provider and discuss the issue. If your diet is poor, you need to improve it with real food. If you feel ill, you need a thorough investigation to discover why. Vitamins are medicines and should not be a substitute for a full medical analysis or a complete diet.

Fiber

Many misconceptions exist about fiber—what it is and its role in the diet. In simplest terms, fiber is largely indigestible plant material that provides no caloric value as it passes through the intestine. Contrary to popular belief, salads, prune juice, and the common breakfast cereals (except those that contain bran) actually provide very little in the way of dietary fiber. People often eat these foods to keep them regular, but in reality they do little in this regard.

Bran and other foods high in fiber will help in promoting normal, regular bowel movements, as well as digestion in general. Fiber is filling without adding calories and, as mentioned, it may help in weight reduction. Diets that are low in fiber (those common in Western industrialized countries) are associated with an increased incidence of diverticulosis, cancer of the colon, hemorrhoids, and gallstones. The link is not completely understood, but it is cause for concern. Most of all, constipation, extremely common in people over fifty-five, is associated with a diet low in fiber.

The average person needs a fiber intake of 2.8 to 5.2 grams each day. This can be supplied by a few tablespoons of bran each day. You can sprinkle it on cereal and vegetables, bake it into breads, and add it to blenderized drinks, breaded fried or baked foods (like chicken or fish), and stuffings. The accompanying chart lists common foods and their fiber content.

Reading Labels

Since many people eat processed or canned foods, it is essential that you know what you are getting from these products. You can learn this from the label on the can, frozen food package wrapper, or from an insert that comes with the product. Processed foods must, by law, list the basic nutritional information, and reading the label will educate you as to the value you are getting for your food dollar. You will be able to make comparisons of products to get the best nutrition for your budget and personal taste.

All of the ingredients in the product must be listed in the order they appear by weight. In other words, if the product is mostly sugar, that must be the first ingredient listed on the label. Sometimes this is deceiving. By using three or four different sugars, like sucrose, dextrose, and lactose, and listing them separately, the manufacturer can obscure the total amount of sugar in the product. This device can be used with different kinds of fats as well. As you become used to reading labels, you will learn to evaluate the ingredients and will soon recognize what is really in the product.

The nutritional information on the label is based on the laboratory analysis by the manufacturer. The Food and Drug Administration (FDA) is responsible for checking all of the products on the market. Although this does not necessarily mean that the information is inaccurate, as consumers, we should be aware that this information does not come from an independent source. The chart on page 44 demonstrates how to read a label.

Some foods, such as ice cream, mayonnaise, and catsup, have additives that are not listed. A product sold under these names must contain certain ingredients. The name ice cream, for instance, is a registered product term: all the individual ingredients therefore do not have to be mentioned. The words *All Natural* on ice cream are misleading, because ice cream has stabilizers and other additives registered under its name. If you are uncertain whether a product has additives, write the manufacturer via the distributor. If you do

Fiber Content of Common Foods

I. Beans and legumes

These foods contain protein as well as being high in fiber. Meats, on the other hand, contain little fiber.

Food	Fiber (grams)
Baked beans, with pork & tomato sauce, 1 cup	3.6
Black beans, dry, 1 cup	8.8
cooked, 1 cup	3.0
Chick peas, dry, 1 cup	10.0
cooked, 1 cup	2.5
Kidney beans, dry, 1 cup	8.4
cooked, 1 cup	2.3
Lentils, dry, 1 cup	6.6
cooked, 1 cup	2.2
Lima beans, dry, 1 cup	7.0
cooked, 1 cup	2.9
Pinto beans, dry, 1 cup	8.6
cooked, 1 cup	2.3
Split peas, dry, 1 cup	2.4
cooked, 1 cup	1.0
White beans, dry, 1 cup	8.6
cooked, 1 cup	2.2

II. Snacks and Sweets

Nuts, seeds, and popcorn are rich in fiber. Candies, commercially prepared baked goods made with refined flour and sugar, and ice cream, however, have almost no fiber.

Food	Fiber (grams)
Brownie with nuts, 1 med.	0.1
Coconut, shredded, 1 cup	2.0
Cookies	
choc. chip, 1	trace
fig bar, 1	0.3
macaroons, 1	0.5
Fruitcake 2 in. sq., ½ in. thick	0.2
Nuts	
almonds, whole, 13–15	0.5
Brazil nuts, ½ cup	3.1
cashews, ½ cup	0.7
peanuts, roasted, ½ cup	1.1
pecan halves, ½ cup	1.0
Peanut butter, 1 tsp.	0.3
Pickles, dill, 1–4 in.	0.5
Pie, 1/7 of 9 in. pie	
apple	0.5
blueberry	0.9
pumpkin	0.7
Popcorn, popped, 1 cup	0.1
Pumpkin seeds, ¼ cup	0.7
Soynuts, roasted, ¼ cup	1.0
Sunflower seeds, ¼ cup	1.3

III. Fruit

Fruits with edible skin and/or seeds are highest in fiber. Juices, like orange juice, have less fiber because most of the pulp has been removed. Eat the fruit rather than drinking the juice. Eat the skins of fruits like pears, apples, and plums. Frozen and canned fruits have the same fiber content as the fresh version unless they have been peeled.

Food	Fiber (grams)
Apple cider or juice, ½ cup	0.1
Apples, 1 med.	1.5
Applesauce, canned, ½ cup	0.7
Apricots, canned, 4 halves	0.5
raw, 3 med.	0.6
Avocados, ½ or eight oz.	1.6
Bananas, 1 med.	0.8
Blackberries, ½ cup	3.0
Blueberries, ½ cup	1.1
Cherries, sweet; raw or canned, ½ cup	0.4
Cranberry sauce, jellied, ¼ cup	0.1
Dates, pitted, ½ cup	2.1
Fruit cocktail, canned, ½ cup	0.4
Grapefruit, ½ med. or ½ cup of sections	0.2
Grapefruit juice, ½ cup	trace
Grape juice, ½ cup	trace
Grapes, seedless, ½ cup	0.5
Honeydew, 2 in. × 7 in. wedge	0.9
Orange, 1 med.	0.8
sections, ½ cup	0.4
Orange juice, ½ cup	0.1
Peaches, canned, 2 halves	0.4
raw, 1 med.	0.6
Pears, canned, 2 halves	0.4
raw, 1 med.	2.8
Pineapple, canned, 1 slice	0.3
Pineapple juice, ½ cup	0.1
Plums, purple, canned, 3	0.3
Prunes, pitted, ½ cup	1.2
Prune juice, ½ cup	trace
Raisins, ¼ cup	0.4
Raspberries	
black, ½ cup	3.8
red, ½ cup	2.0
Strawberries, ½ cup	1.0

IV. Vegetables

The skin and seeds of vegetables contain the most fiber. Figures listed are for raw vegetables and include both skin and seeds. Cooking does not remove significant amounts of fiber, but does usually deplete overall volume and vitamin content.

Food	Fiber (grams)
Asparagus, 4 spears	0.4
Beans, green, 1/ cup	0.6
Beet greens, ½ cup	1.1
Beets, diced, ½ cup	0.7
Broccoli, ½ cup	1.1
Brussels sprouts, ½ cup	1.1
Cabbage, shredded, ½ cup, uncooked	0.4

(continued)

Fiber Content of Common Foods (*continued*)

Food	Fiber (grams)
Carrots, 1 med.	0.8
diced, ½ cup	0.6
Cauliflower, ½ cup	0.6
Celery, 3 small stalks	0.3
diced, ½ cup	0.3
Coleslaw, ½ cup	0.8
Corn, kernels, ½ cup	0.7
cream style, ½ cup	0.6
Cucumbers, 1 med.	1.7
pared, 1 med.	0.6
Eggplant, pared & diced, ½ cup	0.9
Lettuce, raw, ½ head	0.3
Mushrooms, canned, ½ cup	0.6
Okra, sliced, ½ cup	0.8
Onions, 1, 2½ in.	0.6
chopped, raw, ½ cup	0.6
Peas, ½ cup	1.6
Peppers, sweet, ½ cup	1.0
Potatoes, baked, 1 med.	0.7
diced, ½ cup	0.4
french fried, 10 pieces	0.5
mashed, ½ cup	0.5
Radishes, 4 small	0.3
Rutabagas, ½ cup	1.1
Sauerkraut, ½ cup	0.9
Spinach, ½ cup	0.6
Squash, acorn, ½ cup	1.6
zucchini, ½ cup	0.5
Sweet potatoes, 1 small	1.0
Tomato juice, ½ cup	0.8
Tomatoes, 1 med.	0.8
Turnips, ½ cup	0.6

V. Breads, Cereals, Pasta, Rice

Breads and cereals with bran have the highest fiber content. Whole wheat, rye, corn, and oat products are also high in fiber. Brown rice has the hull left on, and this is high in fiber content as well. Products made with white flour have had the fiber milled out. Figures listed below are for one-ounce servings unless otherwise indicated.

Food	Fiber (grams)
Bagel, 1 med.	0.1
Biscuits, 1 small	trace
Breads, 1 slice	
cracked wheat	0.1
French	trace
pumpernickel	0.4
raisin	0.2
rye	0.1
white	0.1
whole wheat	0.4
Cereals, cooked, ¾ cup	
cream of rice	0.1
farina	0.2
Maltex	0.3
oatmeal	0.4
Wheatena	0.5
Cereals, ready-to-eat, 1 ounce	
All-Bran, ⅓ cup	2.1
Bran Buds, ⅓ cup	2.0
Bran Flakes, ¾ cup	1.0
Grape Nuts, ¼ cup	0.4
Grape Nuts Flakes, ¾ cup	0.5
Life, ⅔ cup	0.4
Nature Valley Granola, ¼ cup	0.3
Pep, 1 cup	0.3
raisin bran, ½ cup	0.9
shredded wheat, 1 biscuit	0.5
Total, 1 cup	0.5
Wheat Chex, ⅔ cup	0.8
Wheaties, 1¼ cup	0.5
Cornmeal, dry 1 cup	0.8
Flour, 1 cup, sifted	
all purpose	0.2
cake	0.2
rye	0.3
whole wheat	2.8
Grits, cooked, ½ cup	0.1
Macaroni, dry, 8 oz.	0.7
cooked, ½ cup	0.1
Muffins	
blueberry, 3 in.	0.1
bran, 3 in.	0.7
corn, 3 in.	0.2
English, 1	0.2
plain, 1	0.1
Noodles, dry, 8 oz.	0.7
cooked, ½ cup	0.1
Pancakes, 4 in.	0.1
Rice, brown, ½ cup	
dry	0.8
cooked	0.2
Rice, white, ½ cup	
dry	0.2
cooked	0.1
Rye Krisp, 1	0.2
Rolls, white (dinner)	0.1
whole wheat	0.6
Saltines, 1 cracker	trace
Spaghetti, dry, 8 oz.	0.7
cooked, 1 cup	0.1
Waffle, 1, 7 in. size	trace

VI. Main Dishes

Most main dishes, because they are principally meat, are low in fiber. Listed are some dishes in which the fiber content is increased because beans have been added. A few dishes low in fiber are included for contrast.

Food	Fiber (grams)
Beef stew, 1 cup	1.2
Chicken noodle soup, canned	0.1
Chile con carne, 1 cup	1.8

(*continued*)

Fiber Content of Common Foods (*continued*)

Food	Fiber (grams)
Chow mein, chicken, 1 cup	1.1
Clam chowder,	
Manhattan style, canned, 1 cup	0.4
Franks and beans, 1 cup	2.6
Hamburgers (McDonald's)	
Big Mac, 1	0.9
hamburger, 1	0.5
Quarter Pounder, 1	0.6
Macaroni and cheese, 1 cup	0.2
Minestrone soup, canned, 1 cup	0.7
Pizza, 1 slice of 14 in. pie	0.2
Split pea soup, 1 cup	0.5
Tomato soup, 1 cup	0.4

not get the information, write the Food and Drug Administration, Washington, DC 20204.

Two terms used on labels and in describing basic nutritional requirements are Recommended *Dietary* Allowance (RDA) and Recommended *Daily* Allowance (U.S. RDA). Both are generally considered to be in excess of what one needs to maintain a healthy body. Hence, for most people either of these terms can be considered a safe, minimum nutritional level.

These terms are presented on labels in terms of percentages. For example, you will get 35 percent of your daily calcium need from an eight-ounce glass of skim milk. The carton tells you that amount provides 35 percent of your U.S. RDA. Use these figures to help you plan complete meals.

Diet and Cancer

Studies of cancer, especially of the stomach, intestine, bladder, breast, and prostate, have led researchers to believe that diet may play an important role in these diseases. For instance, diets high in fat have been implicated in cancer of the breast. Nitrates and nitrites found in processed meats, sausage and bacon, and also contained in beer, may be associated with increased risk of stomach cancer. Saccharin has been shown to produce bladder cancers in laboratory animals. BHT, a preservative found in many processed foods, is also a suspected carcinogen. Aflatoxins, molds that are sometimes found on nuts and grains, can produce tumors in laboratory animals.

In general, it is extremely difficult to say whether a food additive or a particular dietary factor causes cancer. But data that implicate chemical additives, as well as fats, as potential dangers are piling up. Many people are consequently trying to avoid processed foods that contain additives.

All of us can ask ourselves whether we actually need, or want, to take the risk of eating foods that have been sprayed with pesticides or contain chemical additives. Often with just a small amount of effort and some added awareness, we can eliminate these substances from our diet and thereby reduce our potential risks. For instance, it is possible to lose weight without using saccharin or diet beverages. We can be more careful to buy foods without preservatives and minimize the amount of smoked meats in our diet. As yet, no firm guidelines exist as to what is best. Yet prudence is

Reading Labels

Nutritional labeling is mandatory on processed foods if something has been added or if the manufacturer makes a claim about the nutritional value. This typical label provides the following valuable information to help you make wise consumer choices:

1. The weight of the product in the container. This aids in comparing price. Be aware that the net weight includes the water in which the product is packed.
2. Ingredients are listed in order of concentration by weight. Check to see that you are getting the food you want, not sugar or filler.
3. Serving size, number of servings per container, protein, fat, carbohydrate, and caloric content of *each serving*.
4. Percentage of Recommended Daily Allowance (US RDA) allows you to assess your basic nutritional intake.
5. The name and address of the distributor must be listed. If you wish additional information, such as salt content or the nature of additives, you can write the manufacturer through the distributor.

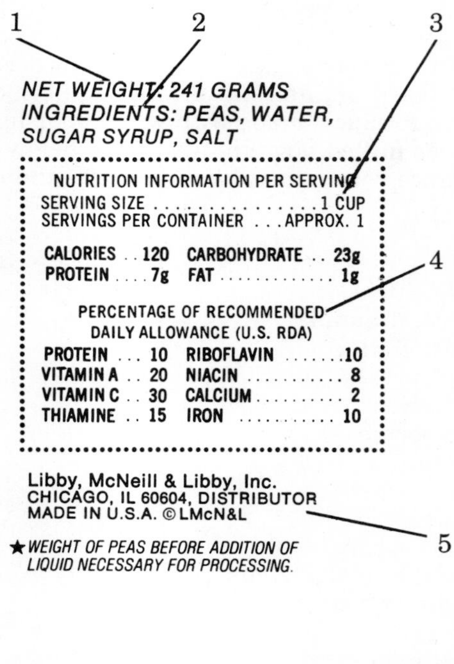

(Reprinted with permission: Libby, McNeill & Libby, Inc.)

clearly the best strategy in the face of the rising number of cancer deaths.

Special Diets

A few common medical problems require special diets. If you have had bowel surgery or diseases of the digestive tract, you will need a more complicated set of dietary guidelines provided by your physician or registered dietician. The diets presented here are for people with high blood pressure, diabetes, and hyperlipidemia (high cholesterol and fats in the blood). Information about these medical problems is also available in Part 3, *Medical Manual.*

Some general diet guidelines should be followed by everyone. We should all limit our intake of salt. By and large we consume far more salt than we need, and excess salt contributes to high blood pressure. Unfortunately, after many years of eating highly salted foods, many of us find foods without added salt have little taste. Substituting herbs, garlic, peppers, dried mustard, and other seasonings will help us kick the salt habit.

We need to reduce the amount of fat we consume, mostly from eating red meats. Diabetes and heart disease are related to this form of dietary indiscretion. Carbohydrates were once considered dangerous for people with diabetes, but now fats are indicted as equally (if not more) dangerous. Most people, including diabetics, should get the bulk of their caloric needs from unrefined carbohydrates like whole grains, rather than from fatty foods and refined carbohydrates.

The information that follows should be added to the advice and counseling of your medical provider. Work out specific diets for your own needs and food preferences. This is an area where you can be a responsible agent, if not prime mover, in your own health care.

High Blood Pressure (Hypertension)

High blood pressure, or hypertension, and salt are intimately linked. The sodium in salt causes your body to retain water. This in turn increases the fluid volume of your blood and raises your blood pressure. Some people with mild hypertension can completely normalize their blood pressure without medication by restricting their salt intake. For others salt restriction helps to reduce the amount of medication they need.

Some sodium is a necessary part of the diet, probably about 230 milligrams per day, or about one-tenth of a teaspoonful. The average American, however, takes in about twenty times that amount, in the form of table salt and in the processed foods that have some salt added to them.

It is not always easy to know which processed foods contain large amounts of salt. For instance, did you know that, ounce for ounce, cornflakes contain more salt than cocktail peanuts? Or that two slices of white bread have more sodium than one ounce of potato chips? Or that a half cup of instant chocolate has more sodium than three slices of bacon? Or that one large dill pickle has six times the amount of sodium of the cornflakes mentioned above? It is a good idea to get used to reading labels for the salt content of processed foods. If you are keeping a food diary, you might want to add a column for the sodium content. You are likely to be surprised at the amount of salt you consume. The following chart lists some forms of hidden salt found in foods.

Hidden Salt

Sodium may be "hidden" in many foods that do not say *salt* on the label. They contain chemicals that have sodium, which act to raise blood pressure in the same way that table salt does. These sodium compounds are usually used as preservatives. Watch out for the following ingredients:

brine (salt and water)
sodium saccharin
sodium alginate
sodium benzoate
sodium hydroxide
monosodium glutamate (MSG)
disodium phosphate
sodium proprionate
sodium sulfite
sodium caseinate

Prepared foods, such as mayonnaise, bouillon powder and cubes, olives, and garlic and onion powders are loaded with salt. So are kosher meats, canned tuna and crab, and canned asparagus and beans. The next chart lists some sample processed foods that are high in salt content and, hence, should be avoided whenever possible.

Highly Salted Foods to Avoid

Many commercially prepared foods are extremely high in salt content even though salt is not listed on the label. The following are common foods that should be avoided if you are on a salt-restricted diet.

- commercial soups, broths, and bouillon cubes
- potato chips, saltine crackers, salted nuts, pretzels, salted popcorn
- olives, pickles, and sauerkraut
- ham, bacon, frankfurters, corned beef, chipped beef, pastrami, sausages, luncheon meats, meats that are canned, smoked or cured
- fish or poultry packed in brine like tuna, shrimp, lobster, and crabmeat; tuna packed in water is permitted
- commercial gravy products, meat tenderizer, catsup, mustard, relish
- soy sauce, Worcestershire sauce, and steak sauces; may be used sparingly in cooking, but should not be liberally added at the table
- Chinese food, if cooked with a lot of soy sauce
- commercially prepared pizzas
- most cheese; use in moderation

Dining out can also be difficult if you want to watch your salt intake. You can ask to have your food prepared without salt, soy sauce, and Worcestershire sauce, but restaurants cannot take the salt out of prepared foods that they purchase. Vegetables, desserts, and sauces that are purchased already prepared by the restaurant probably have large amounts of added salt.

Salt substitutes are available. Potassium is a common sodium substitute, but it tends to taste bitter as well as salty. It also has some physiological effects that can be troublesome. If you are going to use potassium salt substitutes extensively, you should discuss this with your medical provider.

You can also learn to cook with and enjoy other

Salt Substitutes

People with hypertension often take diuretics to reduce their blood pressure. In addition to reducing the amount of water and sodium in the body, some diuretics deplete potassium. The thiazide diuretics, for instance hydrochlorothiazide (HydroDIURIL), have this effect. The salt substitutes presented below are valuable for two reasons: they are lower in sodium than table salt and higher in potassium. They can be used as a seasoning in food, and at the table, instead of table salt. Consult with your medical provider before using these salt substitutes.

Salt products	Potassium content per gram	Sodium content per gram
Co-salt	476 mg	1 mg
Adolph's salt substitute	323 mg	2 mg
Morton's salt substitute	493 mg	1 mg
Morton's lite salt	195 mg	240 mg
Table salt	0 mg	393 mg

Foods that are *high* in potassium include:
Juices: orange, prune, pineapple, grapefruit
Fruits: oranges, grapefruit, raisins, bananas, prunes, strawberries, avocado, tomatoes, apricots, dates, watermelon, cantaloupe
Meats: beef, turkey
Vegetables: artichoke, brussels sprouts

Seasonings to Substitute for Salt

In recent years interest in cooking has increased, resulting in a new and added variety to the number and types of seasonings available. People are willing to enjoy and experiment with spices other than salt. This is especially important for people with high blood pressure, who need to kick the salt habit and learn to appreciate other tastes.

Try the following:
Beef spiced with bay leaf, dry mustard, diced onion and green pepper, thyme, sage, marjoram, chili powder, rosemary, nutmeg, garlic
Poultry spiced with cranberries, orange, paprika, poultry seasoning, sage, thyme, oregano, coconut, garlic
Pork spiced with apples, applesauce, garlic, chili powder, cinnamon, cloves
Lamb spiced with curry, garlic, mint, pineapple, rosemary, thyme, ginger
Fish spiced with bay leaf, curry, dry mustard, ginger, paprika, lemon juice, diced onion, green pepper, mushrooms
Eggs spiced with curry, dry mustard, chopped green pepper, onion and mushroom, paprika, parsley, tomato
Beans spiced with chili powder, cumin, tomatoes, diced green peppers, onion, garlic, dry mustard, brown sugar, savory, thyme
Asparagus spiced with lemon juice or vinegar
Broccoli spiced with lemon juice or vinegar
Carrots spiced with mustard, parsley, mint, brown sugar and butter
Green beans spiced with marjoram, lemon juice, nutmeg, vinegar
Tomatoes spiced with basil, marjoram, oregano, dill
Rice spiced with saffron
Soups spiced with parsley, pepper, tarragon, thyme, lovage, onions and leeks, dill

REMEMBER:

- Do not add salt at the table.
- Whenever possible, decrease the amount of salt in a recipe in favor of increasing the amount of other spices.
- Wine can add flavor to sauces in addition to the spices mentioned.
- Do not use garlic salt and onion salt. Use either fresh garlic and onion, or garlic and onion *powder*.

kinds of seasonings. Be inventive. Getting out of the sodium habit can be an opportunity to experience a whole new array of wonderful tastes.

Diuretics (water pills) used to treat high blood pressure tend to deplete the body's stores of potassium. The salt substitutes listed in the chart will replace this loss. If you are taking a diuretic for high blood pressure, consult your medical provider about these salt substitutes.

Diabetes Mellitus

Adult onset diabetes is intimately involved with diet, both in the acquisition of the disease and its control (see also Chapter 21, *The Hormones*). People with diabetes have an abnormally high concentration of sugar (glucose) in the blood, which has a complex effect on many of the organs of the body.

The more that is learned about diabetes, the more unanswered questions arise. It was once thought that carbohydrates were bad for diabetics, but now the focus has shifted to the elimination of *refined* carbohydrates, such as table sugar and white flour products. In addition, saturated fats—those found in meats and dairy products—seem to aggravate blood sugar abnormalities. In the past people with diabetes were advised to compose their diet of 40 percent carbohydrates, 20 percent protein, and 40 percent fat. It is now felt that 50 to 60 percent of calories should come from carbohydrates, 12 to 20 percent from protein, and only 30 to 38 percent fat. In other words, calories should come from complex, natural carbohydrates like whole grains, and fat intake should be reduced. There should also be an ample amount of fiber, which, along with the complex carbohydrates, seems to improve blood sugar control.

The amount of insulin needed appears to be related to the number of calories consumed and body weight. Most people with diabetes have a weight problem and may resolve their diabetes with weight reduction. A good goal for overweight diabetics is to lose 1 1/2 to 2 pounds weekly. This may mean eating only 1,000 to 1,200 calories each day—a difficult diet to maintain. A regular, vigorous exercise program will, however, allow a somewhat greater number of calories and make weight reduction easier.

Weight reduction should be based on the same principles discussed earlier. The one difference is that insulin takers must space out their calories over three meals, plus three snacks. Not only will this aid in losing weight and keeping it off, but it will avoid the potentially dangerous problem of *hypoglycemia,* or low blood sugar (see Chapter 21, *The Hormones*). This occurs when the level of sugar (glucose) in the blood falls between meals. It may produce serious effects on the body and can even be fatal.

Diabetics should avoid some foods entirely, including sucrose and other refined sugars. In addition, processed foods often have refined sugar(s) added to them. Be wary and read labels carefully. Shake and Bake coating mix and catsup (29 percent sugar), for instance, contain considerable amounts of sugar, as do Russian dressing (30 percent sugar), nondairy creamer (65 percent sugar), and "100% natural" cereal (24 percent sugar). The following chart lists some common foods that should be avoided; however, this is only a partial list. We should all get into the habit of reading the label of every product we buy. If uncertain about a product's ingredients, contact the manufacturer via the distributor or your supermarket.

Foods Diabetics Should Avoid

- cake
- candy
- condensed milk (sweetened)
- cookies
- fruits in heavy syrup
- jam
- jelly
- pie
- honey
- chewing gum
- soft drinks (soda, tonic)
- syrup
- meat coatings for baking

One of the serious complications that occurs in diabetes is the development of rapid and premature atherosclerosis (see Chapter 13, *The Heart*). Although nothing can reverse this condition, eating a diet with lowered intake of cholesterol and saturated fat may be helpful in preventing or forestalling some of the potential complications of this process. It therefore seems prudent for people with diabetes to limit their intake of foods rich in saturated fat. Reduce consumption of red meat (beef and pork), butter, cream, whole milk, and whole milk cheese.

Additional information concerning the role of diet in diabetes may be obtained from:

American Diabetes Association
18 East 48th Street
New York, NY 10020

The American Dietetic Association
620 North Michigan Avenue
Chicago, IL 60611

Hyperlipidemia

Hyperlipidemia is abnormally high levels of cholesterol and triglycerides in the blood. Although both of these substances are necessary for the body to function normally, higher than normal levels increase the risk of heart disease, stroke, and other medical problems.

In recent years the exact role of diet in controlling hyperlipidemia has been mired in controversy. Some researchers have suggested that most cholesterol is produced by the body and cannot be significantly altered by diet. Most medical scientists still feel, however, that dietary control is worthwhile. Studies of people who eat diets low in cholesterol and saturated fats and maintain high levels of exercise and "ideal" body weight generally demonstrate very low levels of cholesterol and triglycerides in their blood. Thus, whereas hereditary makeup probably plays a role in the level of these substances in the blood, we can still alter things for the better by watching the foods we eat.

Foods High in Cholesterol

If high cholesterol is a problem for you, you should avoid the following foods:

egg yolks
bacon, pork
luncheon meats—bologna, salami, wursts
poultry skin
organ cuts of meat—liver, kidney, heart
cream cheese made from whole milk
regular ground beef (use extra lean)
heavily marbled cuts of meat
canned beef
duck and goose
whole milk, cream, butter, lard

Low-cholesterol substitutes include:

fish—cod, haddock, perch
chicken with the skin removed
vegetables
whole grains
vegetable oil and margarine
beans and other legumes
tofu

Basic Dietary Guidelines for Hyperlipidemia

	Type I	Type IIa	Type IIb, III	Type IV	Type V
Diet	low fat, 25–35 gm	low cholesterol; increase polyunsaturated fat	low cholesterol; eat approximately 20% of calories from protein, 40% from fat, 40% from carbohydrate	control carbohydrates; restrict calories	restrict fat to 30% of daily calories; 50% of daily calories should be carbohydrates; moderately restrict cholesterol
Calories	not restricted	not restricted	achieve and maintain ideal weight	achieve and maintain ideal weight	achieve and maintain ideal weight
Protein	not limited	not limited	high protein	not limited	high protein
Fat	restricted to 25–35 gm per day	limit saturated and polyunsaturated fat	limit fat to 40% of daily calories; use polyunsaturated fat	not limited; use polyunsaturated fat	restrict to 30% of daily calories
Cholesterol	not restricted	as low as possible	less than 300 mg per day	moderate restriction, to 300–500 mg per day	moderate restriction, to 300–500 mg per day
Carbohydrate	not limited	not limited	restrict concentrated sweets	restrict concentrated sweets	restrict concentrated sweets
Alcohol	not recommended	use in moderation	limit to 2 servings per day	limit to 2 servings per day	not recommended

1. Your medical provider can tell you the type of hyperlipidemia you have based on your blood tests.
2. Discuss a diet appropriate to your particular type of hyperlipidemia.
3. Remember: foods of animal origin, such as meat, cream, butter, and cheese, contain cholesterol. Oils like safflower, corn, and peanut that are liquid at room temperature contain polyunsaturated fat.

There are five forms of hyperlipidemia, classified according to the levels of cholesterol and triglycerides in your blood. A physician can identify different forms based on a blood test. The particular diet one follows depends on the type of hyperlipidemia one has. The chart on page 48 lists the dietary guidelines for each type of hyperlipidemia.

Be aware that dietary cholesterol always comes from foods of animal origin. Beef and pork products are generally much higher in cholesterol and triglycerides than fish and poultry (except eggs: the yolk is very rich in these substances). Foods containing vegetable oils do *not* contain cholesterol. The chart on page 48 lists foods that are usually high in cholesterol and should be avoided whenever possible.

Saturated fats are high in triglycerides and should also be avoided or eaten in limited quantities. They are also usually found in fats of animal origin, such as butter, cream, lard, whole milk, and cheese. Certain vegetable fats are saturated by nature, including coconut oil, cocoa butter, and palm oil. As a general rule, an oil is saturated if it is solid at room temperature.

Polyunsaturated fats come from plants. These are the types of oils that should be used to replace the saturated fats for people with hyperlipidemia. Some of the more common polyunsaturated oils that can be purchased are corn oil, safflower oil, soy oil, and olive oil.

Remember that the number of calories in a given amount of fat is more than twice that in the same amount of protein and carbohydrate—one gram of fat has an average of nine calories, whereas, one gram of protein or carbohydrate averages four. Most of us do not need the extra calories, nor do we need the fat. Almost everyone in a Westernized nation would benefit from eating less cholesterol and saturated fat and consuming fewer calories in general. Here are strategies for reducing fat intake, as well as some sample low fat menus.

A Fat-Controlled Diet Sampler

Almost everyone can benefit from a diet that is low in fat. This is particularly true for people with elevated cholesterol and triglycerides. Eating less beef and pork, and substituting poultry and fish will help. Consuming more grains and vegetables and less animal protein will reduce your daily fat intake even more.

Below is a three-day diet sampler that provides an idea of how to plan low-fat meals. Only three days are included, since I have found that people quickly become bored with any prearranged meal schedule. Find out for yourself the kinds of foods you enjoy that are low in fat and cholesterol, and change your dietary patterns to emphasize these foods.

DAY 1

Breakfast
orange juice
oatmeal
whole wheat bread with cottage cheese
skim milk, coffee, tea

Dinner (Lunch)
pot roast (round or chuck)
boiled potatoes with margarine
boiled carrots
fruit gelatin
skim milk, coffee, tea

Supper
homemade fat-free soup
water-packed tuna made with salad dressing, on whole wheat bread; lettuce and tomato
fresh fruit
skim milk, coffee, tea

DAY 2

Breakfast
grapefruit half
cold cereal with skim milk
english muffin with margarine
skim milk, coffee, tea

Dinner (Lunch)
hot sliced turkey sandwich
one teaspoon of cranberry jelly
tossed salad with oil and vinegar dressing
fresh fruit
skim milk, coffee, tea

Supper
baked fish with lemon
oven-baked potatoes
stewed zucchini and tomatoes
angel-food cake
skim milk, coffee, tea

DAY 3

Breakfast
grapefruit juice
poached egg
whole wheat toast with margarine
skim milk, coffee, tea

Dinner (Lunch)
homemade fat-free soup
cottage cheese fruit plate
raisin bread with margarine
homemade pudding with skim milk
skim milk, coffee, tea

Supper
baked chicken without skin
baked potato with margarine *or* rice
mixed fresh vegetables
tossed salad with oil and vinegar dressing
fresh fruit
skim milk, coffee, tea

Vegetarian Diets

Since the late 1960s, vegetarian eating has become very popular. Rising costs of meat, greater availability of fresh fruits and vegetables, and increased health awareness have promoted vegetarian eating. We want to look thin and feel energetic, and we are increasingly limiting our meat intake to promote these goals.

Misconceptions concerning vegetarian eating abound. The most prevalent is that vegetarians cannot provide enough protein to their bodies. Actually, most Americans eat more protein than is probably good for them. This may be increasingly true with aging, since the kidneys may lose some of their ability to handle a high protein load (protein is excreted by the kidneys). In any event, many vegetarians eat some amount of egg and cheese (they are called lacto-ovo vegetarians), which makes insufficient dietary protein intake even less likely. One can eat an adequate amount of protein, even without eating eggs and dairy products, although it is somewhat more difficult.

Eating a good vegetarian diet means eating *complementary* proteins (see the accompanying chart, which describes complementary protein foods). All foods are in part composed of amino acids, the building blocks of proteins. Adults need certain essential amino acids (actually eight of them) to make the necessary proteins for body functions; some grains lack one or more of these amino acids. Hence, grains must be combined to provide the essential amino acids for a *complete* protein meal.

Mixing grains, nuts, seeds, and legumes (such as beans) has provided sufficient protein since the dawn of humankind. For instance, Mexican peasants have eaten beans and rice together as the dietary staple for centuries. Both rice and corn lack isoleucine and lysine, two essential amino acids, which can be supplied by the beans. The beans, however, lack tryptophan and methionine, which are supplied by the rice or corn. Hence, the mixture provides a complete protein meal.

Vegetarians who eat cheese, milk, or eggs have less to think about when planning meals. Since these foods come from animals, they have all of the essential amino acids. Even small amounts of these foods, when added to nuts, grains, and seeds, will help provide a complete protein complement.

Thus, a casserole of green vegetables with a topping of grated cheese and toasted grains (like oats or wheat flakes) provides a complete protein combination, as well as a good supply of vitamins, minerals, and energy stores. Vegetarian eating is healthy, light, and satisfying. It is especially good for losing weight, since it does not contain fat, as meat does.

More information on vegetarian eating can be obtained from *Diet for a Small Planet*, by Frances Moore Lappé (Ballantine Books, New York), and *Recipes for a Small Planet*, by Ellen Buchman Ewald (Ballantine Books, New York).

Complementary Protein Sources for Vegetarian Eating

A vegetarian diet can provide all the amino acids necessary to make complete, usable protein. To do so, it should consist of nuts, seeds, vegetables, grains, and legumes (beans) that complement each other, so that each food supplies the amino acid(s) its complementary food lacks. Eating some milk, cheese, or egg eliminates the need for this complementary food eating, since these foods of animal origin have the essential amino acids. It is, however, possible to eat a protein-complete diet with only vegetable sources by mixing foods as follows:

Grains

rice and legumes (beans)
corn and legumes
wheat and legumes
rice and brewer's yeast
rice and sesame

Legumes

legumes and rice
legumes and wheat
soybeans, rice, and wheat
legumes and corn
soybeans, wheat, and sesame
soybeans, peanuts, wheat, and rice
soybeans, sesame, and wheat
soybeans, peanuts, and sesame

Nuts and seeds

peanuts, sesame, and soybeans
sesame and beans
sesame, soybeans, and wheat
peanuts, sunflower seeds

Vegetables

lima beans, green peas, brussels sprouts, cauliflower, broccoli } and sesame seeds or nuts
greens and millet, or rice

✽

Older people may have some significant disadvantages when trying to maintain a healthy diet. They may live alone and not feel interested in cooking complete meals for themselves. Supermarkets package meats, produce, and other items in family-size quantities that may not suit their needs. Sometimes there may be problems with teeth or dentures, or there may be a feeling of depression around meals because eating is often a social event. For some the cost of food may limit choices.

Despite these difficulties—or your basic food preferences—eating better will make you feel better. The time, money, and effort you spend in this area, like that of formulating a basic exercise program, will contribute enormously to your overall health and wellbeing. Sound nutrition is essential for everyone, regardless of age, financial status, or zest for cooking.

Part III

Medical Manual

This manual covers the more common and important medical problems that affect people over fifty-five. Although it is not intended to replace the medical and dental advice of professionals, it will present basic information in a form that the average person can understand and use to take better care of his or her own body and be a more astute consumer when medical care is needed.

The manual begins with advice from Dr. Michael Glenn on how to choose a medical professional and use the medical system most effectively. The patient-physician relationship has been undergoing increasing scrutiny and criticism in recent years. On the one hand, medicine and dentistry have become increasingly technical and specialized; on the other hand, patients are calling for more personalized, prevention-oriented care. Often these two forces conflict. Dr. Glenn suggests some basic strategies for finding a care giver who can be both personal and competent and offers advice on dealing with the health care system.

The manual is then organized by organ system and by the medical or surgical specialty that usually treats a particular problem. Thus, infections of the ear are discussed in the chapter on problems of the ears, nose, and throat. This is because otolaryngology, the specialty of ear, nose, and throat, is a recognized branch of medicine that treats these conditions. That does not mean that a family medical practitioner cannot handle the common problems presented in this manual. Where a problem is best handled by a specialist, this has been noted. In most other areas, your family medical or dental provider should be able to treat the problem.

There is a common confusion about cancer, its nature, and treatment. Not all cancer is the same; cancers differ in underlying cause, treatment, and the overall prognosis of the victim. Not all people with cancer die of their disease, and the survival time for many types of cancer is improving with better detection and treatment. To a large extent, the type of cancer depends on the part of the body from which it originates. For that reason the types of cancer are discussed in the chapters of the manual that relate to the part of the body from which they arise. Thus, cancer of the lung is discussed by Dr. Fanta in Chapter 14, *The Lungs;* cancer of the uterus is covered by Dr. Bowling in Chapter 17, *The Genitourinary System,* and so on.

Four terms that relate to cancer are often misunderstood: *tumor, benign, premalignant,* and *malignant.* An explanation of these terms will help remove some of the confusion often present in discussions of cancer. A tumor is a general medical term for growth or swelling. Hence, a tumor may be benign, premalignant, or malignant.

With cancer the normal pattern of cell growth is disturbed. The underlying reason for this change is not well understood, and in all likelihood no single factor causes cells to become cancerous. The extent of the change from normal to abnormal defines how malignant a tumor is.

Benign tumors tend to grow more slowly than malignant ones. They are usually not fatal because of this slow growth and because they tend to spread in a fairly well-defined or encapsulated mass. When they produce damage to normal tissue, it is because of localized pressure in a circumscribed area—they are taking up more room than the body can tolerate.

Malignant tumors grow more rapidly than those that are benign and have the potential to spread throughout the body. Malignant cells do not resemble normal cells and do not grow in a defined or encapsulated mass. They may invade and damage tissues throughout the body. This form of spread is called *metastasis,* and it makes malignancies lethal.

Premalignant growths tend to fall somewhere between benign and malignant. They are not yet fully invasive or capable of metastasis; nor are they extremely atypical in their cellular appearance. Nonetheless, they possess the capability of becoming malignant and thus require medical care. This may mean removal, medical treatment, or careful observation at regular intervals by a trained medical professional. The point is that cancer is a continuum, not a single disease entity. Some malignancies are more aggressive than others; some benign growths require immediate medical attention, while others can be watched.

In addition to learning more about one's body and about the medical problems that can affect it, it is important to forge a relationship with a medical professional whom you can trust and work with. That person can see you for your basic medical needs and refer you to a specialist when specialty care is needed. When you need hospitalization or specialty care, he or she can act as an intermediary, advocate, and interpreter of the medical care system. This is discussed by Dr. Michael Glenn in Chapter 9.

Chapter 9
Dealing with Doctors and the Health-Care System

Michael L. Glenn, MD

No matter how healthy you are, the day will come when you need a doctor or when you find yourself in a hospital. It is in your interest to know how to use the medical system to *your* benefit, not *its* benefit. The consequences can be life or death.

You should have a physician who knows you well before you need him or her badly. You should also know how to choose a physician, what to demand of him or her, and what your rights are.

One-third of my family medical practice is made up of people over sixty-five. Another considerable proportion is between fifty-five and sixty-five. Most medical practices are made up the same way. Many illnesses develop as the body ages, and a wide variety of chronic ailments are common over fifty-five. For this reason people over fifty-five require medical care more often than younger people. But not only do they need the physicians; the physicians need them too.

Most physicians, working on a fee-for-service basis, rely on people over fifty-five for a good portion of their income. Hospitals house mainly older people. An entire nursing home industry has been built up to make money by caring for the elderly infirm. And the companies that manufacture medicines, medical appliances, wheelchairs, heart monitors, dentures, and the like all depend on people over fifty-five for a hefty part of their profit.

It is important to remember that medical care is a two-way street. Although people need and have always needed medical care, physicians need patients to survive. Unfortunately, the various health-care industries rely more on illness than they do on maintaining health for their incomes. But patients do have rights. Though some physicians may try to act like gods, it is helpful to remember that they are all essentially well-paid hirelings, selling their skill to earn their bread.

The health-care system has expanded dramatically in the past two decades. Close to 10 percent of the gross national product now goes to health care, and the figure mounts yearly.

The mid-1960s saw enactment of both Medicaid and Medicare laws. The former provides health care assistance to the poor through state and federal funds. The latter provides health care services for those over sixty-five through the Social Security Act. Because of these programs, billions of dollars of public money have been poured into the health care industry.

In spite of such programs, few people over sixty-five obtain free medical care. Through an intricate system of deductibles and coinsurance payments, as well as through expenses not covered by Medicare, those over sixty-five actually pay between 35 and 50 percent of their own bills. Many health care needs—dentures and eyeglasses, for example—are not covered. Other available programs are so entangled in red tape or so poorly advertised that many people do not take advantage of them. How many of you, for example, get free transportation to and from a doctor's office? Meals on Wheels? Reimbursements for money spent on medicines? Did you know they might be available? Most of the burden is put on the patient to find out information, fill out forms, mail in receipts, and so on.

Like most bureaucracies, the medical system—whether hospitals, physicians' offices, or welfare bureaus—operates "by the book" rather than in each particular patient's interest. Often the patient's interests are the last to be considered. And, of course, recent cuts in state and federal budgets have severely jeopardized the programs that do exist. As a result, even though health care is commonly thought of as a right, it is in fact a commodity for sale to those with money. Two classes of medical care are available: one for those with money and another for those without. Those with money have access to the best private care in the world. Those without are sometimes given over to second- and third-rate clinics, municipal hospitals, overcrowded offices, or neglect.

This means patients have to find out as much as possible about their rights and about any available programs that can help them out. Often they may have to fight hard to get what they deserve. At times, weakened by illness and unwilling to get into a fight, an individual may withdraw, feeling helpless. I think this is a tragedy. All of us have an obligation to prevent this from happening, whether to ourselves, our families, our friends, or our patients.

Most people agree that a family physician is important. In a crisis the physician's familiarity with a problem can be life-saving. But medical care involves more than acute problems. As we grow older, we all develop a number of chronic complaints and chronic conditions. We also have questions that need to be answered about diet, sex, exercise, and many other health-related issues. And all of us experience changes and loss that strain our capacity to continue as we had before. Often we need the help and support of a personal physician to help us through these tough times.

People with chronic medical conditions need to be seen regularly by a doctor. High blood pressure, for example, should be checked at least once every three or four months. People taking medications often need to be checked for side effects or changes in their blood and body chemistry. Routine office visits are thus a necessity for many people with illnesses.

But even for those over fifty-five who are basically healthy, a regular visit every six months, or at least once a year, makes sense. These periodic checkups should include tests for high blood pressure, diabetes, anemia, and other conditions such as changing bowel or bladder habits, persistent cough, and weight loss. Urine and stool should be checked once a year, and a yearly rectal exam for men and a breast exam for women should be done as well.

More important than these tests, however, the regular visit gives the patient a chance to assess where he or she is in life. The conscientious physician will always ask, "And how are things going with you?" and sit back, listening for an answer. Debilitating effects of change and loss can be discussed even though no illness is present.

Help with problems of living should be simply sought and honestly given. In this sense, your personal physician becomes a member of your family, functioning very much like an aunt or uncle, a brother or sister, a parent, and at times even like one of your concerned children. A caring relationship develops, which you should be able to count on when you need it.

Finding such a doctor, though, is no easy matter.

Physicians today are divided and subdivided into many specialties. In some parts of the country it is hard to find a family doctor, a general practitioner. In other parts of the country, the family doctor is being revived as a medical specialist.

People over fifty-five thus must choose from a confusing array of physicians. Some choose a family doctor, who may also be treating their husband or wife, their children, and perhaps even their parents. Others feel more at ease with an internist, a specialist in disorders of the heart, the lungs, and the other inner organs. Some find a specialist in geriatric medicine more suitable.

“ I was born in Ashland, Kentucky, in 1923, and was raised there. I have done various kinds of work, as a machinist, a truck driver, a post office clerk, and a building and maintenance worker. Most of my life I have held more than one job at a time. From 1943 to 1947, I was in the Marine Corps in the Pacific and in Japan.

I am married and have three children, aged thirty-eight, thirty-two, and twenty-six. They are all healthy, and I know of no hereditary problems that they have. They live near me, and we see each other quite a lot. But I let them run their own family life, and they do the same for me.

I didn't have any medical problems until I was forty-four years old. I mean, I did not know what it was like to be sick. At that time I discovered that I was diabetic and had high blood pressure. I have been doctored for diabetes, high blood pressure, and atherosclerosis ever since, but it has not affected my work. At one point they said that I should not lift more than fifty pounds, but this has never been true. Lifting has never bothered me, even to this day.

In 1973 I discovered that I had bone spurs in my neck, in the third and fourth vertebrae. I was put in the hospital in traction. While I was in traction, I completely lost the use of my right arm. It may have been because of a pinched nerve, but to this day I do not really know what the cause was. I was operated on and had a fusion of two of the discs in my neck.

After the fusion I could hardly use my arm. About four or five months later, the doctor told me that I probably had about all the use of my arm that I was going to get. At that time I could only raise it up against my body, about halfway up my chest.

When the doctors told me that I would have only limited use of my arm, I thought that they must be wrong. The main reason why I felt that was that I could not remember ever having to ask someone, "Will you help me?" or "Will you lift this for me?" I had never had any hesitation to do anything.

That was the worst thing that I had to face, but I was determined. With my son's ingenuity and my family's persistence and my own, I got the use of my arm back. My son built an exercise machine for me that I used on the porch. It helped me strengthen my arm. Now I swim and work all the time. I have about 95 percent use of my arm. There is a slight deterioration of my right shoulder muscle, but I have evidently developed new muscles to take care of the one that I lost.

I have been told that my diabetes, high blood pressure, and atherosclerosis all work together. I am on Tolinase for my diabetes, but not insulin. I take 1,000 milligrams a day, but it is not working. I was told to lose weight, and I went down from 214 pounds to 174 pounds, but my diabetes is still not under control.

I believe that you have to listen to the doctors and then doctor yourself. I do not believe that every doctor understands every case. Just because a doctor says that you will be immobile does not mean that you will be. I do not believe that the medicine today works the same on everybody.

What I mean is that you listen to doctors and hear what they have to say, but you also have to determine for yourself what your problem is and how to handle it. There is no doctor who can tell everyone how to handle their problems.

My advice is that everyone should stay active. I am a past Master of the Masonic Lodge. I have gone through the Chairs in the Masonic Lodge and the Odd Fellows. I have been active in the Eastern Star and been an officer in the Veterans Administration; and I was state vice-president of the American Postal Worker's Union. I have a shop for sharpening all kinds of blades. Even though I can't work eight hours straight, I keep on working. When I am tired, I stop for awhile, but I don't think I will ever completely stop. ”

—Alben Kouns, 57

Whatever field a physician comes from, he or she should possess certain characteristics. (Although I use the masculine pronoun in the following, a good physician may of course be a woman or a man.)

First, the physician should be **empathic.** He should show concern for your suffering and life conflicts. You should feel a "fit" between yourself and your doctor or else the relationship will be strained.

Some people feel more at ease with a physician close to their own age or with one who shares their ethnic, religious, or racial background. Some are more comfortable with a physician of their own sex; others may prefer the opposite sex or feel it does not matter. Others seem to relate more to the particular traits the physician brings to them—an ability to talk openly about difficult problems, for example. You may feel more at ease with a physician with a rosy, optimistic disposition. Or you may feel more assured by a serious-minded, soft-spoken person. You may want a physician who tells you the truth or one who spares you it.

Whatever your particular bent, be honest to yourself and trust the feeling of "fitness" between you and the doctor.

The physician should be **accessible.** If not in his office, he should be available by phone. If on vacation, he should arrange for another doctor to be available for your calls and questions. He should have provisions for emergency service and urgent queries, and he should be able to see you in a matter of hours or days when a problem arises.

The physician should be **competent.** This is often hard for a patient to evaluate. The physician should be able to draw out the history of your complaints and follow it up with an appropriate, thorough physical exam (including blood or X-ray tests) to see what the matter may be.

Often you can get a sense of how competent the doctor is by how quickly he is ready to reassure you. Too-hasty reassurance is *not* reassuring: it only makes you suspect the physician is not taking you seriously. On the other hand, an overly extensive and expensive workup for a simple problem belies an immature, uncertain physician.

If you have questions about what the doctor is looking for, ask him. His response will tell you a lot more than the simple answer to your question.

Competence is usually judged by past success, which is as sound a test as any. Look, too, for affiliations with a reputable hospital, as well as recommendations from other physicians or people you trust. You may even want to schedule a "look-see" appointment, giving the physician a chance to get to know you and yourself a chance to see if you like him.

The physician should be both a **good listener** and a **good explainer.** Listening keys the physician into the problem. A doctor who monopolizes the conversation usually has delusions of self-importance and tends not to be so keen an observer of how *you* feel.

When you have a question, you deserve an answer. The answer should be in language you can understand. If your doctor does not appreciate this, you will find yourself very frustrated from time to time.

The physician should **accept your financial situation.** Discord over fees can sabotage the relationship between you and your physician. Openness about fees is essential to good communication.

Frequently, however, physicians demand pay in advance or set fees that are difficult to pay. Many doctors do not accept Medicaid or Medicare assignments. You should know your doctor's policies. Will the doctor accept your insurance? Will you be seen without being humiliated if you are on welfare? These are important questions to be dealt with in an initial interview.

The physician should be **family-oriented.** He should be willing to talk to concerned members of your family, and he should enjoy it, not view it as a bother. This

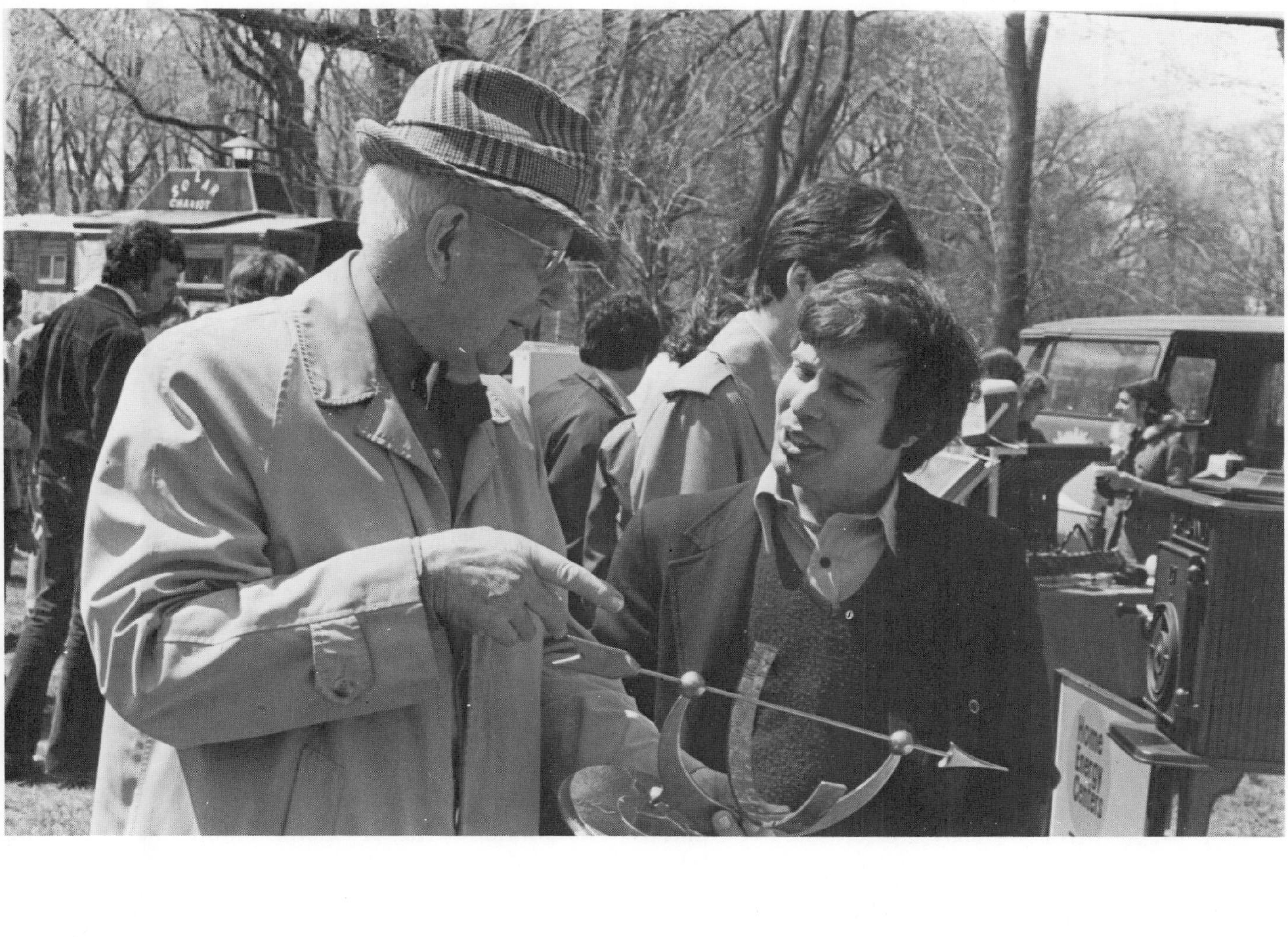

will be critically important when a problem involves a serious illness, but it can be extremely beneficial at other times too.

I have repeatedly run across questions from patients that I would like to answer.

Is it better to be treated by a medical group, or should you have your own personal doctor?

Medical care is organized in a number of ways today. You have to choose from what is available to you and what suits you best.

The majority of medical care is still performed by the office-based solo practitioner. For many people this fits both their image of a doctor and their needs for medical care. The drawbacks occur when the doctor is away or if he becomes ill. Some people, too, feel more confident knowing that other physicians besides their personal one are easily accessible.

Two-person and three-person groups have become increasingly common among physicians. Some groups run as large as fifty or so physicians. Many of these groups are organized on a fee-for-service basis and simply represent an alternative to solo care. Others offer financial alternatives as well. They may be prepaid plans, in which the patient purchases care at a fixed premium, regardless of how intensively the program is actually used.

There is a lot of controversy about such prepaid group plans, called HMOs (Health Maintenance Organizations). Some people believe that they are the most efficient, rational means of providing care, encouraging health rather than profiting from illness. Others argue that, under our system, the HMOs still pursue profit, by *discouraging* patient's visits or by using a number of paraprofessionals rather than physicians.

Often, too, the larger groups of HMOs make it harder for you to see the same physician every time. Thus, you may have to choose between adequate, predictable care (as opposed to irregular and uncertain care) and your wish for personal continuity of care (as opposed to seeing different medical personnel.)

If you are facing such a choice, *ask around.* Listen to other people's accounts of their experiences with different arrangements. Get as much information as you can before committing yourself.

Is it wrong to be an assertive patient? Won't that just make the doctor mad and make him think I don't respect him?

I think the patient always has a right to ask questions, demand explanations, request a second opinion, and so on. To me, this is not being assertive in a negative way. It is the patient exercising his right to know. After all, it is *your* body, *your* problems, and *your* concerns that the doctor is concerned with. You should not have to worry about his or her false pride.

I think it is always appropriate to ask honest questions, to request generic medicines if you want to have them prescribed, to ask for referrals, and so on. Most physicians I know would appreciate that and would not get angry.

What about clinics?

Often people without money are relegated to clinic care. To make matters worse, many big city hospitals and neighborhood clinics are in dire financial trouble now. More are shutting down than opening up.

Some clinics, it is true, especially those associated with teaching hospitals, offer by and large excellent care. You should not hesitate to seek care at such places if you are ill, although you will probably have to wait a long time for your visit, may see different doctors each time, and so on. I believe in being realistic. If you are ill and need treatment and cannot afford private care, go to the best available clinic. Do not—as many have done—refuse to go anywhere because of uneasy feelings about clinic care. Remember that it is not *your* fault that two systems of medical care exist in this country. If you are ill, get yourself to the best place available.

Some clinics have a reputation for being "Medicaid mills." They accept Medicaid and welfare, but their staffs are ill-trained. You will have to find out for yourself whether local clinics are reputable or not; stay away from those that are not.

Aren't medicines really bad for you? Do I have to take them?

When prescribed correctly, medicines ease your symptoms or attack the cause of your malaise. All medicines do, of course, have side effects because they affect your whole body, not just the part of your body they're aimed at.

If a medication makes you uncomfortable or if you feel uncomfortable while taking a medication, tell your doctor. Do not just stop taking a pill, though, without telling him or her. Usually another medication can be prescribed for the same problem, with a different chance of that specific side effect.

Periodically, you should review your medications with your doctor. If you do not need one any longer, it should be stopped. If you need it for a long time, it should be renewed. Some medicines, like digitalis or diuretics, should routinely be monitored in your blood.

Trust your body to tell you if it cannot tolerate a medication. Do not be afraid to mention any adverse reaction to your doctor.

When a medication is correctly given, do follow the instructions. It is not a sign of weakness if you happen to need a certain medicine or two to feel better.

How can I afford to be sick?

The cost of illness, even for those with insurance, can be staggering. Catastrophic illness, which strikes unexpectedly—as in an auto accident or from a stroke—can wipe out your savings in a few months.

The best advice about financial matters is to examine whatever insurance options are open to you. Check into your policy carefully. If you can afford Medex as well as Medicare, for example, it is probably in your interest to do so. But, in any case, try to find the best coverage you can afford.

Once again I must point out that many of us feel medical care should be a person's right. Until this is actually so, in the law of the land, people will ask questions like the ones I am now answering and people will have terrible experiences with the costs of illness. The solution to this problem is beyond the scope of the book you are reading now.

Chapter 10
The Eyes

Lynn Zashin, MD

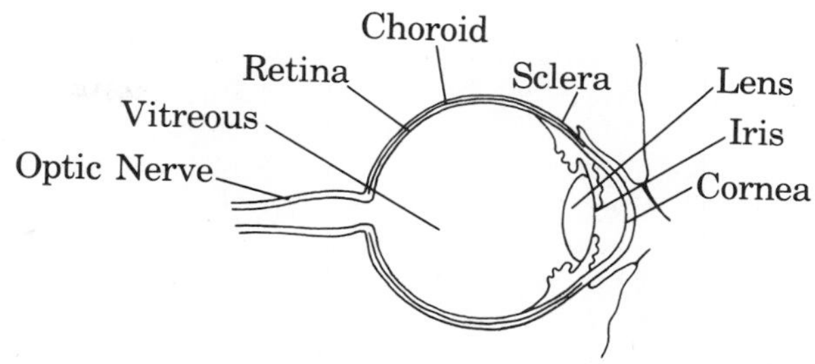

Anatomy of the eye, side view.

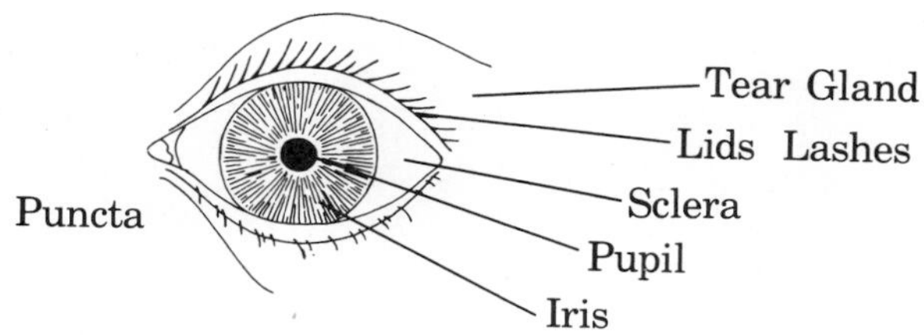

Anatomy of the eye, front view.

Of all our senses, vision is often the one most dear to us. It provides information that protects us from injury, helps us communicate with others, and aids in our appreciation of the world around us. Unfortunately, many of the problems that affect vision occur more frequently as we age. They can be quite frightening but can, in many cases, be remedied with medical treatment.

It is worthwhile to make a distinction between needing glasses and eye disease. Being unable to see clearly—whether the object is close or far away—does not necessarily mean one has eye disease, nor does it mean eventual loss of sight. *Refractive error,* the technical term for needing glasses, is quite common at any age. It is *not* a disease in any sense of the word, and it can be readily corrected with properly fitting lenses. It is a fact, however, that more older people need glasses than actually wear them. One of the main points of this chapter is that all of us should have our eyes examined by a trained professional and should seek, and wear, properly fitting lenses if we need them.

Among diseases of the eyes, the most common for older people are cataracts, glaucoma, and diabetic retinopathy. In the pages that follow, you will find explanations of the causes, effects, and possible treatments for these conditions. Use this information to help you understand how to deal with these problems if they affect you or those you care about. In general, eye problems do not lend themselves to self-care or self-diagnosis. You should rely on an ophthalmologist, a physician who is a trained eye specialist.

Normal Vision

The eye is made up of an eyeball (called the *globe*), *lids* and *lashes, bones* around the eye (the *orbit*), *tear glands* (*lacrymal apparatus*), *conjunctivas* (which cover the eyeball and inside of the lids), and the *muscles* that move the eyeball. The "white" of the eye is called the *sclera.* It is a hard covering to which the muscles that move the eye are attached. The *choroid,* a chocolate-colored membrane composed primarily of blood vessels, lies beneath the sclera. Toward the front of the eye, the sclera forms the *cornea,* a clear membrane through which light passes to enter the eye. Tears drain from the eye through the *puncta* into the nose. Use the accompanying diagrams of the anatomy of the eye along with the text to help you understand eye problems.

The eyeball has a complex, minute anatomy. The *iris* works in the eye, as it does in a camera, opening and closing to control the amount of light entering the eye. The *lens,* which sits behind the iris, focuses the light onto a structure at the back of the eye called the *retina.* The eyeball is filled with a clear, gellike substance called the *vitreous humor,* through which light passes.

Seeing is a complex process in which the light that strikes the retina is converted into electrical impulses by the *rods* and *cones.* From there the signals are transmitted to the brain and decoded into vision. Thus, seeing is a product of the proper functioning of both eye and brain.

The cornea, lens, and vitreous all cloud somewhat with aging, reducing the amount of light that enters the back of the eye. The process begins around age twenty, but we become aware of it around age sixty. This is not eye disease, but it does require that we work, read, drive, and perform many other activities that require clear vision with ample illumination. Using good lighting overcomes this normal aging change and allows any task to be performed safely and efficiently.

Normal vision requires both eyes to work together. Blurred or double vision may occur if movement of the two eyes is uncoordinated, often because of a problem with the muscles. It may, however, result from changes in the ability of the lens to focus, faulty coordination or decoding by the brain, or eye disease. Therefore, *any* change in vision should be promptly investigated by a trained medical provider.

The reduced ability to see near objects—for example, the words on a page—that occurs with aging is called *presbyopia.* It is a normal change in vision that most people experience by the time they are over fifty. It is one of the refractive errors spoken of earlier and can be corrected with glasses. Because presbyopia is so common, more people should be wearing glasses than actually do.

Caring for Your Eyes

Caring for your eyes is not very different after age fifty-five than it was when you were younger. Wear protective goggles when playing sports, working with machinery, painting, and doing repairs around the house. If you wear glasses, be sure the frames fit properly. Have the prescription checked at regular intervals, and have your eyes tested for glaucoma once every five years or so.

Three kinds of professionals are specially trained to deal with the eyes, but often there is confusion about their roles. *Ophthalmologists* are physicians who perform eye surgery and diagnose and treat eye disease. They also prescribe glasses. *Optometrists* are trained doctors of optometry, who measure your eyesight and prescribe glasses. Although they are trained to a large extent to recognize diseases of the eye, they generally do not treat them with medical or surgical procedures. *Opticians* are not doctors. They are trained to fit and sell glasses. They should not be relied upon to determine the proper lens prescription or to diagnose and treat eye disease.

Some preliminary parts of an eye examination may be performed by your family doctor, as well as by an ophthalmologist or optometrist. The ability to see distant objects will be tested with the Snellen Chart, familiar to most people with its letters gradually decreasing in size from top to bottom. Normal vision is expressed as 20/20. This means that you can read at twenty feet what a normal person reads at that distance. If your vision were, say, 20/200, however, this would mean that you would have to be twenty feet from an object to see it with the same clarity as people with normal vision do at two hundred feet. If your vision is not 20/20, you should be referred to an ophthalmologist for a complete eye exam. In addition, a simple test to screen for glaucoma should be performed. This can be done by your family medical provider or optometrist.

The ophthalmologist can distinguish eye disease from refractive error, which can be corrected with glasses or contact lenses. Organic diseases of the eye may have many causes, so that a complete examination is necessary. If, after seeing an ophthalmologist and getting an appropriate prescription for glasses (if needed), your vision remains the same and you have no eye pain, redness, or discharge, visits to check your eyes and glasses may be performed by an optometrist every two to five years. After age forty almost everyone should probably be screened for glaucoma every five years. If you do not see someone to have your glasses checked, have your eyes checked for glaucoma by your family doctor.

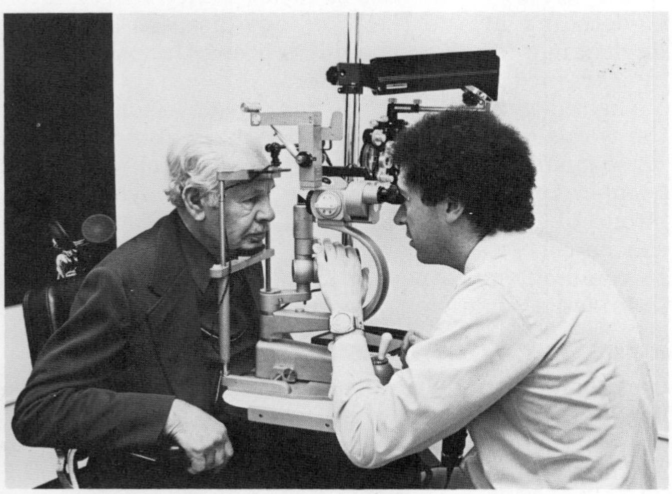

Refractive Error

If you have difficulty seeing clearly, either for objects that are far away or close, you may benefit from having properly fitted glasses. This problem, refractive error, is caused by a fault in the way light is focused onto the retina in back of the eyeball. The three types of refractive error most common in people over fifty-five are *myopia, hyperopia,* and *presbyopia.* The first two normally develop during the growth period (up to age twenty); the last is a development of the mature years.

Myopia and Hyperopia

For light to strike the retina and make a clear image, the incoming rays must be bent and focused by the lens. In myopia (nearsightedness) these rays are focused *in front* of the retina; by the time the light rays reach the retina, they have gone out of focus again, making it difficult for one to see clearly objects that are at a distance. In hyperopia (farsightedness) the opposite is true: the light rays are focused at a (theoretical) point behind the retina; that is, when the rays reach the retina, they are not yet in focus, so that viewed objects are blurred. The illustration shows how both myopia and hyperopia occur.

Neither myopia nor hyperopia are diseases. They can be corrected with glasses or contact lenses. The corrective lens for myopia is concave so that the focused visual image is moved backward onto the retina. The lens for hyperopia is convex, which moves the focused image forward.

Presbyopia

In the course of life, the lens gradually loses its elastic ability. Although this process begins early in life, not until usually age fifty has it progressed far enough to require corrective lenses. The limitation that most people develop with presbyopia is such that reading

Hyperopia and myopia.

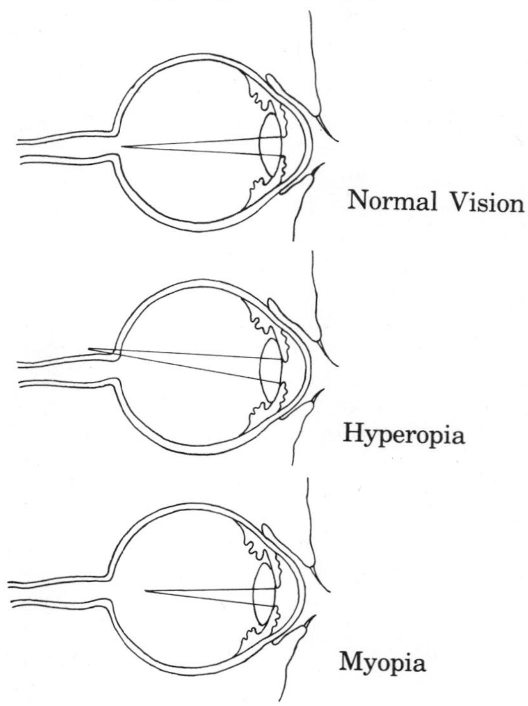

material has to be held about one to two feet away to avoid blurring. Since many people cannot see small print at that distance, it is extremely important to have glasses to magnify and help focus. This refractive error affects any work done on near objects, and corrective lenses should be worn when repairing things and measuring, as well as reading and doing other close work.

The changes in the lens that occur in presbyopia take place whether or not glasses were needed before. Though presbyopia is not an indication of eye disease, it is a reason to wear glasses.

Sometimes when myopic (nearsighted) individuals develop presbyopia, the two processes cancel each other out for a period of time. For awhile these people may be able to read without any glasses at all. As the presbyopia progresses, however, glasses are often needed.

Although individuals with presbyopia and no other refractive problem need only plain convex reading glasses, some of them prefer bifocals with a clear portion on top for seeing objects at a distance and the prescription lens on the bottom for reading and working on small, close objects. Using bifocals in this fashion is purely for personal convenience, enabling one to converse with others and work or read without continually removing and replacing glasses. Half-glasses will also do this.

Medical Problems of the Eyes

Eye disease can begin abruptly or gradually. The changes that occur in vision may be subtle at first. If you notice *any* change in your vision, if your eyes are tearing or red, or if you have pain, seek immediate medical attention. Early medical treatment can prevent irreparable damage. In the pages that follow, we will be looking at three eye diseases most commonly associated with advanced age, and a fourth condition (the red eye) that frequently occurs at any age.

Glaucoma

Glaucoma is the third leading cause of blindness in the United States and the most common cause of blindness in people aged forty to sixty-five. It is really a group of diseases all caused by increased pressure within the eye. The technical term for this is *increased intraocular pressure,* or *ocular hypertension*. It should not be confused with high blood pressure or hypertension and has nothing to do with nerves or eyestrain.

The pressure within the eye is normally fairly constant. It is maintained in the normal range by a balance of production and flow of fluid (*aqueous humor*) within the eye. If the flow of this fluid is impaired, pressure will build up within the eye. Eventually damage will occur to the ocular structures, especially the optic nerve, which transmits visual signals to the brain. If glaucoma is allowed to progress without appropriate treatment, extensive damage to the optic nerve will result in blindness.

There are two types of glaucoma: *open-angle* and *closed-angle*. Open-angle glaucoma develops gradually over time, while closed-angle glaucoma occurs more rapidly. The symptoms of closed-angle glaucoma are pain (often excruciating), loss of vision, excessive tearing, and a very hard and red-looking eyeball. Because open-angle glaucoma develops more slowly, these symptoms, if they occur at all, do not appear until late in the course of the disease. By then damage that may have been prevented has already occurred, and it cannot be repaired. That is why it is wise to have glaucoma testing as part of your medical checkups.

Testing intraocular pressure is easy, safe, painless, and can be performed in the office of a family physician, ophthalmologist, or optometrist. The simplest test uses a *tonometer,* an instrument that measures tension, which is placed lightly on an eyeball anesthetized with drops. Although placing an object on the eyeball may seem frightening to you, it is completely safe and painless. Ocular pressure can also be tested with a special apparatus that measures the pressure by blowing a puff of air onto the eyeball. As part of the glaucoma testing, your visual fields should also be checked for small areas of vision that have been lost (blacked out); such loss would indicate irreparable damage to the optic nerve.

Open-angle glaucoma is treated medically with eyedrops or oral medication. Pilocarpine drops make the pupil smaller, thereby aiding the drainage of the aqueous fluid. Epinephrine eyedrops (Epitrate) and acetazolamide (Diamox), taken orally, decrease the production of aqueous humor, as well as aiding its flow. Timolol (Timoptic) reduces intraocular pressure without constricting the pupil or blurring vision. It should not be used by people who have asthma or severe heart problems. None of the treatments cures glaucoma; they

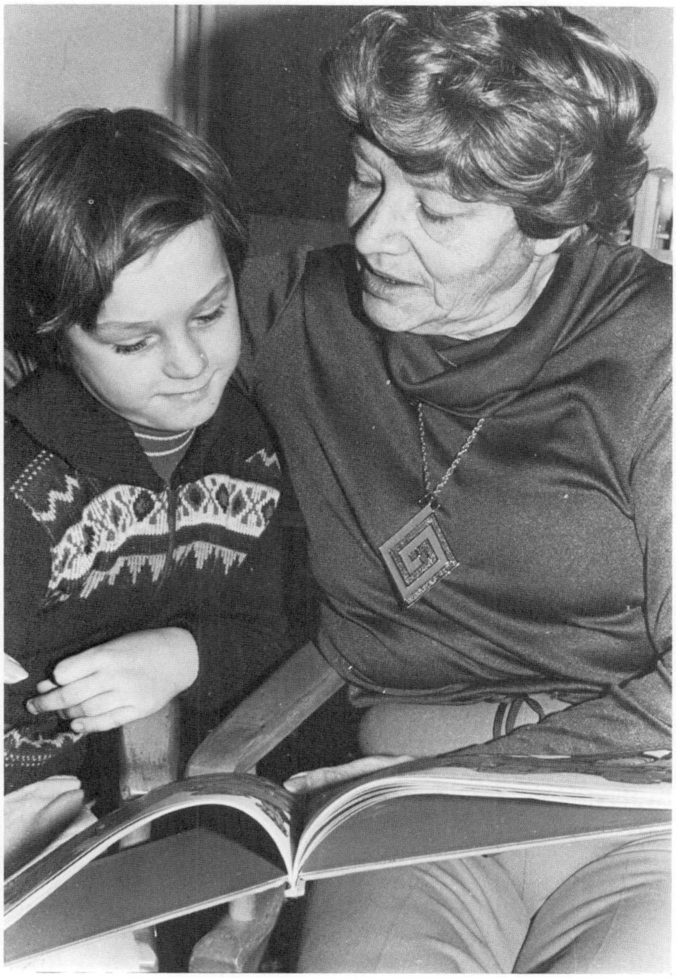

simply correct the condition *while* the medication is used. If medication is prescribed, it must be used regularly for the rest of one's life.

Closed-angle glaucoma, also called acute glaucoma, comes on suddenly. Its symptoms include a pupil that reacts poorly to light and may be somewhat dilated, as well as profuse tearing, a "steamy" or cloudy cornea, nausea, vomiting, and headache. It is an emergency that should be treated immediately or blindness may result. If your family has a history of glaucoma, you are at greater risk of having an acute attack. Be particularly careful to have your ocular pressure checked regularly.

It is unfortunate that few physicians perform tonometry as part of a regular physical examination for people over fifty-five. With age the lens tends to increase in size slightly, thereby increasing the likelihood of glaucoma. In addition, glaucoma is more common in people with diabetes, which also occurs more frequently in older people. Ophthalmologists recommend that intraocular pressure be checked at least every five years, more frequently if there is a family history of glaucoma or if one is diabetic or has had increased ocular pressure in the past.

Cataracts

Cataracts are the most common disabling eye problem of older people. A cataract is the gradual clouding of the lens, which reduces the amount of light that is transmitted to the retina. At birth the lens is virtually transparent, but with age the lens fibers lose their transparency and become yellow or yellow-brown in color. As cataracts progress and limit the amount of light that enters the eye, one experiences a gradual but progressive loss of sight.

We do not know the cause of age-related cataract formation, although some consider it a normal process of aging on the level of the cell and its biochemistry. Some conditions increase the risk of developing cataracts, including diabetes, X-ray exposure, severe eye trauma, prolonged eye inflammation, and high doses of steroids.

The symptoms of a cataract develop slowly and imperceptibly over the years. A cataract cannot be seen with the naked eye. Generally there is no pain or inflammation. When the cataract is fairly advanced, one may have the sensation of looking through a waterfall. Sometimes double vision may be experienced in one eye, but this commonly disappears as the lens continues to cloud.

The appropriate treatment for cataracts is surgical removal of the cloudy lens. (You may have heard of treating cataracts with drops, but that is not curative. The drops dilate the pupil, which lets more light in, and that may help vision for awhile. These drops should not be employed by people who have glaucoma.) In general, people choose to have their cataracts removed when their vision is so impaired that it interferes with normal daily activities. It is most common to have one eye operated on at a time, giving the eye several months to heal and adjust before operating on the second eye.

Cataract surgery may be performed under local or general anesthesia and takes about one hour. People are usually walking about on the same day as the operation. A number of possible surgical procedures can be used, and the risk of complication is only about 5 percent. It is a very successful and safe type of operation.

After the removal of the cataract, eyesight is very poor because there is no lens to focus the light. By no means, however, is one blind. The loss of the lens can be corrected in a number of ways. Some ophthalmologists implant a plastic lens, whereas others prescribe glasses or contact lenses to be worn externally. In each case a manmade lens replaces the natural one.

If glasses are chosen after cataract removal, a period of adjustment in vision will be necessary. The glasses will be rather thick and are most effective when viewed through their center. Objects seen in the peripheral areas will appear quite blurred. Separate corrections for viewing near and far objects will be necessary, which means bifocal or trifocal lenses. Distortions in depth perception will probably occur until the eyes adapt to the glasses. Objects at a distance may seem overmagnified, so that wearers may tend to step too high for stairs and not reach far enough for objects.

If contact lenses are chosen, these distortions will not be so great, but the difficulty many people experience with handling and inserting contact lenses will have to be overcome.

All of these problems require a period of adjustment. With time, however, most people learn to adjust quite well. Cataract surgery has improved the quality of life for many people who would otherwise have been functionally blind.

Diabetic Retinopathy and Other Diabetes-Related Eye Problems

Diabetes is the single largest cause of blindness in the United States. Although only a small percentage of diabetics suffer blindness, the sheer number of diabetics in this country (over 4 million) causes this high occurrence. For people over fifty-five, diabete's effect on the eye is especially important, since the longer one has diabetes, the more likely that eye difficulties will develop.

The most common problem faced by people with diabetes is blurred vision. This may be either transient or chronic. Transient blurring, which comes and goes suddenly, probably results from changes in blood sugar levels. Chronic blurred vision may be indicative of cataract formation or of swelling in areas of the retina.

Because diabetes accelerates atherosclerosis and because the blood vessels of the eye are among the first to be affected, yet another visual impairment often results. As blood flow through the vessels becomes blocked, new vessels tend to form on the retina and in the gellike vitreous humor. Although this may sound like a good thing, the result is an interference with the transmission of light through and to these structures. In addition, the thickening and narrowing of the vessels characteristic of atherosclerosis impedes the normal flow of blood. As a result, the blood vessels are more likely to hemorrhage, and sudden loss of vision or a sensation of seeing floating spots may occur. This may also be a sign of detachment of the retina.

Using a hand-held instrument called an *ophthalmoscope,* your medical provider can spot and analyze in the office the eye problems that result from diabetes. A more precise image of the eye's blood vessels may be obtained by injecting a harmless dye into the vein of an arm and taking pictures as it courses through the vessels. Some people may become nauseated or, more rarely, may vomit after administration of the dye. In twenty-four to forty-eight hours, the dye is excreted by the kidneys.

The medical community is still debating whether strict control of blood sugar prevents or delays the development of diabetic eye disease. Although no one is certain, most people feel that good control of blood sugar with diet, exercise, and insulin (if necessary) is a worthwhile goal. Additional information about the treatment of diabetes can be found in Chapter 21, *The Hormones*.

Laser therapy, photocoagulation, and removal of blood-filled vitreous humor are other treatments that may be employed by the ophthalmologist to help maintain sight. Because the effects of diabetes on the eye can be devastating, it is extremely important for diabetics to have regular examinations by an ophthalmologist. This will make early treatment possible and increase the likelihood of preserving sight.

The Red Eye

Red eye is both a medical and lay term that describes exactly what you see in a reddened, bloodshot eye or eyes. Some of the causes of the red eye are serious and require prompt medical attention by an ophthalmologist if blindness is to be prevented; others will get better spontaneously without treatment.

Although laypeople should not try to diagnose the cause of red eye, it is helpful to understand what can be wrong and what should be done about it. In general, the kind of problem depends on the part of the eye that is affected. Inflammation of the eyelids and sinuses is different from reddening of the conjunctiva

The Red Eye

1. Red eye may or may not be serious, but it should not be self-treated repeatedly with over-the-counter eyedrops unless you have had a medical evaluation.
2. If you have blurring of vision or pain, seek medical care *immediately*.
3. Have your eyes regularly screened for glaucoma.

Condition	Symptom					
	Blurred Vision	Pain	Sensitivity to Light	Discharge	Halo	Itching
Acute glaucoma	yes	yes	maybe	rarely	maybe	no
Subconjunctival hemorrhage	no	no	no	no	no	no
Bacterial conjunctivitis	no	no	no	yes—matted or caked lids	no	no
Viral conjunctivitis	no	no	no	yes—matted or caked lids	no	no
Allergic conjunctivitis	no	no	no	maybe, usually clear	no	yes
Sty	no	maybe	no	no	no	maybe
Chalazion	no	no	no	no	no	maybe
Blepharitis	no	no	no	maybe	no	maybe
Dacryocystitis	maybe	no	no	yes	no	maybe

(the clear covering of the eyeball and inside of the lids). Injury to the cornea is distinctly different from inflammation of the conjunctiva, and so on.

After ascertaining the source of the redness, a medical provider will check to see if vision is normal or impaired. This can be done before visiting the doctor by trying to read the letters on a poster or street sign at varying distances. If any change in vision is perceived, emergency medical care should be sought. By determining the site of the injury and visual acuity, and by doing some other simple tests, a medical provider should be able to tell whether the problem is a simple one or one that requires care from an ophthalmologist.

Many drops can be purchased without a prescription to treat red eyes. These prescriptions cause short-term shrinkage of the blood vessels on the surface of the eye. They are *not* a substitute for an accurate medical appraisal of a problem, and they should be used only after the sufferer is certain the underlying cause does not require professional attention. The following sections describe common causes of the red eye condition.

The Conjunctiva

The conjunctiva is the clear membrane that covers the eyeball and the inside of the eyelids. Infection, allergy, exposure to fumes and smoke, and rupture of the small blood vessels that supply the conjunctiva are extremely common causes of red eyes.

Subconjunctival hemorrhage is a rupture of the very small blood vessels that course through the conjunctiva. It can occur spontaneously, with very minor trauma, or even during such innocuous activities as crying or straining to have a bowel movement. Sometimes high blood pressure or bleeding tendencies such as hemophilia can produce it.

In general, these hemorrhages look much worse than they are. This is because the conjunctiva is clear, and the blood vessels are very close to the surface. A subconjunctival hemorrhage that involves the entire "white" of the eye (the sclera) after a head injury is, however, a more serious sign. It may mean that there has been a rupture of the back of the eyeball or a fracture of one of the bones of the eye socket (orbit).

Small subconjunctival hemorrhages do not require treatment and will fade on their own within two weeks. If vision is blurred, however, prompt medical attention is necessary to make certain that there is not a serious medical problem.

Conjunctivitis is a general term for inflammation of the conjunctiva. It may be caused by bacterial or viral infections, as well as exposure to toxic fumes and smoke.

Bacterial and viral infections produce a sense of fullness and grittiness (like having a foreign object under the lid), itching, and a yellowish discharge from the eye. You may awake with caked material sealing your lids.

Although many bacterial infections will clear without treatment because your tears contain natural antibacterial substances, antibiotics are a useful form of therapy. They will eradicate the infection rapidly and may prevent scarring of the cornea that sometimes results from untreated infections.

If the infection does not clear within three to four days, contact a medical provider to see if a change of prescription is needed. Antibiotic drops should be applied on the lateral side (ear side) of the eye. Blinking and tears will wash the medication across the eyeball. Antibiotic ointments should be applied in a thin ribbon on the lower lid and will also be naturally spread over the conjunctiva by the action of blinking and tearing.

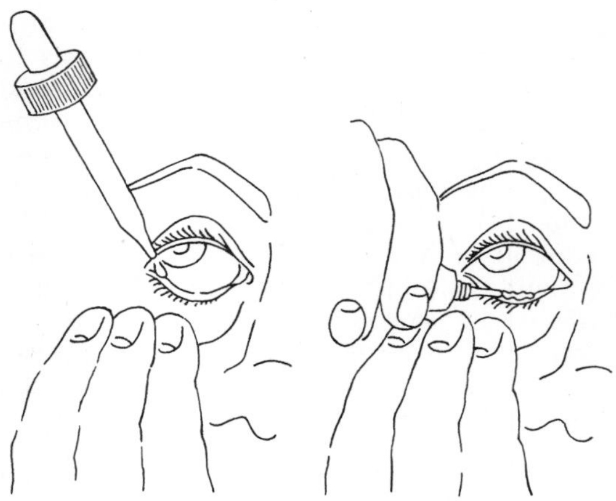

Applying eyedrops and ointment.

Viral conjunctivitis has the same symptoms as bacterial infections, and the two cannot be told apart merely by physical examination. In general, most medical providers will prescribe antibiotics even though they do not help viral infections. This is because the medications are relatively inexpensive and rarely have unpleasant or dangerous side effects. The only medication that should not be used in viral infections of the eye is steroids. These medicines will exacerbate certain viral infections, most notably herpes infections.

The symptoms of allergic conjunctivitis are itchiness, tearing with a watery discharge, and a swollen, red eye. Treating allergic reactions involves removing oneself from the offending substance. For some this may mean pets in the household, whereas for others it may mean chemical exposure on the job. If the source cannot be found—or, like plant pollen, cannot be easily avoided—symptoms can be relieved with antihistamines.

The Lids and Tear Ducts

Chronic inflammation of the eyelids, called *blepharitis,* can produce burning, itching, and redness. The eyelids appear red, thickened, and swollen, and they may be denuded of lashes. Other lid problems include pussy infections called *sties* or chronic infections of a gland in the lid, called *chalazia.*

Dandruff and scaly skin frequently contribute to blepharitis and should be treated along with it. The treatment for these problems involves careful cleaning of the eyes with warm water and a lint-free cloth, warm compresses to the sty or chalazion, and an antibiotic ointment like Bacitracin applied to the affected area with a cotton swab at bedtime. Although this treatment can be performed by the layperson, it is probably wise to do so in conjunction with a primary care medical provider who can follow the condition's progress.

The tear sac is located under the upper eyelid in the corner nearest the ear. Inflammation of this sac is called *dacryocystitis,* and it may produce blockage of the tears and symptoms of the red eye. Sometimes, however, swelling occurs without redness. Treatment involves oral antibiotics and hot compresses applied to the eye.

Other Causes of the Red Eye

Injury, infection, exposure to chemicals and medicines, X rays, and even some nutritional deficiencies can produce problems in the cornea, iris, or the bones around the eye. All of these problems require immediate medical attention or loss of sight may result. Similarly, glaucoma can also produce a red eye. Most of these problems, except for glaucoma, are rather rare. Because our sight is so important to us, however, it is essential that sufferers find out why the red eye is occurring. Eyedrops and other home remedies should not be substituted for prompt medical attention.

Chapter 11
The Ears, Nose, and Throat

Amy Jacobsen, PA-C

The ears, nose, and throat are related anatomically and are the concern of a special branch of medicine called *otolaryngology,* or *ENT*. These three parts of the body lie close to each other in the skull and are all connected. The ears are connected to the mouth by the eustachian tube; the nose and throat are connected at the back of the pharynx. In this chapter the common ear, nose (and sinus), and throat problems of people over fifty-five will be discussed, beginning with ears, then proceeding to nose and throat.

Many problems of these structures are normally handled by a family medical provider. Sore throats, nosebleeds, allergies, ear infections, and accumulation of ear wax plugs occur frequently and can be handled by a general medical practitioner. More complicated problems, such as hearing loss, tumors, and persistent infection, require more specialized care by the otolaryngologist, a physician who has surgical training in ENT. Another specialist, the *audiologist,* is trained to test hearing. This person is usually not a physician but will often work with a physician to determine what kind of hearing problem exists and what may be done about it.

The Ears

Our sense of hearing allows us to communicate with the world we live in. Without it we lose essential cues for safety—the wail of sirens, the noise of approaching cars, the shouted warnings of others, the ring of the telephone. It also provides us with stimulation on a subconscious level. Even in a quiet environment, the gentle sounds of the world impart a sense of well-being. That is why loss of hearing often brings with it depression and withdrawal. All the same, support with counseling, good medical care, and properly fitted hearing aids may prevent hearing loss or at least mitigate the negative emotional responses that accompany it.

Unfortunately, the number of people who have lost some or all of their hearing is growing, possibly because of high levels of noise pollution from cars, industry, and urban activity. Moreover, the number of people with hearing loss in the United States is proportionately higher than in other Western industrial nations. It is estimated that one-third of those over sixty-five have some degree of hearing loss that creates problems with safety, work, or in relating to others.

We have generally been more concerned with air and water pollution, chemicals, and smoking, than with noise pollution, yet the effects of too much noise are also harmful. In societies that have fewer machines and less electronic media, traffic, and firearms, people do not lose much of their hearing as they age. In our society, however, noise pollution is a major source of disability for over four million people.

The hearing loss that occurs with aging is called *presbycusis.* Some of this loss may result from normal changes in the anatomy. It is likely, however, that this condition is further aggravated by an environment of excess noise.

Normal Hearing

Sound begins as energy created by movement. This can be the vibration of vocal cords, the rolling wheels of a vehicle, or the impact of objects striking each other. This energy sets particles in motion, usually air, but solids and water can also conduct sound.

Sound energy then enters the *pinna* and is transported and amplified in the *external ear canal,* also called the *auditory canal.* Here it is magnified by resonant vibration of the bone that surrounds the canal. This bone resonates most efficiently in the frequency of sound we hear best (3,000 to 4,000 hertz).

The vibration sets into motion the *tympanic membrane,* or *eardrum,* which in turn conducts the sound energy to the three bones, or *ossicles,* of the middle ear, the *malleus, incus,* and *stapes* (hammer, anvil, and stirrup). The malleus is fixed to the eardrum, so that each movement of the tympanic membrane produces movement in the malleus. The sound is magnified in the middle ear approximately a thousandfold.

The sound energy now passes into the inner ear. Here it is converted into electrical impulses in the *cochlea,* where movement of the fluid within the cochlea stimulates the tiny hair cells of the *basilar membrane* that lines the organ. These hair cells convert the vibratory signal to an electrical signal. The *au-*

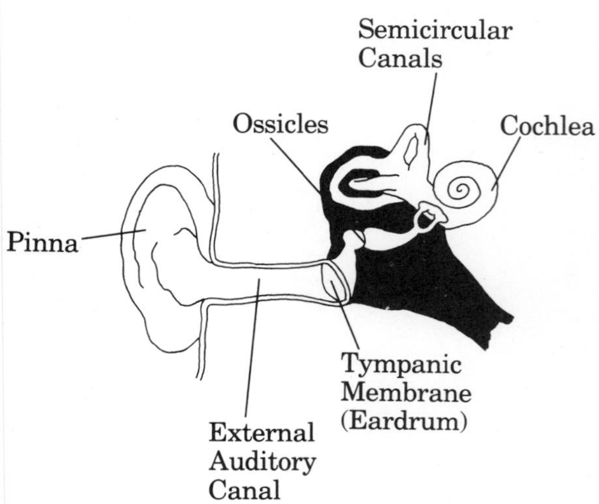

Anatomy of the ear.

ditory nerve carries this impulse to the brain, where it is decoded into sound.

Presbycusis

Like many of the changes that occur throughout the body, hearing loss generally begins in the late twenties and thirties, but because we have a considerable reserve of hearing potential, it is not until after age sixty-five that people become aware of the loss. The cumulative effects of years of changes occurring in the inner ear are then felt. By age eighty most people will have approximately 25 percent hearing reduction; some will have significantly greater impairment.

Because we commonly lose the ability to hear in the upper frequency range, the range in which the human voice falls, the perception of speech is most seriously impaired. That is why presbycusis has serious social implications. Hearing is an essential part of communicating with others, and any impairment produces feelings of frustration and a natural tendency to withdraw from social contact.

Four kinds of presbycusis have been identified, each caused by anatomic and physiologic changes in the inner ear. Although the reasons for these changes are not completely understood, it is fairly well accepted that noise exposure is an important contributing factor. Diminished blood supply to the inner ear and infection may also be factors in some people.

It is important to realize that hearing loss comes on very subtly. At first there may be only a difficulty hearing soft sounds like whispers or the rustling of leaves. Then it may become difficult to understand or hear what people are saying unless their faces can be seen. Pay attention to these signs and make an appointment for a hearing exam. This can be done initially by a family medical provider. If he or she suspects a problem, an audiologist should perform an examination. The audiologist is trained to give a complete hearing exam, plus help with the nonmedical aspects of hearing loss, such as obtaining a hearing aid and training to get cues from the environment. One of these cues is lipreading, but many other strategies can be learned as well. Medical aspects of hearing loss, such as an infection, will be treated by a family medical provider or an otolaryngologist.

Hearing Aids

Those who suffer from hearing loss may benefit from a hearing aid. Not all hearing loss will improve with hearing aids, however; therefore, a complete medical evaluation by a trained medical provider and an examination by an audiologist are necessary. If, after both evaluations, a hearing aid is recommended, it is worthwhile to understand how hearing aids work. A number of types of hearing aids are available; and knowledge about them will help in choosing the kind best suited for a hearing loss sufferer.

Hearing aids differ in style and size, but they all have the following components:

1. A *microphone* to transform sound waves like speech or street sounds into an electrical signal
2. A *battery,* which supplies the power to make the electrical signal
3. A *receiver,* which converts the electrical signals back into sound waves
4. An *earpiece* (ear mold), which holds the receiver in the ear

Hearing aids can be purchased from an audiologist or hearing aid dispenser. Many possible sizes and styles are available; choose one in conjunction with the advice of the person dispensing the product. Work with this person to find the type of appliance that best suits individual needs. If an appliance seems uncomfortable or unsightly, it may spend more time in a drawer than on the wearer.

Hearing aids may be worn in the pocket (body aid); behind the ear; completely within the ear; or incorporated into the frame of eyeglasses. Purchase an eyeglass aid only if glasses are worn at least 80 percent of the time. Be aware that if any part of the eyeglass aid needs repair, both glasses and hearing aid will be out of commission. If possible, have a second set of both.

The fit of the earpiece, called the ear mold, is especially important. The mold should be custom-made for each individual. A plastic impression should be taken and used by the lab to make an ear mold that fits the ear exactly. Improper fit can produce painful irritations, infection, or damage to the ear canal.

There are some technical considerations to be aware of when using hearing aids. Distortion occurs when the sound is amplified excessively. This is the squeak or feedback sound, like that from a microphone during a speech or concert. It means that the appliance is turned up too high or that the earpiece does not fit properly. If this occurs repeatedly, an audiologist or hearing aid dispenser should check the appliance.

Some people may find the controls of the hearing aid difficult to operate. "In the ear" hearing aids have a cosmetic appeal, but since the instrument is small,

A typical hearing aid. (Courtesy of Maico Hearing Instruments, Inc.)

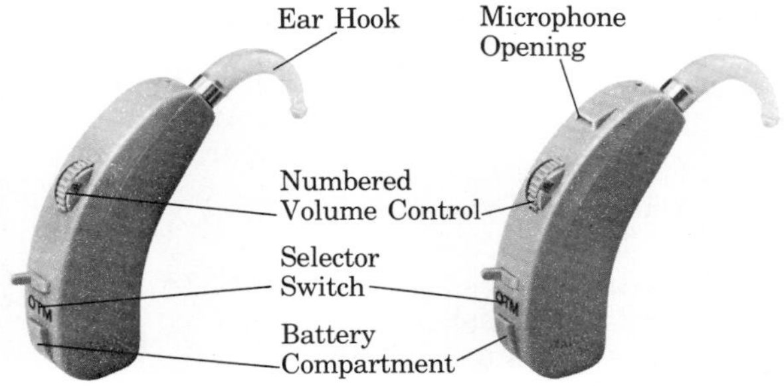

people with poor mobility of their fingers (for instance, those with arthritis) may have problems. When purchasing an aid, avoid those on which the controls are too small and those in which the volume wheels are difficult to reach. Since social situations often demand volume adjustment fairly often, the appliance chosen should be easy to work.

Battery life varies with the amount of volume needed. The higher the volume, the faster the batteries wear out. To get the most out of a battery, be certain to turn off the hearing aid when not in use. Some people put a sign next to their bed or on the bathroom mirror to remind them to turn off the appliance when they retire.

Infections of the ear canal may be a problem for hearing aid wearers, especially in the summer or in warm climates. Moisture can accumulate in the ear canal, creating an ideal environment for bacterial growth. Discharge from the ear is a sign of infection. Pain or redness are additional warning signs. Report these to a medical provider immediately.

A hearing aid can be purchased for $300 to $500. Buy one only after a thorough examination by both a medical care giver and the audiologist. If buying from a hearing aid dispenser, feel that person out for their reliability. The appliance may have to be exchanged or repaired at a later date. The person who dispenses the product should understand and agree to this arrangement before purchase. In addition, the purchase agreement should include the right to a full refund in thirty days if the appliance does not improve hearing.

A family medical provider, audiologist, or otolaryngologist should be consulted a few days short of one month after a hearing aid purchase. During this visit an evaluation will be made to determine whether or not the appliance really improves hearing. Not all people are helped by hearing aids. The ear canal should also be checked for signs of irritation or infection resulting from a poorly fitting earpiece. If the appliance is not helping, it should be returned for a refund. If the earmold does not fit properly, it should be refitted.

The ear mold may need to be replaced every few years if the appliance causes the size and shape of the external ear canal to change. The cost is usually about $25 to $35. In addition, hearing may change over several years, requiring a different appliance. Before purchasing a new one, obtain a hearing aid evaluation from an audiologist.

The hearing aid requires care. It should be kept clean, turned off when not in use, never submerged in water, and kept from extreme cold and heat. The ear mold can be wiped clean with a damp cloth or soaked in soap and water. The hearing aid dispenser or audiologist will provide instructions for care. If properly maintained, the appliance should last five to ten years.

Each year the Veterans Administration performs tests on hearing aids and rates the products. If you are interested in this information, write to: Director of Information Services, Veterans Administration, 810 Vermont Avenue NW, Washington, DC 20420 and ask for a copy of the Hearing Aid Performance Measurement Program data.

An excellent pamphlet is "Facts about Hearing and Hearings Aids," published by the U.S. Department of Commerce ($1.30 from National Bureau of Standards, Washington, DC 20234).

A hearing aid can never fully replace the function of the ear. It is a mechanical compromise that must be augmented by social cues from people's hands and faces and from our other senses. Inevitably, wearers must adjust to the appliance—to wearing it and using the controls. For some this is a frustrating period, but with practice almost anyone can become accustomed to its use.

Medical Problems of the Ears

Of the many possible medical problems of the ears, only a few are more common in people over fifty-five than in other age groups. They are wax buildup (cerumenosis), infections, cholesteatoma, tinnitus, and vertigo.

Wax buildup and most ear infections can be treated by a family medical provider. Vertigo, tinnitus, and cholesteatoma usually require treatment by an otolaryngologist.

Ear Wax (Cerumenosis)

Cerumen, or ear wax, is a normal product of the glands located in the external ear canal. A coating of ear wax protects the walls of the canal by preventing the skin from drying and cracking. In older people the wax tends to be drier than in younger people, and it may cake and clog the canal. Some people simply produce more wax than others. Accumulation of wax can impair hearing. If the external ear canal is exceptionally plugged, a sensation of dizziness or ringing in the ears may result.

Ears should be cleaned routinely with a wet washcloth inserted only as far as the little finger can push it. *Never* put cotton swabs, bobby pins, or other hard instruments into the ear. They may injure the canal or eardrum, force a wax plug farther inward (making it more difficult to remove), or remove too much wax and denude the skin, leaving it vulnerable to drying and cracking.

Use one of a number of products available in a pharmacy without a prescription to remove wax from the ear. Among these are Debrox and Cerumenex. These inexpensive drops loosen the wax, allowing it to fall out on its own. Read the label and use as directed.

If a wax plug cannot be removed in this manner, see a family medical provider. The ear can be irrigated with water at body temperature or be scooped out with a wire loop. Do not try to do this without medical assistance, or serious damage to the ear canal or eardrum may result.

Ear Infections

Infections of the ear tend to localize in one of three anatomic areas: the outer ear, the middle ear, or the inner ear. It is possible also to get an infection in the mastoid bone that sits behind the ear and communicates with the space of the middle ear.

Infections of the Outer Ear (Otitis Externa)

Often called "swimmer's ear" (because it is common in bathers), otitis externa appears as a pussy discharge with pain when the earlobe is moved. Any redness or pain in the earlobe may indicate an infection. It is also more common in diabetics, who should be particularly conscious of seeking prompt medical attention if these symptoms appear.

Treatment usually involves prescription antibiotic drops placed in the ear a few times a day, as directed. Avoid swimming or allowing water to enter the ear while showering. Inserting cotton into the external ear is not necessary.

Infections of the Middle Ear (Otitis Media)

Infections in the middle ear generally cause pain, transient hearing loss, and a stuffy or plugged sensation in the head. The cause is fluid accumulation in the middle ear and resultant increase in pressure. Sometimes the eardrum may burst, and pus from the middle ear will drain out. When the infection clears, the membrane will usually grow back. Persistent infections may cause permanent scarring of the eardrum and hearing loss. These infections should therefore be promptly treated by a family medical provider or otolaryngologist.

This problem is treated with oral antibiotics and occasionally decongestants that open the eustachian tube that connects the mouth and the middle ear. Keeping this tube open allows pressure to equalize between the mouth and ear and clears the stuffy or plugged sensation. If the eustachian tube remains closed, it may be more difficult to clear the infection.

If the infection does not clear with antibiotics, a surgical procedure called a *myringotomy* may be necessary. Performed under local anesthesia, this procedure involves an incision in the eardrum and placement of tubes to drain the pus.

Infections of the middle ear in people over fifty-five may be an indication of diabetes, benign tumors (polyps) of the nose or mouth, or cancer. Therefore, if you have a number of infections, or one infection that persists for more than six to eight weeks, you should have a complete examination by an otolaryngologist.

Mastoiditis and Inner Ear Infections

Much less common is *mastoiditis,* an infection of the mastoid bone, which is the part of the skull behind the ear. It may occur after repeated middle ear infections that do not heal. At one time mastoiditis was quite common and serious. With antibiotics, successful treatment of middle ear infections prevents their spread to the mastoid bone and nowadays mastoiditis is uncommon and amenable to treatment. Pain or redness behind the ear, especially with a fever, is a potential warning sign. Seek medical attention promptly.

Inner ear infections are also uncommon since the development of antibiotic therapy. These infections used to occur because of untreated middle ear infections that spread inward. If a medical care giver suspects an inner ear infection, treatment must be given by an otolaryngologist.

Cholesteatoma

Cholesteatoma is a chronic condition that can result from persistent middle ear infections. Tissue that normally is found in the external ear canal grows inward, into the middle ear. This abnormal growth may destroy the structures of the middle ear and produce hearing loss. Cholesteatomas require surgical removal and, sometimes, repair of the damaged middle ear structures.

Vertigo

The human ear is partially responsible for helping maintain balance. Sometimes dizziness and difficulty maintaining balance are caused by problems within the inner ear, in the *semicircular canals.*

Vertigo is a balance problem in which the world seems to rotate or twirl. Light-headedness without the sensation of the surroundings spinning is often confused with vertigo and most often is *not* caused by problems in the inner ear.

A number of medical problems can produce vertigo. Eighty-five percent of the time the dizziness and poor balance result from disorders in the eyes or ears, and 15 percent of the time the problem exists within the brain. An important sign of vertigo is *nystagmus,* a rhythmic oscillation of the eyes similar to that of a person trying to focus on a series of telephone poles while riding a train. You cannot see nystagmus in yourself, but others can. The motion may be in one or both eyes, in vertical, horizontal, or circular directions.

Persistent or frequent dizziness requires a complete medical examination to rule out serious disease. The exam should include caloric testing, a simple and safe test in which cold and warm water are alternately put into the ears and the eyes are simultaneously observed for nystagmus.

Benign positional vertigo may trouble people over fifty-five. The disorder is not completely understood, but the problem lies within the cochlea of the inner ear. The attacks usually are brief, lasting only seconds, and often occur when the head is held in one particular position—a particular tilt to the head produces the attacks. Usually this problem resolves itself without treatment, but the symptoms may persist for a few months to a few years.

If tests reveal that benign positional vertigo is the problem, the simplest form of treatment is to avoid the positions that produce the symptoms. Some physicians feel that assuming the troublesome posture promotes faster recovery, but most people do not tolerate this form of therapy. Certain medicines, called vestibular suppressants (e.g., Antivert) may be helpful.

Ménière's disease is a condition of the inner ear in which normally present fluid in the ear accumulates and produces ringing in the ears, hearing loss, and vertigo. Nausea and vomiting may occur as well. The spells of vertigo are often severe and may last from thirty minutes to twelve hours. They may occur in clusters or fall months apart. Ménière's disease will show up in both caloric and hearing tests.

Ménière's disease may be successfully treated with vestibular suppressant medicines, antinausea drugs, diuretics, a low-salt diet, and avoidance of caffeine, alcohol, and tobacco. If medical treatment is not successful, it is also possible to surgically drain the excess fluid or perform a more radical surgical procedure called a *labyrinthectomy.*

Tinnitus

Tinnitus, or ringing in the ears not associated with sounds from the environment, is fairly commonly experienced with aging. As with vertigo, there are many possible causes for tinnitus, including changes in the bones of the middle ear; the overuse of aspirin and antibiotics like streptomycin and kanamycin; presbycusis; Ménière's disease; nerve fiber damage from noise exposure; tumors; and some other less common conditions.

Wax plugs and infections may also produce the ringing. Thus, like vertigo, tinnitus requires a complete medical examination; the type of therapy will depend on the underlying cause. Ear wax can be removed, medications can be changed, and infections can be treated. Nonmedical approaches include a device called a tinnitus masker, which resembles a hearing aid but acts by introducing sound into the ear that is less annoying than the ringing and overrides it. Another strategy is to play a radio to provide a pleasant background sound. Since 1972 biofeedback has been used to treat tinnitus. Sufferers learn ways to achieve relaxation and reduction of the anxiety associated with the ringing in the ears. In general, biofeedback does not deal with the noise per se or its underlying cause, although it may effectively help control the symptoms.

The Nose

The nose is an organ of smell, as well as an opening to the airway. Along with the sinuses, the nose modifies the quality of speech by resonating with the passage of air. The hairs in the nose filter out particles in the air, and the mucous membranes warm and moisten the air before it enters the lungs.

The sinuses drain into the nose, as do tears produced in the eye. Because of the latter communication, crying also produces a runny nose. Inflammation of the sinuses produces drainage from the nose as well.

Common problems of the nose and sinuses, such as simple nosebleeds, allergy symptoms, and inflammation of the sinuses, can often be cared for by your family medical provider. These are some of the more common problems that bring one to the doctor. Persistent nosebleeds or infection are a sign of a more serious problem, however, and care by an otolaryngologist may be needed.

Medical Problems of the Nose and Sinuses

Nosebleeds (Epistaxis)

Nosebleeds are extremely common in people over fifty-five, especially in smokers or during the cold months when homes are centrally heated. Both smoke and heated air dry the nose and make it more prone to bleed.

Most nosebleeds occur in the front of the nose, where the tiny blood vessels are close to the skin surface. Drying of the skin that covers these vessels exposes them. Any small trauma, either from picking the nose or sneezing, may produce bleeding. On occasion the bleeding may occur without any prior injury.

Most people are not aware of the dryness that central heating produces during the winter. Many homes are actually drier than the Sahara Desert. Raising the humidity in the home is extremely helpful in preventing nosebleeds. It will also make the room feel warmer and make breathing easier. You can humidify your home with pans of water placed on radiators or the stove, with an electric room humidifier or a humidifier attached to your central heating unit. If you use a humidifier, be sure to clean it regularly according to manufacturer's instructions. A humidifier is a good breeding place for bacteria and airborne fungus.

Bleeding from the front of the nose can be stopped by applying local pressure (see also Chapter 23, *Emergencies*). If the bleeding continues, stop using these measures and contact your medical provider or proceed to a hospital emergency room. The bleeding may stem from the back of the nose and may require medical attention.

A very common cause of nosebleeds is chronic picking of the nose. During the winter, when dried mucus accumulates more heavily, one may tend to use the fingers to clear the nostrils. People with recurrent nosebleeds should avoid inserting anything into the nose. That means no cotton swabs, as well as no fingers.

Any persistent or recurrent bleeding in people over fifty-five deserves a medical investigation. It may be a sign of oral cancer. Smoking and exposure to toxic fumes over the years increases one's risk of oral cancer.

Runny Nose (Rhinorrhea)

The most common cause of a runny nose is the common cold, caused by one of the many cold viruses. Viruses are spread by droplet contact from person to person when we cough, sneeze, and talk. The familiar symptoms include a feeling of irritation in the back of the nose and throat, sneezing, a clear nasal discharge, mild fever, malaise, and headache. In addition, there may be a cough produced either by the virus infecting the

Anatomy of nose and sinus.

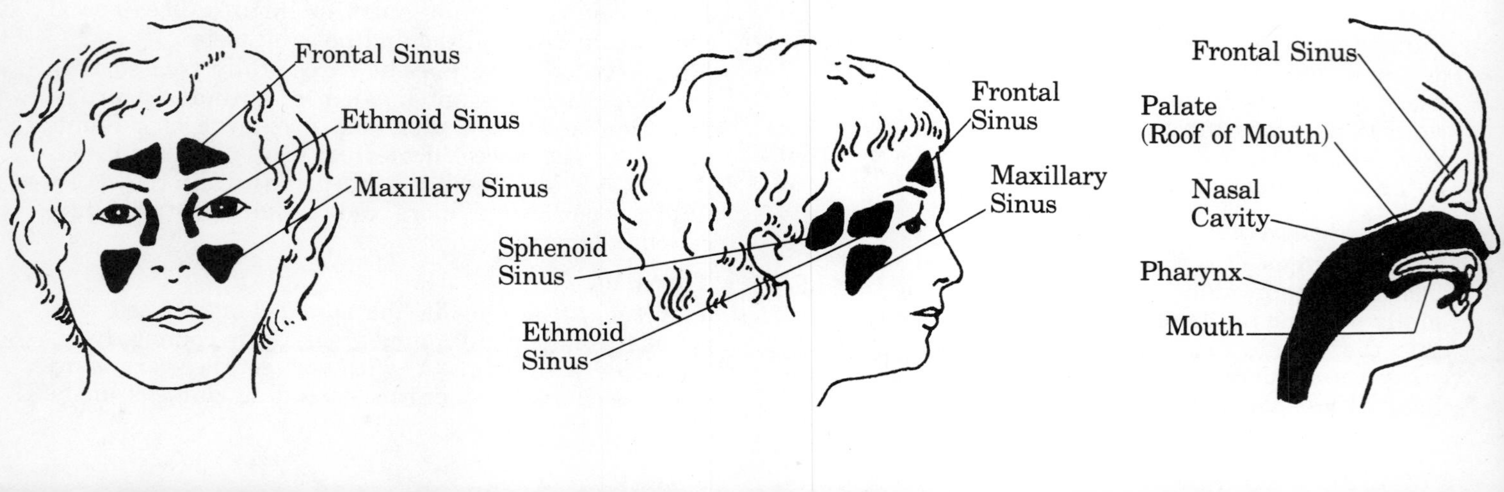

airway or irritation as a result of nasal discharge running down the back of the throat. Usually these symptoms last from four to seven days and disappear without treatment.

Occasionally bacteria will invade during this period of diminished resistance. The result may be *sinusitis* (infections of the sinuses), *bronchitis,* or *pneumonia.* Antibiotics have no effect on viral infections, but they may be helpful against a bacterial infection superimposed on the viral one.

The treatment for viral runny nose or sinusitis is bed rest, fluids, a humidifier or vaporizer in the home (at least in the bedroom at night), and aspirin or aspirin substitute for the headache and fever. Hot showers, (allow the steam to build up and inhale it deeply) may also help break up mucous congestion.

The effectiveness of vitamin C in treating the common cold has been widely debated. Currently, no strong evidence supports the theory that high doses of vitamin C (or any other vitamin) shorten or prevent the common cold. People tend to have strong feelings about vitamin C, however, and if you feel that it is helpful, continue to use it. In general, it has few or no harmful side effects. Vitamin C in excess of body need is excreted in the urine. This is not true with other vitamins (A and E most notably), so care should be taken with large doses of these.

Nosedrops are generally not considered helpful for a runny nose associated with a cold; in fact, when overused, they may have a rebound effect. This means that, after an initial short period of diminished nasal discharge, it will return with a more annoying and copious flow. This vicious cycle may develop in some people after as few as five days of nosedrop use.

The benefits of oral decongestants are also questionable. These are found in the many cold tablets and capsules that can be purchased over the counter. They may provide relief of nasal discharge but probably have no effect on the duration of the cold. It is important to be aware that they produce drowsiness; avoid driving a car or operating dangerous machinery if you take them. They also tend to dehydrate (a general effect of their action to "dry up" nasal discharge), so particular care should be taken to drink fluids when this medication is used. Oral decongestants should not be taken by people with high blood pressure.

Allergies and hay fever also produce nasal discharge, usually not accompanied by the cold symptoms of headache, fever, and cough. Allergic runny nose tends to occur in seasons when trees and plants are in flower. In a more chronic pattern, allergies to dust, newspaper, feathers, wool, animal hair, foods, tobacco smoke, fumes, and many other substances may cause nasal discharge year-round.

The best treatment is to find the allergen and eliminate it from the environment. Allergy shots to desensitize one to an offending substance are a possibility, but these shots do not always work. Moreover, some people find going through a series of shots not worth the expense and trouble.

Whether or not allergy shots are used, certain measures may be helpful in controlling the troublesome symptoms.

1. Cover pillows and mattress with plastic.
2. Eliminate chocolate, milk, and eggs from the diet. After a few weeks, try small amounts of these foods one at a time to see if they produce symptoms.
3. Remove domestic animals from the home, and clean to remove the animal hair.
4. Cover upholstered furniture with plastic.
5. Use nonallergenic cosmetics.
6. Remove wool bedding and substitute synthetics.
7. Air-condition home and office.
8. Use antihistamines for symptomatic relief and to *prevent* symptoms during a difficult season or when the offending allergen is present.

Nasal Polyps

Polyps are benign growths that may appear in the nose. They are small, raised, rounded, and slightly reddened. Most of the time they cannot be seen by looking in the mirror or felt by touching the nose. One needs a light and a nasal speculum to open the nostrils. This can be done in the office of a family medical provider or an otolaryngologist.

Nasal polyps are more common in people who have chronic allergic *rhinitis* (runny nose produced by allergies) and in smokers. Although these growths are not cancerous, they should be removed because they can produce obstruction of the sinuses and added nasal discharge. Some physicians initially employ antihistamines to try to shrink them. If symptoms persist, the polyps should be removed by an otolaryngologist. Unfortunately, polyps do tend to recur because the underlying allergy is often difficult to control.

Vasomotor Rhinitis

Some people suffer from nasal congestion that comes and goes because of hypersensitivity of the glands and blood vessels of the nasal mucous membranes. The precipitating factors differ among people, but commonly smoke, chemical fumes, car exhausts, alcohol, and changes in humidity and temperature will cause the runny nose symptoms. Sometimes headaches, changes in the position of the head, stress, and hypothyroidism will also produce symptoms.

As with allergies, the treatment is to avoid the situations or substances that provoke attacks. Some individuals find that exercise helps. In addition, oral decongestants and antihistamines may be used to prevent attacks if exposure to an offending substance or situation is anticipated. Thus, if smoky rooms are a problem, a decongestant or antihistamine can be used before going to a meeting where contact with tobacco smoke is likely. Finally, if hypothyroidism is a cause of the problem, a medical provider will diagnose this and provide appropriate medical treatment to eliminate this symptom.

Sinusitis

There are four paired sinuses in the skull. The two *frontal sinuses* lie over the eyebrows, the two *maxillary sinuses* above the upper teeth, the *ethmoids* between the upper part of the nose and eyes, and the *sphenoid sinuses* behind the upper portion of the nose. All drain into the nose, and it is through this conduit that infections may be transmitted from the nose to the sinuses. Sometimes dental infections will produce inflammation of the maxillary sinus.

Like the symptoms of a runny nose, sinusitis is a common problem. The sudden attack of sinusitis most often accompanies or follows a viral cold or a sudden drop in atmospheric temperature. Sometimes it may come after swimming, diving, or being exposed to an allergen.

The symptoms of sinus inflammation commonly begin with a feeling of nasal stuffiness, followed by pressure over the involved sinus. Sufferers may also have a headache or fever or feel generally ill. These symptoms often progress over two to three days until severe pain is experienced over the sinus that is inflamed. A thick, copious yellow-green, and possibly blood-tinged nasal discharge will probably develop. Secretions that drip down the throat (postnasal discharge) may cause a sore throat.

The site of the pain and inflammation will provide valuable information about which sinus or sinuses are infected. Pain over the eyes is likely to indicate an infection in the frontal sinuses; pain over the teeth, the maxillary sinuses; pain behind the eye, the ethmoid or sphenoid sinuses. X-ray films of the sinuses may be needed to provide information as to the site and extent of an infection.

Treatment of sinusitis includes pain medications, application of wet heat (compresses) to the affected area, and hot showers or steam baths to promote nasal drainage and pain relief. Nosedrops may be useful to keep the nasal passages clear. (Nosedrops may, however, exacerbate the symptoms if abused. Use them only as directed by a medical provider.) Antibiotics are useful to control bacterial infection. Untreated sinusitis may produce serious complications that affect the skull bones or brain and therefore requires prompt medical treatment.

Ordinarily surgical procedures to drain the sinuses are not employed during the acute phase of the illness.

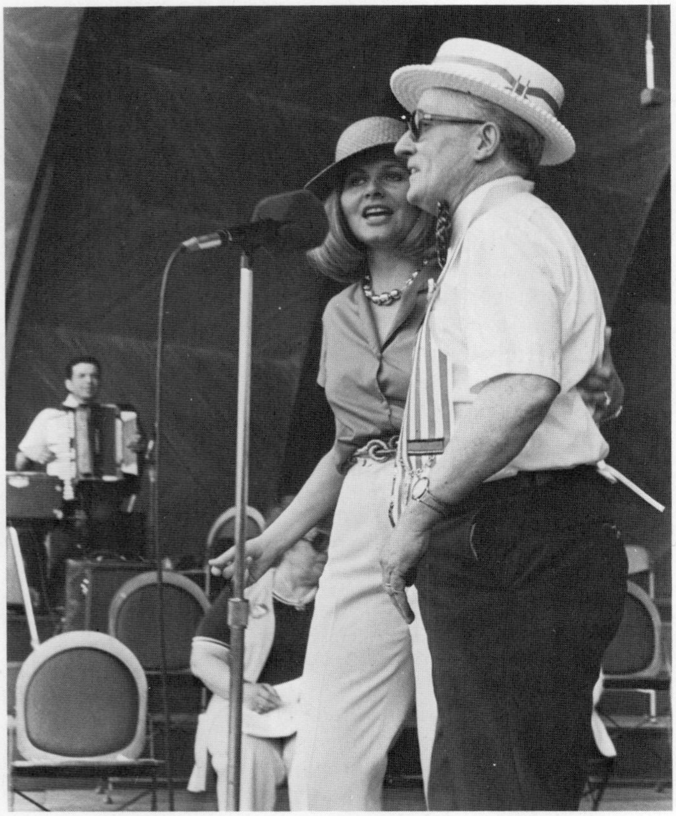

If the sinuses do not drain, however, or if X-ray evidence indicates invasion of the sinus bones, a surgical procedure may be necessary. This usually involves a special cleaning of the infected sinus through the nose but may also mean an operation to clear out areas of abscess or diseased bone if an infection exists in these structures. Early and effective medical treatment generally makes surgery unnecessary.

Chronic sinusitis may occur if the problem is neglected. Sometimes incomplete medical treatment may also cause a chronic problem. When this happens, the sinus tissue often thickens irreversibly, and a continual thick, yellow nasal discharge develops. This may also happen if the nose or sinuses are continually inflamed by allergy. Treatment often involves surgery to remove the diseased bone and tissue.

The Mouth and Throat

The mouth and throat are organs of both digestion and respiration. The *taste buds* line the *tongue,* providing sensual and safety information concerning the food we eat. Proper coordination of the *pharynx, epiglottis,* and *vocal cords* prevents food from entering the lungs when we swallow. In the *larynx* the vocal cords are essential to producing speech.

The mouth and lips are important for facial expression and beauty. The lips, teeth, tongue, and mouth convey feeling and sensuality equalled perhaps only by the eyes.

The mouth or throat do not undergo a normal aging process similar to presbyopia or presbycusis for the eyes and ears. In the absence of illness, the swallowing mechanism, speech production, and taste remain remarkably intact with advancing years. Therefore, lesions on the mouth, tongue, or lips; changes in the voice quality; a persistent cough; difficulty in swallowing; or a change in the taste of food should always be considered abnormal and potential signs of illness. They require prompt investigation by a medical provider.

Medical Problems of the Mouth and Throat

Lesions and Sores in the Mouth

Leukoplakia is a general medical term for a white lesion seen in the mouth or throat. Some physicians consider it to be premalignant (precancerous), so any whitish spot in the mouth should be examined by a medical provider. This includes whitish areas on the palate, tongue, lips, gums, or cheek.

Because it is difficult to distinguish benign from malignant lesions with the naked eye, a biopsy is often helpful. This means removing the tissue with a local surgical excision and having it examined under the microscope by a pathologist.

Leukoplakia of the larynx or mouth is caused by chronic irritation, usually by heavy smoking. It is more common in men, presumably because they have traditionally been the heavy smokers. But now that more women are smoking, it is increasingly likely that they too will have these lesions. When leukoplakia involves the larynx, a white membrane forms on one or both of the vocal cords, producing a persistent painless hoarseness. There is also a tendency to cough more than usual in an attempt to remove the secretions that accumulate on the vocal cords.

Since leukoplakia and smoking are more or less entwined, smokers who find a lesion should stop smoking. A much higher than average risk of cancer of the oral cavity results if smoking is continued.

Lichen planus is a skin disease that can occur in the mouth. It usually appears on the inside of the cheek as fine white lines in a lacy pattern. Sometimes it may appear on the tongue or lip. The underlying cause of the lesion is not fully known. It is not painful, serious, or precancerous. It will get better without medical treatment.

Canker sores (*aphthous stomatitis*) are small, painful, yellow-white, usually round ulcers that may appear on the tongue, palate, gums, and inside tissues of the cheeks. The cause of these lesions is not known. They regress on their own. An oxidizing mouthwash composed of one part hydrogen peroxide to two parts water may sometimes help in reducing the painful symptoms. Gargle with this mixture two or more times a day if you have the ulcers.

Infections

Viral and bacterial infections commonly appear in the mouth and throat. Contrary to popular thought, strep throat (caused by the streptococcus bacterium) is not common in adults unless they have had recurrent strep throat beginning in childhood. When it occurs, however, it should be treated with antibiotics to prevent potentially serious complications to the heart and possibly the kidney. In adults the overwhelming number of sore throats is caused by viruses that are spread by coughing, breathing, and speaking.

A strep throat cannot always be diagnosed just by looking at the throat. Sometimes patchy white areas of pus in the back of the throat are present with strep, but they may also occur in viral infections. If you have a fever, sore throat, and swollen glands in your neck and you are concerned that you may have a strep throat, see your family medical provider for a throat culture. This is safe and inexpensive, and the results should be available in two days.

Herpes virus can infect the mouth, tongue, lips, inside of the cheeks, and throat, as well as the nasal passages and the eyes. It usually appears as blisters that eventually rupture and leave shallow craters. Herpes infections are painful. The virus lives in the nerves that supply the mouth area, and becomes active in many, often unpredictable, situations. Colds, stress, changes in temperature, dental procedures, and anxiety can all produce outbreaks of herpes.

Unfortunately, no treatment is yet available to cure the infection. The sores will go away in seven days to two weeks, but they often recur. Herpes is extremely common, and because so many people are affected, many researchers are working on a form of treatment. It is hoped that results will soon come from this effort.

Some simple measures can help tide one over during a herpes attack. Aspirin and gargling with an oxidizing mouthwash (for example, one part hydrogen peroxide to two parts water) can help with the pain. It is sometimes helpful to apply viscous xylocaine directly to the affected area with a cotton swab. During painful attacks avoid spicy foods, smoking, and hot foods and liquids. Avoid using a toothbrush if you have sores inside your mouth. (For additional information on herpes, see also the discussions in Chapter 17, *The Genitourinary System* and Chapter 22, *The Skin, Hair, and Nails.*)

Cancer of the Mouth and Throat

Oral cancer is increasing in frequency. It is seen most frequently among heavy smokers, those with poor oral hygiene, and often in association with excessive alcohol consumption. Most of these tumors are visible in the mouth. That they often come to the awareness of the physician late therefore indicates that people avoid early diagnosis and treatment.

Any lesion in the mouth, gums, or lips should be examined by a trained medical person, as should a lump that you can feel in the neck; pain in the mouth, throat, ears, or face; difficulty swallowing or chewing; or a change in the quality of your voice. Tumors of the nasal portion of the throat may appear first as nasal blockage, a sensation that the ears are plugged, ear pain, hearing loss, ringing in the ears, or a mass in the neck.

Tumors of the larynx usually begin with hoarseness or a change in the voice that does not go away. If medical attention is sought early, the overall prognosis is good and the treatment is not very disabling. Unfortunately, most people do not consult a health provider early, so many of these cancers prove to be fatal. The symptom of hoarseness is especially common in smokers, who often feel that this is an inevitable result of cigarette abuse. If you smoke, you should not regard a change in your voice as normal. Get prompt medical attention. You may be developing a malignancy.

Surgery is the principal curative treatment of these cancers, although very small tumors may be treated through laser or radiation therapy. Chemotherapy with anticancer drugs is not very helpful and can provide only limited palliation.

The surgery involves partial or total removal of the larynx and formation of a tracheostomy, a hole placed in the neck through which one breathes. Most people who have lost their voice through the surgery learn to communicate by esophageal speech. For people who do not learn this technique, mechanical and electrical devices are available to produce speech.

Much of this chapter has provided information about common problems of the ears, nose, and throat in people over fifty-five. The overall point that we should be aware of is that many of these problems can be prevented or remedied with simple measures: humidifying the home, reducing or stopping smoking, avoiding irritants in the environment. Regular checkups with a medical provider will uncover hearing loss or suspicious lesions. Hearing aids can help many overcome hearing loss. Aging does not mean that we necessarily have to lose normal functioning of the ears, nose, and throat.

Chapter 12
The Teeth

Peter Lockhart, DDS

With proper care your teeth should last a lifetime. Unlike other medical problems that occur with aging, the loss of teeth should not be considered normal or inevitable. Both periodontal disease, which affects the gums and supporting tooth structures, and caries (cavities) can usually be prevented with proper and conscientious home care of the teeth and regular care by a dentist. If this chapter has any single message, it is that you yourself can prevent the majority of oral disease and eliminate the need for time-consuming, unpleasant, and expensive treatment.

The importance of a healthy mouth cannot be overemphasized. Although humans may be the only animals that can live without the teeth nature gives them, the loss of their teeth makes good nutrition more difficult, and it compromises speech, facial expression, personal appearance, and self-esteem. Even if you have had dental problems in the past, good oral hygiene will likely prevent or control these problems in the future. Except in certain unusual situations, there is little excuse for dental disease or loss of teeth.

The normal adult has thirty-two teeth. Each jaw, upper and lower, has four *incisors* located in the front of the mouth for cutting, two *canines* (important to our ancestors for ripping meat), and four *premolars* and six *molars* for grinding food. All human teeth are basically alike, in that they have an outer shell or *crown* covered by *enamel,* the hardest substance in the body, which gives them a white appearance, and an inner layer of *dentin,* or ivory, which surrounds and protects the *pulp chamber*. This chamber is important because it contains the nerves, blood vessels, and other cells that enable teeth to increase the thickness of dentin in the face of progressing caries. The thickening also occurs as a normal process of aging.

The *root* of the tooth, normally located deep in the jawbone, is composed of dentin with a yellowish covering of *cementum.* Within the root is the *root canal,* through which blood runs to carry oxygen and nutrients to the cells within the tooth.

Completely surrounding the root is the *periodontal membrane,* a fibrous network of cells, rich in nerves and blood vessels, that attaches the tooth to the jawbone. It also allows for the small amount of tooth movement that occurs with chewing food.

At the junction between the gum (*gingiva*) and the neck of the tooth is the *periodontal pocket.* Lining the pocket is a thin layer of *mucosa* (the "skin" of the mouth) that acts as a barrier between the mouth and the bloodstream. When we floss and brush our teeth, we clean *plaque* (bacteria, dead cells, and food) and *calculus* (tartar) away from the periodontal pocket. Allowing the plaque and calculus to collect around and within the pocket produces periodontal disease and ultimately loss of teeth.

Oral Disease

Two main types of oral disease afflict adults: *caries* (tooth decay or cavities), which destroys the enamel and dentin of the tooth, and *periodontitis* (pyorrhea), which affects the gums and eventually the underlying tooth support. *Gingivitis* refers to inflammation and swelling of the gums from the accumulation of plaque, producing bacteria and calculus around the teeth.

Caries (Cavities)

Dental caries is the major cause of tooth loss in children and young adults and affects over 90 percent of all individuals in this country. Over two hundred species of bacteria and other organisms live in the mouth, more than in any other area of the body. Only those few bacteria that live by fermenting sugar and refined carbohydrates, however, produce tooth decay. These bacteria prefer the easy-to-digest sucrose or table sugar that is so liberally added to our food and beverages. During the process of fermentation, these bacteria excrete acid, which demineralizes and erodes the tooth enamel. Furthermore, bacteria that are allowed to remain on teeth multiply rapidly and combine with saliva and food debris to produce a dense sticky plaque. This plaque formation produces a cycle of tooth erosion, more plaque formation, and eventually tooth loss from infection that spreads to the jawbone.

Tooth decay can begin in three areas. First, the biting surfaces of the back teeth (premolars and molars) have natural pits and fissures. The depth of these fissures is determined largely by heredity. For many of us, these surfaces are self-cleaning, but tooth brush bristles cannot reach the bottom of these deep pits and fissures, and plaque is therefore not removed. The second area is below the point where the teeth touch each other, or just above the gingiva. So-called smooth surface caries occurring here are usually preventable with regular flossing and brushing. The third area is the root surfaces of teeth that have been exposed, usually because of loss of gingiva from periodontitis. The root surface, composed of cementum, is much softer than enamel and readily erodes under acid-forming bacteria.

In most instances decay of any surface of the tooth can progress to the pulp chamber or root canal of the tooth. If the infection reaches the pulp, it may destroy this vital area of the tooth. It is then important that a "root canal" be performed or the tooth be extracted; otherwise the infected pulp may eventually infect the jawbone. This, in turn, may cause a serious infection of the face and beyond.

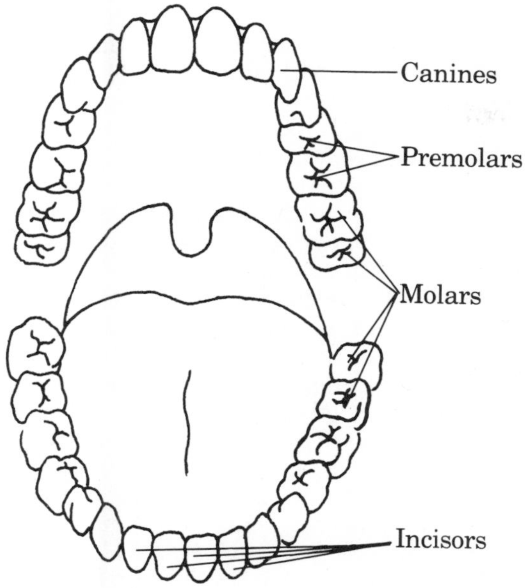

Normal human dentition.

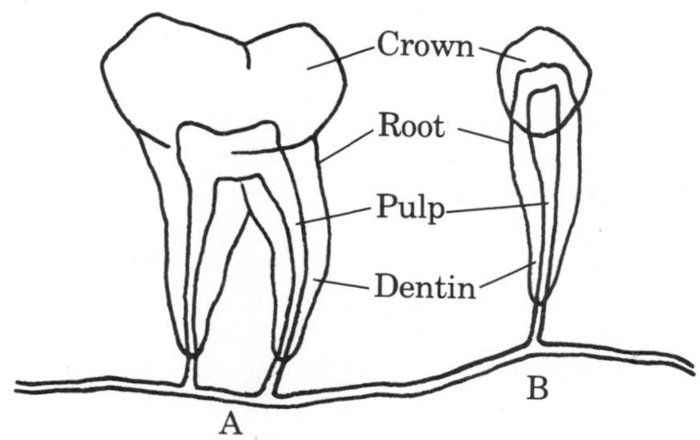

Anatomy of individual teeth: (A) molar; (B) canine.

Oral hygiene and reduction of sugar in the diet may inhibit or totally prevent this process. In people over fifty-five, root surfaces are often exposed, the diet may contain greater quantities of refined sugar and carbohydrates, and less attention may be paid to oral hygiene; the incidence of tooth decay therefore increases.

Gingivitis and Periodontitis (Pyorrhea)

Gingivitis is the inflammation (swelling) of the gums caused by the accumulation of plaque and calculus; periodontitis refers to the loss of bone resulting from this process. Together, they affect over 90 percent of the adult American population. Because of this disease process, an estimated 20 percent of adults have no teeth at all and the majority of adults require some treatment for a variety of dental problems.

Once plaque has "matured" for several days to a week, it may begin to calcify (become hard) by extracting calcium salts from the saliva. The resulting calculus acts like sandpaper on the gingiva and starts a vicious cycle of increased inflammation and destruction. Periodontal disease is often painless and may not be noticed until an acute infection (abscess) forms or bleeding occurs with toothbrushing. This bleeding is a cardinal sign of gingivitis or periodontitis, indicating that significant disease exists and that treatment should be sought to prevent additional loss of tooth support. If left unattended, the gingiva will become more inflamed and the periodontal pocket will enlarge, creating an environment where more destructive bacteria will accumulate and multiply. Eventually the bone and ligament around the root will be damaged.

Periodontal disease.

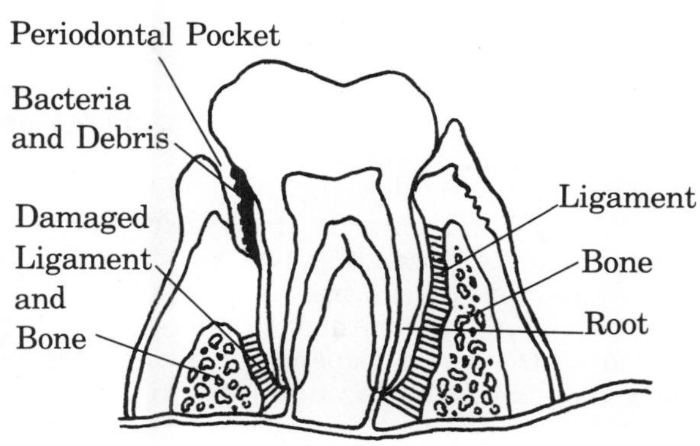

Caring for Your Teeth

The key to maintaining healthy, attractive teeth and gingiva is in the hands of the individual. Both caries and periodontitis are preventable. Proper flossing and brushing, along with modification of our diets and routine visits to a dental hygienist will go a long way toward preventing tooth loss throughout life. There are four steps to a healthy mouth.

Step 1: Reducing sugar consumption

Most of us should reduce the amount of sugar and refined carbohydrates in our diet. The incidence of caries in the world is directly proportional to the amount of sugar in the diet and is largely a problem of modern and Western cultures. This not only means decreasing the amount of sugar added to coffee, cereal, and other foods, but also avoiding processed juices, prepared salad dressings, canned fruits and vegetables, and other foods to which large amounts of sugar are added.

It is essential to realize that the frequency of sugar consumption is more important than the amount consumed. Sugar raises the acid level in the mouth. The level stays high for about an hour and then slowly drops. Amazing as it may sound, therefore, it is less harmful to your teeth to eat a box of candy in one sitting than to spread out a smaller amount over a whole day (although it is not recommended you do either). If sugar is consumed every hour or two, the level of acid in your mouth will remain high for a much longer time. This can destroy your teeth in a matter of months. If you do eat sugar-containing foods, brush your teeth or rinse your mouth vigorously with water to wash the sugar off your teeth. This will lower the acid level.

Step 2: Flossing

Daily flossing is perhaps the single most important thing an adult can do to maintain healthy gingiva. Periodontal disease is present to some extent in nine out of ten adults, but it can be controlled, if not eliminated, with regular oral hygiene.

Flossing teeth, although a tedious chore at first, is essential to prevent periodontal disease. Some dexterity is needed to floss between all the teeth, and it takes time to master the technique. You may find it helpful to floss in front of a mirror at first to avoid missing spaces, but after awhile you should no longer need to look to see what you are doing. There is no uniform opinion on whether it is better to use waxed or unwaxed floss. It is a good idea to keep several rolls of floss around the house (for example, on top of the television) as a reminder and convenience, since flossing need not be accomplished only in the bathroom; although perhaps unpleasant to watch, it serves as a good example for younger people in the household.

Here is the best way to floss. Cut off a section about twelve inches (30 cm) long and wrap it around your middle fingers, leaving about six inches (15 cm) between. Do not wrap so tightly that you cut off circulation. Starting in the same location each time (behind the last tooth in the upper right jaw is a good place to begin), hold the floss taut between thumb and index fingers, and gently "saw" the floss through the contact between the teeth. Move the floss up and down several times along the surface of the tooth under the contact point. Then do the same to the adjacent tooth without removing the floss through the contact point. Move on to the next space between the teeth and repeat. Remember to get the back side of the last tooth in each jaw, and do not move the floss so hard that you injure the gum. If the floss breaks or frays, this may indicate a faulty restoration or buildup of calculus. Bring this to the attention of a dentist or hygienist during the next visit. After flossing all surfaces between the teeth, rinse vigorously with water to remove the loosened bacteria and food from the mouth. Avoid toothpicks. They often do more harm than good.

What about oral irrigating devices? A variety of these devices are on the market. Although they may be useful as a cleaning aid for patients with orthodontic bands or other prosthetic devices, they should not be used as a primary method of oral hygiene. They may further trap food between the teeth and are considered dangerous for patients with certain types of heart problems because they may force bacteria into the bloodstream. Consumer's Union reported the uncommon problem of electrocution with pulsating varieties that employ an electric water pump.

As a dentist, I try to encourage both brushing and flossing, but if I have to choose between one or the other, I would say that flossing may be more important. Periodontal disease is a more common cause of tooth loss in adults than caries, and it usually begins between the teeth where toothbrush bristles cannot reach.

Step 3: Brushing

The toothbrush is an essential item in the maintenance of oral hygiene. Although many types of brushes exist, a soft, polished nylon bristle is generally recommended. Stiff bristles, improperly used, can damage teeth and gingiva and should not be used unless recommended by your dentist. Brushing techniques vary. Your dentist or hygienist may recommend a certain technique. For people with limited dexterity, an electric toothbrush is an alternative.

Brushing should be done in conjunction with flossing. It is important to spend several minutes a day brushing all surfaces of the teeth, especially the areas where tooth and gingiva meet. Brushing should ideally be done at night just before retiring so that no food (and therefore no acid) will remain on the teeth overnight. If done properly, one thorough brushing per day is adequate to prevent disease. People particularly susceptible to oral disease may need more frequent brushing.

The kind of toothpaste you use is of little importance. Toothpaste has some cosmetic value, and its taste may promote more frequent brushing, but the ingredients of toothpaste have little effect on either caries or periodontitis in people over fifty-five. It is the mechanical action of the brush and floss in removing plaque that is beneficial.

Toothpastes and powders differ mostly in their abrasiveness. Tooth whiteners tend to be more abrasive and can damage exposed or sensitive root surfaces of teeth. Most of the claims concerning one toothpaste over another are unfounded scientifically.

Fluoridated toothpastes do have some benefit for adults in that the fluoride is incorporated into the surface of the enamel and makes it harder. There is some question as to the extent of benefit of fluoride in older people. A well-conducted scientific study has never shown any harmful effects from fluoride for older people, however, and there is some indication that it may strengthen bones. Fluoride rinses are felt to be helpful for all age groups. They may be particularly beneficial to adults with root surfaces exposed from periodontal disease or its treatment. A daily one-minute swishing of one of the over-the-counter fluoride solutions may prevent or slow down the problem of root caries. Ask your dentist about the usefulness of this therapy for you.

Mouthwash has cosmetic value only. In spite of advertising claims, it does not significantly improve oral hygiene. In fact, overuse of mouthwashes may alter the delicate balance that exists between different bacteria in the mouth and cause problems of its own. Use of toothpaste or mouthwash in conjunction with inadequate brushing and flossing leads to false security and has been likened to pouring perfume on garbage. What keeps plaque from forming is the mechanical action of brushing and flossing, along with consuming less of the sugar and refined carbohydrates that acid-producing bacteria thrive on.

Step 4: Professional cleaning

Dental hygienists are trained to remove plaque and calculus from the teeth. Depending on the amount of plaque and calculus that accumulates in your mouth, you should avail yourself of this service every three to twelve months. Hygienists are also trained to examine your mouth for oral disease and may alert you to the need to be seen by a dentist. Cleaning by the hygienist can help prevent more serious and expensive procedures that might be performed by a dentist.

An increasing number of physicians and public health analysts feel that routine physical examinations, laboratory tests, and X rays are unnecessary for most people. With dental disease, however, just the opposite is true. Caries and periodontal disease are usually painless processes until significant damage has been done. It is false economy to avoid regular oral hygiene at home, dental cleaning by a hygienist, and regular oral examinations. In general, proper care, regular cleanings, and periodic professional checkups can preserve the teeth for a lifetime.

Choosing a Dentist

Choosing a dentist involves finding a person with whom you feel comfortable who is trained in the area for which you need help. A general, or family dentist will treat your regular dental needs and refer you to a specialist if you need one. In general, specialists are not for routine care.

Like the rest of medicine, dentistry has undergone considerable specialization since World War II. Dental specialties are offshoots of general dentistry. Many general dentists have received pre- and postdoctoral training that allows them to practice most of the specialty areas listed below. The American Dental Association recognizes eight dental specialties, five of which may be of value to people over fifty-five.

Periodontists are primarily concerned with the prevention and treatment of diseases of the tooth-supporting structures. They use surgical curettage (cleaning the teeth with scalers) and periodontal surgery (removal of diseased gum, tooth, or bone) to stop the progression of bone loss around teeth. They also treat problems related to improperly aligned teeth and oral habits that may contribute to periodontal disease.

Endodontists treat root canals that have become infected through caries or periodontal disease. Once a root canal becomes infected with bacteria, it must be cleaned out and obliterated, as the body cannot, on its own, eliminate an infection in this location. Obliteration involves packing the cleaned out space with a synthetic material.

Prosthodontists restore and replace broken-down or missing teeth. They make crowns, bridges, and full and partial dentures. They may also construct appliances for parts of the face that are missing because of serious accidents or cancer surgery.

Oral surgeons remove teeth, treat broken bones of the face, reconstruct facial deformities, and perform complex surgical procedures necessary before the construction of prosthetic devices like bridges and dentures.

Orthodontists align teeth to make a more normal bite. In the past this has been considered a specialty for children, but many adults now seek their services, especially prior to construction of prosthetic appliances.

Replacement and Restoration of Broken-Down and Missing Teeth

The major oral problems encountered by adults are the preservation and the replacement of existing teeth and the replacement of those that are missing. Although a missing tooth or teeth need not always be replaced, the resultant malocclusion or empty space can create a situation where the remaining teeth suffer increased trauma from chewing and are more likely to be subject to caries or periodontal disease.

Restorative materials such as silver alloys and tooth-colored fillings (resins) have advanced to the point where teeth that used to require crowns (caps) may now often be restored in a less expensive and less time-consuming manner. Nevertheless, once teeth become so broken down that they will not hold a filling, or when there is a risk of the tooth breaking, a crown may be necessary.

Crowns are made from a variety of materials. Preformed stainless steel crowns provide strength and protection against breakage. Less expensive than other types of crowns, they are difficult to fit over the tooth in such a way as to avoid periodontal problems. Most crowns are custom-constructed in the laboratory to fit exactly over a tooth that has been cut down to provide room for the crown. These crowns may be all porcelain for front teeth, all gold or nonprecious metal for back teeth, or gold and porcelain or acrylic bonded together. Different situations dictate different types of crowns. Your dentist is best able to explain why one is better than another for your specific case.

Replacement of missing teeth can be accomplished in a variety of ways. The most desirable, although most expensive, is with fixed bridgework. This involves cutting down teeth on either side of the missing tooth or teeth for crowns and fusing a false tooth or teeth to the crowns on either side. These multiple-unit fused crowns are then cemented in place. A fixed bridge cannot be installed in all situations, however, because teeth on either side may not be healthy enough to support the bridge. In addition, there may not be a tooth on each side to support the bridge. Finally, fixed bridgework is expensive, and that may be deemed an obstacle. A partial denture is an alternative. Partials involve a metal framework with clasps attached to it that grasp the teeth and hold it in place. Only one tooth, however, may be needed to clasp onto. False teeth that match the existing teeth are fused to this metal or plastic framework.

People missing all of their teeth in the upper or lower jaw require full dentures. Dentures may be placed in the mouth right after the remaining teeth are removed or may be constructed after several weeks to allow healing of the extraction sites. The advantage of immediate dentures is that aesthetics are maintained for people who do not want to be without teeth during the healing phase. They may be difficult to tolerate, however, because of painful areas that exist after surgery. Although a more minor consideration, immediate dentures must be relined at some point following the extractions, as the bone and tissues shrink, leaving a space between denture and supporting tissue. Discuss the issue of immediate dentures with your dentist.

The ability to tolerate full and partial dentures varies among people. Partial dentures are more desirable than full dentures because they are held in place by natural teeth. Full dentures require an adequate-sized jawbone to provide for suction or other form of retention that prevents movement during speech and eat ing. Suction is not usually obtainable on lower dentures; the denture merely sits on the lower ridge or jaw, relying on gravity to hold it in place. People who experience difficulty with the fit of full dentures should be evaluated by their dentist to see if anything can be done to improve the retentions. If not, one of a variety of denture adhesives available over the counter may be tried. Experiment with a few of them until you find the one that is best for you.

Care of Dentures

Cleaning

Dentures should be cleaned regularly. This is most easily accomplished by holding the appliance over a sink filled with water (this lessens the risk of breaking them if they should be dropped) and cleaning them with a toothbrush. It is helpful to rinse them with water after eating to remove food trapped under and around the appliance. Failure to clean the appliance may promote infection or halitosis (bad breath), because plaque and calculus build up on appliances just as they do on normal teeth.

If you have a partial denture, be certain to clean your remaining teeth by flossing and brushing. Every effort should be made to keep those teeth healthy, as they are the necessary support for your partial denture.

Dentures and partials should be kept in water when out of the mouth. This prevents the denture acrylic from drying out and warping. Denture cleaners for use while soaking are available, but they are probably not as effective as a denture brush. Many of these denture cleaners are dangerous if swallowed and should be kept away from children.

Night Wear

In general, removable appliances should be taken out of the mouth at night. Like wearing shoes twenty-four hours a day, keeping your dentures in around the clock is not a good idea. It can cause mouth ulcers and other problems. If leaving the appliance out at night is socially unacceptable, they should be removed for about eight hours at some other time of the day. This provides a time when the tissues in the mouth can recover from the stress of having a foreign body pressing on them.

Denture Adhesives

Denture adhesives are often employed to help with a loose denture. Although a dentist may recommend an adhesive for long-term use, adhesives should be thought of as a temporary solution to the problem until dental advice can be obtained. Prolonged use of ill-fitting dentures can cause ulcers and accelerated bone destruction that may rule out the possibility of dentures in the future.

Sore Spots

Sore spots under and around dentures and partials, especially new ones, are common. They are not likely to go away on their own, however, and they should not be ignored. The denture will usually require readjustment by a dentist. These sore spots are not only distracting, but in the face of alcohol and/or smoking, are thought to increase the possibility of oral cancer.

Relines

Whereas some people can wear dentures or partials for many years without having them relined, most are not so fortunate. Over a period of time, there is usually some loss of jawbone, and remaining teeth can shift position. When this happens, a space is formed between the denture and the supporting hard and soft tissues. Full dentures become loose, and partial dentures may place added stress on the remaining teeth and shorten their life span. Periodic checks with your dentist are necessary to prevent this situation.

Denture Reliners, Cushions, and Repair Kits

Use of these over-the-counter products is to be discouraged. They may be used in an emergency or to repair a broken denture over a weekend, but their use invites severe problems with bone loss and oral ulcers. Most dentists have seen often irreversible problems from the use of these products.

Dental Warning Signs

Mouth Pain

Tooth sensitivity to cold or sweets should alert you to the possibility of caries. As decay approaches the center of the tooth, the pulp tissue becomes inflamed and sensitive to cold or to the acid produced by bacteria. Leaking or faulty fillings, exposed roots caused by loss of surrounding gingiva, and fractured teeth may also produce pain and sensitivity. Sensitivity to cold, however, is common in teeth following the placement of silver fillings, but this should decrease with time.

Sensitivity to hot foods may indicate that the pulp has partially or completely died. Heat causes expansion of the contents of the pulp chamber and stimulates the remaining nerve tissue. Spontaneous pain, or pain on chewing that is not temperature related, may be a sign that infection has spread to the jaw.

Pain in the soft tissues of the mouth may be of bacterial, fungal, viral, or traumatic (i.e., ill-fitting dentures), or other origin. Often there may be an accompanying sore. Space does not permit a discussion of all the possibilities for mouth pain and sores, but any sore that remains for over a week should be seen by your dentist.

Bleeding

The most common cause of oral bleeding is periodontitis. Bleeding of the gingiva during tooth brushing or awakening in the morning to find blood on your pillow are not uncommon occurrences, but they should not be ignored. There are other causes of bleeding from the mouth, including oral cancers and certain bleeding disorders. If you have any mouth pain or bleeding, see your dentist. Delay in diagnosis and treatment may result in more serious, if not more expensive, problems.

Dental Patients with Special Medical Problems

Diabetes

It is not known whether diabetics have a higher frequency of oral infections, but they often have more difficulty handling infections when they do occur. It is therefore important for a person with diabetes to maintain good oral hygiene and obtain regular dental care to avoid the risk of infection that may complicate the management of their diabetes.

Heart Disease

Individuals with certain heart problems, such as rheumatic heart disease, have a higher risk of getting infections of the heart than the average person. In people with periodontal disease, brushing, flossing, and eating may cause a shower of bacteria to enter the bloodstream. For most people this is harmless, but those who have recently undergone heart surgery or who have a pacemaker, a faulty heart valve, a prosthetic (replacement) heart valve, or a particular type of heart murmur may require special management of any dental treatment.

Those people who are scheduled to have heart valve surgery should receive dental care prior to the procedure, so that the mouth is restored to the healthiest state possible. Individuals with any of the above mentioned heart problems may need antibiotic medicines prior to any dental procedures. Persons with a heart condition should discuss anticipated dental treatment with both their physician and dentist to prevent problems from arising.

Kidney Disease

People who have had kidney transplants and are on medications to suppress rejection of the organ, as well as individuals on dialysis, are at some risk for acquiring serious kidney or shunt infections that originate from the mouth. Like the heart patients mentioned before, they may require special dental consideration.

Orthopedic Joint Replacement

There is evidence that replacement joints can become infected because of poor oral hygiene or from dental treatment. It is my feeling that people undergoing orthopedic joint replacement require special consideration in their dental treatment. The surgeon should be consulted about the timing of any dental procedures.

Cancer

Patients receiving radiation around the neck and face have special dental needs. Salivary glands may be destroyed and bacteria may accumulate around the teeth as a result. Not only does the risk of losing teeth because of periodontal disease and caries increase, but there is the chance of acquiring a serious infection in the jaw. Radiation also reduces the blood supply to the jaws, making it more difficult to eradicate infections.

Cancer patients receiving chemotherapy commonly have some level of suppression of their immune system. Consequently, a high percentage of chemotherapy patients risk painful ulcerations of the gingiva and other soft tissues, as well as serious mouth infections. The chance of having these problems is partially related to the state of oral hygiene prior to chemotherapy. Anyone who is scheduled for chemotherapy should be examined by a dentist prior to treatment and should be monitored while they are on medication.

Many of the problems that are encountered during and following cancer therapy are preventable, or at least treatable, if the dentist and physician work together.

Medications

Problems in receiving dental care can arise if the patient takes antiinflammatory medications (like steroids), anticoagulant drugs (like Coumadin), certain psychiatric medications, Dilantin, and even aspirin in some cases. Dentists should be aware of all the patient's medications, any allergies, all other aspects of medical history, and any changes in health since the last visit.

A large number of other physical and emotional disorders and therapies increase the risk of oral problems that can threaten the patient's general health and well-being. The home management of these problems is the same as for the general public. Excellent home care and other preventive measures, along with periodic and thorough oral exams and cleaning, will go a long way toward preventing problems that range from a simple nuisance to those that may result in seriously compromised overall health.

Oral Cancer

Oral cancer comprises only 5 percent of all cancers, yet it is particularly tragic because it is a disease that often can be prevented. An overwhelming amount of research demonstrates the direct relationship between smoking and oral cancer. Moderate to heavy alcohol consumption further increases the risk, especially when combined with smoking.

These tumors can often be seen and cured in their early stages. Unfortunately, people who are moderate to heavy smokers and drinkers may also tend to have poor oral hygiene habits and generally do not seek routine dental care.

Less than half of the adults in this country seek the services of a dentist in any given year. People generally fear the expense or pain of dental care. Although the cost of regular dental care may seem high, it is relatively small when compared to the cost of procedures that are needed when oral disease reaches an advanced stage. Moreover, there is no accurate way of accounting for the cost of losing teeth in the social terms of daily living.

Unfortunately, many people who have dental insurance still tend to go to the dentist only when their problems are far advanced. Cost is therefore only one factor in accounting for our reluctance to seek dental care. Because of recent advances and innovations in dental care delivery, it is now possible to undergo dental care with minimal or no discomfort. Local anesthetics to numb the area of treatment and various forms of sedation can combine to make dental treatment at least very tolerable. My point, therefore, is that you can have healthy teeth throughout life if you spend a little time and effort taking care of them.

Although most people seek dental care from a private dentist, alternatives do exist. Dental schools often take large numbers of patients into their student and postdoctoral clinics. Here the fees are often considerably lower, and the work is closely supervised by the faculty. Treatment, however, usually proceeds more slowly, so that if saving time is important to you, do not seek care in dental schools. Many hospitals offer dental services to outpatients, and many towns and cities have other types of clinics and public health facilities.

You should try to find a dentist who will work with you in a considerate, thorough, and relatively painless manner. Discuss your treatment plan with that person, and be an active participant in your own oral health.

Chapter 13
The Heart

Ann Stewart, RN, NP

An awareness of the normal aging process commonly brings fears concerning chronic and life-threatening heart disease. You should not assume because you are entering the sixth, seventh, or later decades of life that you are destined for severe debilitating heart disease. Although the incidence of heart disease is higher with increasing age, many adults aged fifty-five and older have healthy hearts and enjoy full, active lives.

Nonetheless, we should all learn about the heart, heart disease, and how to help better take care of this organ. The figures speak for themselves. Heart disease is the leading cause of death for men over forty. Women have about one-third the heart disease rate of men until they reach menopause. After that, their risk increases, and it is similar to men by age seventy.

The heart is a pump that delivers blood to the tissues of the body. It is slightly larger than your fist and weighs less than a pound. The frequency of beating and the force of contraction are regulated by the nervous system, and although we are generally unaware of this regulation, it is essential for maintaining normal life.

The heart is divided into four chambers: two *atria* and two *ventricles*. In addition, it is divided into two sides: right and left. The right portion receives blood that has come from the tissues and pumps it through the *pulmonary artery* to the lungs, where it receives oxygen. Oxygen-rich blood returns to the heart via the *pulmonary vein* and is pumped to the body via the *aorta*. The four valves, *mitral, aortic, tricuspid,* and *pulmonary,* keep blood flowing in the correct direction.

Heart disease not only produces fatal heart attacks, but is responsible for hospitalizations, limitation on activity, and sometimes permanent work disability. Strokes affect approximately 500,000 persons annually in the United States. Statistically, it is the third leading cause of death. In over 50 percent of stroke victims, the cause can be related to a disease process called atherosclerosis. Atherosclerosis is a process each individual can help to prevent.

Atherosclerosis

Atherosclerosis is the cause of most heart attacks and strokes. This process may begin as early as infancy and childhood and increase in severity with age. The walls of the arteries become thickened with plaques composed of cholesterol and fats. The thickening of the wall progressively narrows the artery and reduces the amount of oxygen-carrying blood reaching the heart, brain, and other parts of the body. The artery may become completely blocked from atherosclerosis or from a clot lodged in the narrow vessel. Complications occur when there is interference with blood flow to the tissues of the body.

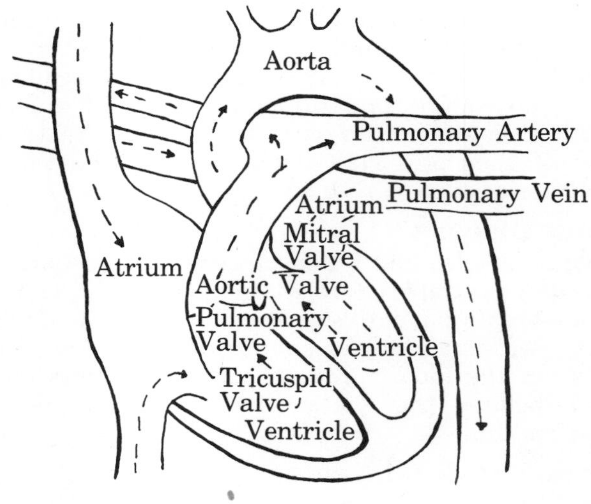

Anatomy of the heart. Blood flow is shown by arrows. (Adapted with permission: The American Heart Association.)

Cholesterol deposited from the blood forms atherosclerotic plaques. Although it is true that our own bodies produce cholesterol, evidence from animal studies supports the connection between atherosclerosis and high dietary intake of cholesterol and fats. In general, the lower the cholesterol level, the less the likelihood of heart disease; the higher the cholesterol level, the greater the risk. Significant coronary artery disease is rare in areas of the world where the average blood cholesterol level is less than 170 milligrams per 100 milliliters of blood, expressed as 170 mg/100 ml. In the United States, the average cholesterol level for adults is approximately 245 mg/100 ml. It is not difficult to see from these figures why the incidence of coronary artery disease is so high in this country.

The relationship between heart disease and triglyceride levels is not clear. High levels of triglycerides in the blood *may* increase the risk of heart disease, especially if present with other risk factors.

Hyperlipidemia

Hyperlipidemia refers to an abnormally high concentration of fats in the blood, most commonly cholesterol or triglyceride. The major goal in the treatment of hyperlipidemia is the prevention of early disease to the vessels of the body, especially the coronary arteries. *Lipoproteins,* which contain fat and protein, are normal constituents of the body. In excess, however, they may cause hyperlipidemia and atherosclerosis. The various lipoproteins differ in their role of contributing to atherosclerosis. Low-density lipoproteins

(LDL) cause atherosclerosis because they accelerate the deposit of cholesterol in the arteries. High-density lipoproteins (HDL) may be protective and actually decrease the risk of coronary heart disease. Exercise and modest alcohol intake may increase HDL levels, whereas smoking and obesity may lower HDL.

Dietary control is the most common and safe therapy for all people who have hyperlipidemia. If you have hyperlipidemia, a nutritionist or nurse should be able to create a diet for your particular needs, according to the results of your blood tests and body weight (see also Chapter 8, *Nutrition*).

If the risk of coronary artery disease is very high and diet alone is ineffective in controlling the levels of fat in the blood, drug therapy may be initiated. For some, more than one lipid-lowering medication is necessary. Side effects have been noted with all of these medications. Drug therapy is generally not recommended for people over the age of sixty.

Hypertension (High Blood Pressure)

Everyone has blood pressure. Blood pressure is the force of the blood against the walls of the arteries, generated by the heart, which contracts between sixty and ninety times a minute in order to keep blood moving from the heart to all parts of the body. As the heart relaxes between beats, the blood pressure goes down. When your blood pressure is taken around the large artery of your arm or leg, two pressures are recorded. The higher number represents the blood pressure in the artery when the heart is contracting (*systolic pressure*); the lower number is measured when the heart is relaxed and filling with blood for the next beat (*diastolic pressure*). For example:

$$\frac{120\text{ (systolic)} = \text{heart contracting}}{80\text{ (diastolic)} = \text{heart relaxed}}.$$

These readings refer to the pressure in millimeters of mercury. Both measurements are considered to be of equal significance.

Blood pressure varies from one person to another, and in the same person, it varies from moment to moment. The blood pressure may increase at times of stress, anxiety, and exercise; it may decrease during relaxation and sleep. Therefore, it is the trend of the blood pressure over a period of time that is considered important rather than one single blood pressure measurement.

There is a wide range of normal blood pressures. The systolic may be as low as 90 or as high as 160; the diastolic may be as low as 60 or as high as 90. Age

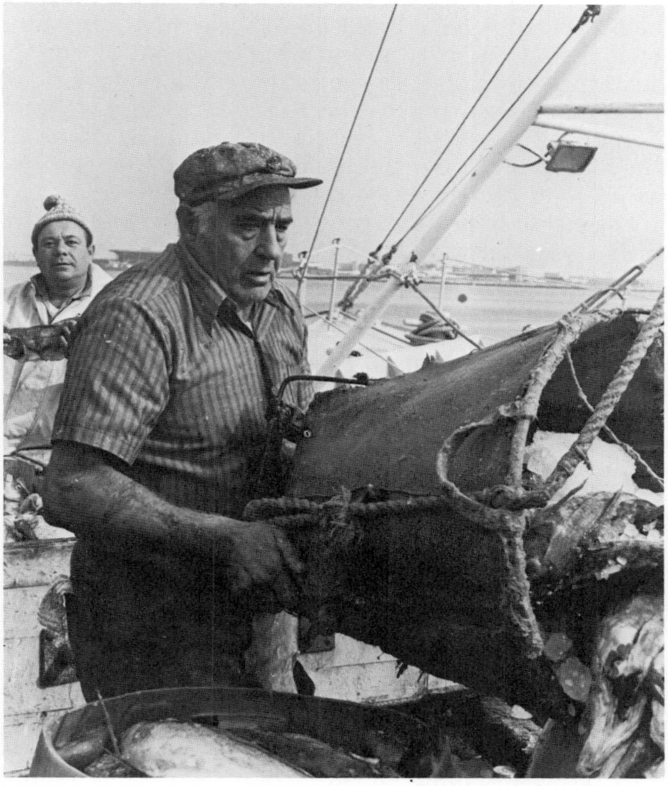

Lowering Cholesterol and Triglycerides

Dietary guidelines to lower cholesterol

1. Limit intake of dietary cholesterol to less than 300 milligrams per day (average American diet has 500 to 800 milligrams per day).
2. Limit intake of animal fat to 30 percent of daily caloric intake.
3. Replace saturated fats with polyunsaturated fats.
4. Reduce to ideal body weight.

Drug therapy to lower cholesterol and its possible side effects

Cholestyramine, colestipol: Constipation, stomach discomfort, bloating; interferes with absorption of Coumadin, digitalis medication, thyroxine, antibiotics—take these medications one hour before taking cholestyramine or colestipol.

Dietary guidelines to lower triglycerides

1. Reduce weight and maintain ideal body weight.
2. Eliminate or strictly reduce alcohol intake.
3. Replace saturated fats with unsaturated fats.
4. Limit fat intake to 30 to 35 percent of daily caloric intake.
5. Reduce intake of carbohydrates.

Drug therapy to lower triglycerides and its possible side effects

Clofibrate: Weight gain, mild nausea, diarrhea, increased risk of gallstone formation; increases the action of Coumadin.

Nicotinic acid: Flushing, nausea, bloating, stomach discomfort, sugar intolerance; may increase uric acid level and produce abnormal liver function values in blood tests.

and past blood pressure measurements should also be considered in any determination of an individual's normal pressure range.

An occasional blood pressure that is higher than normal is nothing to worry about. When the systolic blood pressure is consistently greater that 150 to 155 or the diastolic is consistently greater than 90 to 95, however, the diagnosis of hypertension is justified. An evaluation of the hypertension should be initiated, and a management program should be determined.

Types of Hypertension

Over 90 percent of those diagnosed as having elevated blood pressure have *essential hypertension*. This term means that there is no apparent explanation for the sustained elevation. The sufferer generally has a heart that pumps too much blood or has a normal heart output with narrowed vessels that cause resistance to the blood flow. Essential hypertension cannot be cured at present, but it can be controlled.

Essential hypertension is sometimes classified as mild or moderate. Data now demonstrate that even mild forms of hypertension deserve some form of treatment, although this does not necessarily mean medication.

Secondary hypertension refers to high blood pressure caused by a known organic abnormality, such as kidney disease, obstruction to kidney blood flow, or disease and tumors of the adrenal gland (which lie above the kidney).

Severe hypertension refers to blood pressure readings as high as 200/115. The greater sustained force of pressure on the vessels increases risk of injury to organs supplied by the vessels. When an individual who has had consistent mild or moderate hypertension develops severe hypertension, secondary causes must be investigated.

Accelerated hypertension refers to blood pressure that may be recorded as high as 240/150. This type of hypertension is also called *malignant hypertension*. The term *malignant* in this case is in no way related to cancer. The diagnosis is made by the blood pressure recording, as well as by other tests that indicate such symptoms as increased pressure in the back of the eyes and protein in the urine. Hospitalization is often necessary to control the blood pressure. Accelerated hypertension most frequently affects the black population.

Tendency toward Hypertension

An estimated 35 million people in the United States have hypertension—one of every six persons. High blood pressure affects all ages but is most often noted in people over forty. Blood pressure levels increase as we age because the blood vessels become less elastic.

If other members of your immediate family have high blood pressure, you are at a higher risk of developing hypertension than if your family had no history of hypertension. Environmental as well as genetic factors may be responsible for this tendency.

Hypertension afflicts blacks in greater numbers and with more complications than whites. It develops early in their lives, is generally more severe, and results in a greater number of early deaths from stroke.

Obese individuals also have a greater tendency to develop hypertension. They are more likely to develop diabetes and hyperlipidemia as well. This combination of risk factors influences heart disease and other potential serious illnesses of the hypertensive person.

Other Factors Contributing to the Development of Hypertension

Cigarette smoking has been shown to elevate the blood pressure in some individuals. The hypertensive smoker also has a higher risk of developing other cardiovascular diseases, especially coronary artery disease.

A high sodium intake in the diet seems to be related to the development of hypertension. Salt retains additional fluids in the body, thereby increasing the blood volume and consequently the work load of the heart. A diet high in saturated fats and cholesterol increases the risk of atherosclerosis, which in turn narrows the arteries and arterioles of the body, thereby increasing blood pressure.

Stress also contributes in some ways to the development of hypertension. Psychological, social, environmental, and occupational stresses are a part of everyone's daily life, but one's response to the stress determines the effect it will have on an individual.

Drugs, such as corticosteroids, certain nosedrops, appetite suppressants, decongestants, amphetamines, and cocaine may influence or be responsible for hypertension. People who take birth control pills, other estrogens, or thyroid medication may also have elevated blood pressure.

Signs and Symptoms

Since high blood pressure has no reliable symptoms, this disease often goes undetected. For this same reason, many who are aware that they have hypertension do not follow daily treatments to control elevated blood pressure.

Some symptoms that may or may not occur are a throbbing headache that generally appears in the morning and persists through the day; fatigue and nervousness, dizziness, palpitations, and shortness of breath.

Severe headache associated with nausea and vomiting, blurring of vision, and unexplained weight loss may signal early malignant hypertension. A change in personality with mental confusion and disorientation may also be noticed. Any of these symptoms require immediate medical attention.

Keep in mind that symptoms you attribute to high blood pressure may have nothing to do with your actual blood pressure. These same symptoms may be related to emotional tension or other medical problems.

End Organ Damage

After years of high blood pressure, the heart may enlarge slightly and be less able to meet the demands placed on it. The arteries and arterioles may become less elastic and more scarred earlier than would be expected with the normal aging process. As the vessels become narrowed, they are less able to deliver the amount of blood necessary for a specific organ to function well. A blood clot may lodge in a narrowed vessel and totally deprive that area of a normal blood supply. The organs most affected in this way are the heart, the kidneys, the brain, and the eyes.

Diagnosing Hypertension

Individuals are considered to be hypertensive when an average of three blood pressures, taken on separate

Normal Blood Pressure by Age Group (Upper Limits)

Infants	90/60
ages 3–6	110/70
ages 7–10	120/80
ages 11–17	130/80
ages 18–44	140/90
ages 45–64	150/95
ages 65–older	160/95

days, exceeds that specified for the appropriate age group. The blood pressure should be measured on both arms and occasionally in the legs.

It is important that information about current state of health and social behaviors (smoking, alcohol use, exercise), as well as past history and family history be obtained. A complete history and physical examination, along with specific laboratory studies, should be done to find a curable cause of the hypertension. This evaluation is also necessary to assess the severity of end organ damage and the presence of other silent diseases or risk factors.

Blood studies that should initially be done include a complete blood count (CBC) and measurement of blood electrolyte, blood urea nitrogen or creatinine (to assess kidney function), blood sugar, fasting cholesterol, and uric acid levels. Sometimes thyroid function, triglyceride levels, and calcium levels are also measured. Other necessary studies include a urinalysis, a chest X ray, and an electrocardiogram.

If a secondary cause of hypertension is suspected from the information obtained from the history, physical examination, and laboratory data, additional blood, urine, and radiological studies may be necessary.

Treatment

The goal of treatment for hypertension is to restore blood pressure to a normal or near normal level. It should also be aimed at reducing or eliminating other cardiovascular risk factors. The treatment program is individualized to include necessary education about hypertension and alterations in personal health habits.

Hypertension may be controlled effectively in some people without medication. Weight reduction (if overweight) and decreased intake of salt and saturated fats to lower the blood cholesterol are essential. Regular exercise can also lower blood pressure and tends to reduce the risk of heart attack.

Ideally the sodium intake should be below two grams per day. This means not using salt at the table and consuming fewer foods, beverages, and seasonings that contain salt. Restricting sodium intake will decrease the body's retention of fluid and thus lower the blood pressure.

Smokers are encouraged to stop smoking, taking advantage, if needed, of one of the variety of techniques and programs available to help. Information may be obtained from physicians or other health care providers or by writing for free information from the American Cancer Society or the American Lung Association.

If high-stress situations are identified, efforts to eliminate or minimize these situations should be taken.

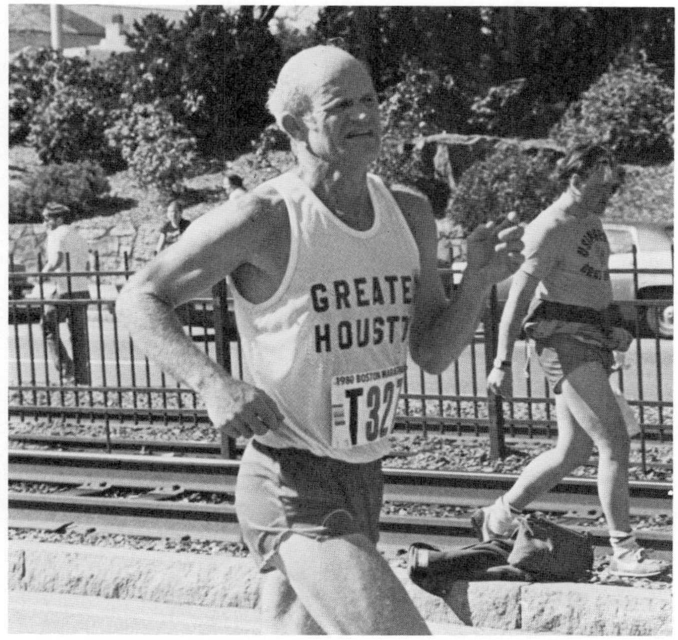

Stress reduction techniques such as relaxation exercises, self-hypnosis, or meditation may be useful tools. A daily exercise program should also be established.

If blood pressure cannot be satisfactorily maintained, medications may need to be added to this program of care. The "stepped-care" approach to treatment is still the most widely used method of treatment with medications. It begins with one medication, generally a diuretic to eliminate extra body fluid. High dosages and additional medications are added if necessary in order to maintain a reasonable blood pressure.

The antihypertensive drugs range from mild to strong in their potency. Most of the drugs produce some side effects, but these are generally mild and do not interfere with normal activities. Common side effects are dry mouth, dizziness, and tiredness. Some medications cause the loss of potassium via the urine, resulting in muscle cramps. Dietary supplements of potassium or a potassium medication may be added to eliminate this effect. A decreased interest in sex and impotence may also occur with some of the antihypertensive medications. If this should occur, the dosage of the medication may be lowered or the medication changed.

The antihypertensive medications generally fall into three categories: those medicines that eliminate extra fluids from the body, for example, diuretics like hydrochlorothiazide (step 1); those medicines that relax the blood vessels by acting primarily on the brain and central nervous system, like propranolol and methyldopa (step 2); those medicines that relax the blood vessels by acting primarily directly on them, for example, hydralazine (step 3). Guanethidine prescribed in large doses, the action of which is the same as the step 2 medications, requires careful supervision by a medical provider.

If a medication is prescribed for you, it is important that you take the medicine every day as directed. It is helpful to establish cues, such as placing the amount of medication needed for the day in a location that reminds you to take it or associating the medication

Medication for High Blood Pressure

Step 1	Step 2	Step 3	Step 4
diuretics: hydrochlorothiazide (HydroDIURIL); spironolactone (Aldactone); triamterene (Dyrenium)	propranolol (Inderal); guanethidine (Ismelin, Esimil)—small doses; clonidine (Catapres); methyldopa (Aldomet); reserpine (Serpasil)	hydralazine (Apresoline); prazosin (Minipress)	guanethidine (Ismelin, Esimil)—200 mg

with an activity that you do daily, such as brushing your teeth.

Remember, the medication helps to *control* blood pressure. It does not *cure* hypertension. Therefore, it is necessary to take the medicine daily for an indefinite period of time, unless advised otherwise by a physician.

Periodic visits to the doctor's office or clinic every four to six months are recommended for those under treatment in order to measure blood pressure and to check for any health problems or side effects from the medications. The dosage or type of medication may be adjusted at this time if necessary.

Most cases of high blood pressure respond to therapy. Not all individuals will require medication—some will be successfully treated by modifying life-style behaviors that are harmful and adding good health behaviors. Most people who are successfully treated live a long and normal life.

It may be annoying or discouraging at times to follow a course of treatment indefinitely for a disease with no symptoms. Keep in mind that these efforts are worthwhile, especially when weighed against the risks associated with and the complications of untreated hypertension.

Risk Factors for Cardiovascular Disease

In addition to hypertension, many factors contribute to atherosclerosis and its major complication, *ischemic heart disease* (lack of oxygen to the heart muscle). It is clear that any one of the following is likely to increase the likelihood of cardiovascular disease. In combination, the risk is significantly increased.

Smoking

Since the 1940s studies have consistently demonstrated that smokers have almost twice the rate of death from heart disease as nonsmokers. This correlation is much greater in individuals under the age of sixty-five.

The risk is proportional to the amount of smoke inhaled and the number of cigarettes smoked. More than twenty cigarettes a day is associated with a three to five times higher incidence of coronary artery disease. Pipe and cigar smokers have only a slightly higher risk than nonsmokers. Substances in the cigarette smoke that are hazardous to the heart are nicotine and carbon monoxide.

A large portion of the smoker's excess risk for heart disease will disappear within two years after quitting. After ten to fifteen years, an exsmoker's chance of early death from a heart attack is no greater than that of someone who has never smoked.

Diabetes

Diabetes is the fourth most important risk factor for cardiovascular disease. Diabetics have twice as many heart attacks, twice as many strokes, and more severe atherosclerosis than nondiabetics. They also are more likely to be overweight and have elevated blood pressures.

Stress

It is not clear if personality types influence the development of atherosclerosis, but they do increase the risk and incidence of heart disease.

The so-called Type A personality, which is competitive, time-conscious, aggressive, and impatient, is the type considered to carry the increased risk. The emotional stress of these feelings is converted into increased blood pressure, increased heart rate, and increased breathing rate. It is difficult to know whether these changes are always harmful, but sometimes they seem to be so.

The Type B personality is more relaxed, easygoing, and relatively noncompetitive. Type B people are less frenzied and preoccupied with time. They seem to be somewhat protected from heart disease.

Additional Risk Factors

Individuals who are overweight or inactive have a higher risk of heart disease since they also tend to have higher levels of fats and sugar in their blood. Overweight individuals may also have elevated blood pressures.

It is believed that a genetic predisposition to heart disease exists. Excess cholesterol in the blood, hypertension, and diabetes are known to be hereditary. Any contribution to risk made by genetic conditions is increased by cigarette smoking, poor dietary habits, and other behaviors that family members tend to have in common.

Angina (Ischemic Heart Disease)

Angina is a symptom of heart disease caused by a decrease in the amount of oxygen to the heart muscle. This temporary pain or discomfort will occur in a person with disease of the coronary arteries when the need for oxygen is greater than what the diseased artery can deliver. It may also occur if the delivery of blood is interrupted by a problem with a valve of the heart or with anemia.

Angina may occur with activity or with rest. For the most part, angina is triggered by an activity or setting that requires the heart to do more work. The pain or discomfort may be experienced as a tightness or a heaviness in the middle part of the chest directly under the breastbone or shoulder area. It sometimes is described as similar to indigestion. A sensation may radiate to the jaw, neck, throat, or arm. The discomfort is usually brief, lasting from two to fifteen minutes. Stopping the provoking activity, resting, and/or using the medication nitroglycerin will generally relieve angina.

You should notify or visit your doctor if:

- chest pain is experienced for the first time
- angina changes in *frequency* (occurs more often every day), *location* (occurs in a different place), or *severity* (becomes more intense or requires more nitroglycerin to relieve it)
- angina is experienced while resting
- angina is not relieved by taking three nitroglycerin pills, each three minutes apart

Angina may be diagnosed after the doctor has taken a full history of symptoms and done a physical examination. An electrocardiogram, a chest X ray, and generally an exercise stress test are necessary. Sometimes a trial dose of nitroglycerin under the tongue is also recommended in order to make the diagnosis. If the medication relieves the symptoms, the problem is very likely angina.

Factors that Commonly Produce an Angina Attack

shaving	combing hair
running	climbing stairs
walking in the cold	playing
athletic events	smoking
sexual intercourse	heavy meals
isometric exertion	shoveling
emotional aggravation	excitement
fear	pain

Nitroglycerin

Nitroglycerin is a short-acting medication that is useful to relieve pain from an acute episode of angina. It works by expanding the walls of the coronary arteries, allowing more blood to flow to the heart muscle. It also causes vessels in other parts of the body to dilate, helping to reduce the oxygen requirements and work load of the heart. Sometimes headache and light-headedness occur with the dilation of the arteries.

A nitroglycerin tablet is taken when the chest discomfort is not relieved by rest. The medication is placed under the tongue, where it dissolves immediately. It is not effective in relieving pain if it is swallowed. Generally, nitroglycerin takes effect within forty-five seconds to three minutes. If the tablet gives no relief after three minutes, a second tablet should be taken. If more than three tablets are needed, a physician should be contacted.

Some people use nitroglycerin before an activity that tends to cause an anginal attack. Taking a nitro tablet three to five minutes *before* engaging in a stressful activity may prevent chest pain. The medication should be effective for ten to thirty minutes.

Common side effects from this medication are headache, flushing of the skin, and dizziness. The standing position should be avoided when the medication is taken and shortly thereafter.

Anginal sufferers should carry a supply of nitroglycerin with them at all times. It should be kept in a tightly closed dark glass container in order to ensure its potency. Additional tablets should be stored in the refrigerator. Heat, light, air, and moisture may decrease the effectiveness of the tablet. A new supply of nitroglycerin tablets should be purchased at least every six months, since the potency of this drug decreases with time. Suspect that the medication has become weak if a burning sensation is not experienced under the tongue when the medicine is taken.

Other Treatment for Angina

Medications such as Isordil and Inderal may be recommended for frequently occurring episodes of angina. These medicines are prescribed for daily use, not for the time of the angina symptom. An ointment formula of nitroglycerin is also available for angina that occurs at night. It is applied directly onto the skin, generally on the arms or abdomen. It is used at night because it is effective for about six hours, allowing for a night's sleep.

Sufferers from angina should also learn strategies for preventing attacks. Among these are reducing emotional stress and tension, avoiding heavy meals, and controlling the other risk factors that have been mentioned. A program of exercise and rest will help reduce tension and improve overall fitness. For instance, a slow walk of three to five minutes, gradually increasing to a mile in fifteen to twenty minutes over a four- to six-week training period can *decrease* the oxygen needs of the heart by 57 percent. This can reduce the frequency of attacks and the need for nitro (see also Chapter 7, *Physical Fitness*). Any program should be designed in consultation with a medical provider.

Heart Attack (Myocardial Infarction)

A heart attack is not primarily a disease of the heart muscle. It occurs as a result of disease in the coronary arteries, which supply blood to the constantly active heart muscle.

Atherosclerosis may severely narrow a branch of a coronary artery, interfering with adequate blood flow to that part of the heart. The diminution of blood supply can cause an area of the heart muscle to swell and die. Sometimes these areas of injury to the muscle are small; at other times they are large and potentially lethal.

As is true with acute injuries in other areas of the body, a healing process will occur if an adequate amount of rest is allowed the heart. Complications sometimes delay the healing process, however. Until the scar forms, the injured portion is very weak. Since the scar formation takes approximately one week, limited activity is very important during this time. New arterial branches called *collateral circulation* are also forming at this time to bring a supply of blood around the injury.

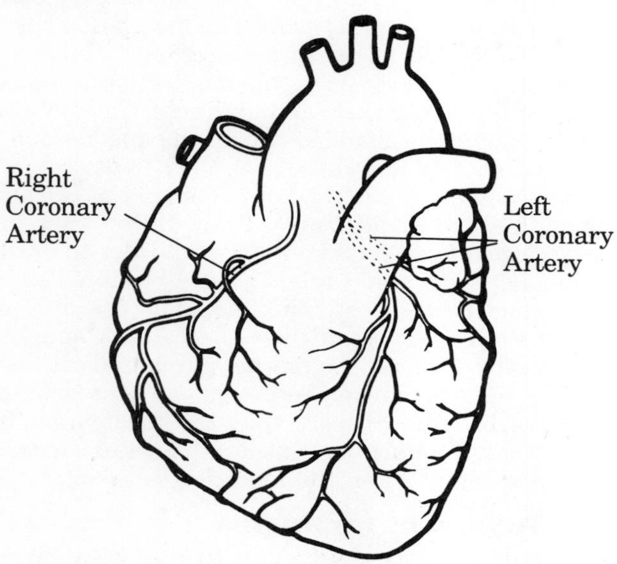

The coronary arteries. (Adapted with permission: The American Heart Association.)

Although the scar may form in the first few weeks, it may take up to two months to become firm and complete the healing. With a gradual and progressive exercise program, most individuals are able to resume their previous activities by this time.

Signals of a Heart Attack

The heart usually gives warning signals if there is a problem. Certain symptoms have been identified that suggest that a heart attack may be occurring. These symptoms may vary from one individual to another, and they may also vary in intensity.

If you believe that you may be having a heart attack, stop *all* activity. Immediately tell someone nearby so that emergency care can be arranged. Many communities have an emergency phone number of 911.

As a result of new technology and research, many people survive a heart attack and return to a meaningful life. The use of mobile coronary care units and the development of the hospital coronary care units, as well as other sophisticated equipment and medications, have made this possible.

In order to determine whether or not a heart attack has occurred, medical personnel in the emergency room will take a history of symptoms and general health state, as well as a physical exam. An electrocardiogram (EKG), a chest X ray, and several laboratory blood studies are necessary to make the diagnosis. Abnormal EKG changes and cardiac enzymes analyzed from the blood that reflect damage to the heart muscle occur during the first three days following the injury. Therefore, a conclusive diagnosis may not be made until that time.

Only a trained medical provider can determine whether an individual has had a heart attack. If you have the slightest hesitation about whether or not you should obtain a medical examination, remember that it is *always* better to be safe than sorry. If you should have any of the symptoms of a potential heart attack, seek medical care immediately.

Care for the Heart Attack Victim

An intravenous access line (IV) and continuous heart monitoring with an EKG will be started immediately if a heart attack is suspected. Oxygen, pain medication, and medications to prevent abnormal heart rhythm may be administered.

Heart attack victims will be admitted to a coronary care unit (CCU) or to a part of the hospital where they

Signs of a Heart Attack

- an uncomfortable sensation, pressure, or discomfort in the center of the chest lasting longer than five minutes
- an uncomfortable sensation, pressure, or discomfort in the shoulders, arm, neck, jaw, back
- sweating that begins before or with the pain described above
- shortness of breath
- nausea and/or vomiting
- generalized feeling of weakness

can be closely observed. They stay here for approximately three to four days, provided that no complications arise. Activity is limited for the first two to three days.

If the heart attack was uncomplicated—that is, if no heart failure, electrical disturbances called *arrhythmias,* or persistent chest pain occurred, the patient will probably remain in the hospital for about ten to fourteen days. During this time the activity level will be increased gradually, so that, by the last two to three days of the hospital stay, the patient will be walking freely and perhaps beginning to climb stairs.

Heart attack victims and their families should get information about the heart and how it functions, as well as some explanation for the cause of the heart attack and symptoms to look for. Careful instructions for medications, diet, rest, and activity will be provided, as well as specific information about when and how to resume household activities, sex, driving, and work. These should be discussed *before* leaving the hospital. Most people should also make plans to stop smoking and find strategies for reducing stress.

Some hospitals offer group sessions where both the patient and the family get information and support from the professional staff as well as from others who have had a heart attack. These groups may meet during the hospitalization and after discharge. They are often extremely helpful in examining questions and feelings that may be difficult to discuss. Every member of the family should be included in these discussions. Often family members develop new attitudes about the heart attack victim's role in the family. They may unnecessarily overprotect a loved one, because they are afraid of precipitating another attack. This is sometimes more detrimental than helpful. After a heart attack, the goal for most people should be to return to a fairly normal life-style. Each family member can help with that goal.

Activity Following a Heart Attack

All activity after a heart attack should be gradual and progressive. It is important to know which specific types of activity and exercise are safe to practice. Knowing the proper frequency, duration, and pace of activities will help build strength and endurance. Initially, however, any activity that demands sudden or short bursts of energy or extensive effort against resistance should be avoided, because these are taxing to the heart (see also Chapter 7, *Physical Fitness*).

Exercise stress testing by a physician may be performed four to eight weeks after the heart attack, provided there are no special complications. This will help the physician prescribe an appropriate exercise program. Exercise is generally recommended two to three times a week for periods of thirty to forty-five minutes, including a warm-up and cool-down period. The heart rate should not exceed 70 to 85 percent of the highest rate safely achieved during the exercise test.

A medical provider can teach how to take a pulse. This can be done at the angle of the jaw (carotid pulse), groin (femoral), or wrist (radial) most easily. Check the pulse rate before the exercise workout, after the warm-up period, during exercising, during cool-down, and finally during the rest period.

If palpitations, dizziness, chest pain, or any irregularity of the pulse rate or rhythm during or following exercise are noted, the exercise should be discontinued and a physician should be notified before resuming the activity. Breathlessness or extreme fatigue for twenty-four hours following exercise, as well as insomnia, are cues that the exercise is too vigorous and needs to be more gradual.

Participation in an active conditioning program produces significant improvement in general fitness, aerobic capacity, blood pressure readings at rest and during exercise, blood cholesterol levels, and the frequency and quality of sexual activity. The psychological benefits include improved self-confidence and self-esteem and less depression and dependency. Eighty-five percent of those in an active exercise program return to work two to three months after their heart attack.

“ I am sixty-two years old. Incredible! I didn't believe I would see the day. Five years ago, I started to feel bad. Those darn kids. They weren't coming out the way I wanted, and my relations with Lynn, with whom I had been infatuated for over thirty years, were at a low ebb. All I could do was ride my bike a lot and think a thousand thoughts about a better world and happy people.

Then it happened. Those insipid morning pains and nausea started intruding in the afternoon at work and when I rode my bike. I was sure that if I could ride fifty miles without dropping dead, I was okay. So, I rode my bike fifty miles without dropping dead and talked the pain away.

At Thanksgiving I gathered the clan and drove four hundred miles to northern Vermont to visit my communing son, who was living the simple, rugged life in the cold north woods. On the way, while driving in a blizzard, I nearly passed out, almost killing all of us. I attributed that little incident to the lousy plastic hamburger I had had for dinner the night before, and we continued on with our celebration of holiday.

How wonderful it felt, all of us together again! The joy of family unity was driving away unpleasant thoughts of the pain inside. Suddenly, I collapsed over the turkey and ended up in Burlington Hospital, barely clinging to life.

The doctors, beautiful guys, split open my chest, tinkered with the pump, bypassed some pipes, and laid me out in bed looking like a zombie. I was hurting all over, still dazed and not fully aware of the reality that had befallen me. They told me they had saved my life, cleaned up my angina, and made it possible for me to keep on living. They couldn't say how well or for how long, but I was alive. I bade my farewells, and went home with my loving Lynn, Stan, Joey, and Danit to try to resume my life.

I went back to work, still hurting all over. What were the pains, though, compared to the reality that I was alive and breathing and able to feel them? I didn't want to return to my boring desk, but the docs wouldn't give me an excuse and were against just about everything else. "Work is good for you, but you are getting old and you have coronary disease, so don't do much of anything else except maybe walk a little."

It wasn't enough. I tried, but I couldn't feel content back at work, walking a little. I had to go out and breathe deeply, and feel once again that I was strong, that my body was able to do what it was made for, to run, to jump, to push my pulse up, with blood rushing, sweat pouring.

So, I started walking and running, running and walking. I read all the gurus of the running revolution—Browerman, Lydiard, Corbett, and Sheehan. Oh, that beautiful Sheehan, who led me into the cosmos!

After a while the cardiologist gave me a stress test, and I ran off his machine. He was flabbergasted by my EKG, my blood pressure, my other vital signs. "How could it be?" he asked as he pondered the remarkable news coming from his medical machines. "How old did you say you were?" We even discussed building a track somewhere and putting all his patients on a running program!

Then, there I was, October 22, 1978, living in Manhattan. I am gone from the double-crossing suburb. I am back with the people I love, and I am running the New York Marathon with 10,000 others.

We pour over the Verrazano Bridge, millions of people cheering me on. I cheer them. Oh, what joy, what love! I prance and I dance. I jump and I jiggle. I chase the men and women in front of me, and look back at those behind me. I feel so good flying through the cheering crowds in the neighborhoods we pass: Bed-Stuy, Williamsburg, Greenpoint, Long Island City.

On to the Queensboro Bridge—my bridge! On I go, up First Avenue to the plaudits of millions. I am going like crazy, out to catch Bill Rodgers! At 72nd Street I am aware of friends, relatives, and everyone else cheering, yelling, kissing, and squeezing orange juice down my throat.

I am passing into Harlem. No pain, but oh, the exhaustion. I can't lift my legs. My shoulders sag. "Oh my, fella, let me hold on to you." (Sure you can hold me, you are my best friend.) From the street: "Come on old man, we are with you. You can make it. You are in, man. Come on, grandpa!"

How beautiful! I am getting the exhaustion under control. Soon, I feel new strength, and I am in the park, nearing the end, making it through the gate . . . Lyndy, Lyndy! Hal, Jane, Stan, Ronnie, Dave, Adele, Frank, Sylvia, Paul, how wonderful for all of us! What an amazing three years—the best years of my life! ❞

—Eugene Schapiro, 62

Sexual Activity

Many people commonly fear that sexual intercourse will precipitate another heart attack. For the active, conditioned person who has had a heart attack, male or female, sexual intercourse involves less risk than for the person for whom sexual activity is his or her *only* form of exercise. The general rule is that intercourse may be resumed with the usual partner when the individual is able to walk two flights of stairs. Provided that no complications arise, this occurs within a four-to-eight week period after the heart attack.

Emotional Response

The heart is a crucial aspect of the body image. It is visualized as a symbol of love and life. Following a heart attack, one must face the reality that the heart is damaged and that, although it is functioning, certain life-style behaviors must be modified.

The emotional reaction to a heart attack is similar to the grief process that follows other experiences of loss. Denial, anger, stoicism, and bargaining are common feelings. During the first months at home following the heart attack, anxiety, depression, weakness, fear of sexual arousal, and disturbed sleep patterns are common. It is normal to fear dying, to feel helpless and to be apprehensive about resuming work and other responsibilities. Support from family members, and sometimes from professional services, is important.

Sexual Activity after a Heart Attack

1. Suggested techniques
   - Lie on your back and have your partner kneel to avoid placing his or her full weight on you.
   - Lie side by side.
2. Resume previous level of sexual activity.
3. Warning signals
   - Rapid heart rate and rapid breathing are normally associated with sexual intercourse. Stop if having extreme breathlessness, chest pain, or disturbing heart rhythm.
   - Stop or slow down if you experience extreme fatigue the day following sexual activity.
   - Notify your medical provider if any of these symptoms occur.
4. Avoid intercourse if you
   - are fatigued;
   - have eaten a heavy meal;
   - have excessive alcohol intake;
   - are under emotional tension;
   - are in an extremely hot or cold environment.

Coronary Artery Bypass Surgery

Bypass surgery is an operation that attaches new blood vessels to the heart muscle in order to bypass areas that are significantly diseased or damaged. The vessel or vessels used are obtained from another area of the body, generally a vein in the leg. Coronary artery bypass surgery is not considered beneficial for all coronary artery disease patients. Selection of appropriate candidates and optimal timing of the operation are important.

A study known as a *cardiac catheterization with arteriography* is used to locate the blocked areas of the coronary arteries. It is extremely useful in identifying suitable candidates for this serious operation. These tests are uncomfortable, hazardous, and expensive. Therefore, the benefit of the information gained from these procedures must exceed the risk to the patient.

Generally, people who have left main coronary artery disease should undergo surgery. A recent study reported an 85 percent thirty-month survival rate following surgery in comparison with a 65 percent survival rate in the medically treated patient with left main coronary artery disease.

Arteriography and bypass surgery are also possibilities for patients with persistently incapacitating angina. Following a heart attack, medical management is the usual course. If angina persists following a heart attack, however, surgery may be considered.

Bypass surgery is not therapy for coronary artery disease. It does not alter or reverse the atherosclerotic process. The atherosclerosis that caused the heart disease initially may reoccur in other coronary arteries or in the bypass graft itself. This risk can be decreased, however, if one follows recommendations regarding diet, exercise, medication use, and smoking.

Congestive Heart Failure

A heart attack is not necessarily heart failure. The function of the heart is to pump sufficient blood to meet the body's needs. Heart failure occurs when the ventricles of the heart are no longer able to deliver an adequate amount of blood to the tissues during rest or exercise. The blood then begins to back up into the lungs and body, producing congestion in the lungs. Imagine that the heart is a pumping station delivering water from a reservoir to a community. If the pump fails, or if pipes to the homes become clogged with debris, an adequate water supply will not be delivered to the households that depend on this source of water. In addition, if water cannot be delivered, a backflow will occur, causing the reservoir to fill up and eventually overflow.

Fatigue and shortness of breath are the most common complaints associated with heart failure. They may at first be noted only with activity. As the heart disease progresses, the symptoms may occur even with rest. A change in one's ability to lie flat (*orthopnea*) or an awakening from sleep (*paroxysmal nocturnal dyspnea*), both caused by a shortness of breath, may also be signs. Swelling of the feet, ankles, lower back, and back of the thighs are possible indications. There are many other potential signs of heart failure, and an investigation by a medical care giver is essential. Some of these may be signs of other medical problems, so that this diagnosis should be made by a trained medical person.

Heart failure is a process, not a single event, which occurs because the heart becomes increasingly unable to pump blood into the body's tissues. Congestive heart failure does not necessarily mean that the heart will stop beating and death will follow. The condition must be treated, however, so that the heart will continue to function and sustain life.

Diagnosis

After gathering data about signs and symptoms of suspected heart failure, a physical examination will be done. Particular attention will be paid to the sounds of the heart and lungs for any changes that suggest failure of the heart to pump effectively. A galloping rhythm or a rhythm with abnormal beats may suggest the problem. Crackling sounds, called *rales,* in the lungs are a traditional clue to the diagnosis.

An examination will also be made to determine if there are other effects on the body from the heart's inability to pump forcefully. These additional findings help determine the seriousness of the failure and its treatment. *Edema,* or swelling as a result of fluid collection, in the extremities of the body and in the lobes of the lungs is commonly found. Tenderness over the liver and distension of the jugular veins in the neck will be present if the right side of the heart is not able to pump blood to the lungs. In extreme cases a large volume of fluid may collect in the abdomen, in the scrotum, or at the base of the spine.

An electrocardiogram will be done to check for lack of oxygen to the heart muscle and irregular rhythm patterns. A chest X ray will identify fluid congestion in the lungs as well as the size of the heart. Studies will be done on the blood to find possible causes of the failure, such as infection or a heart attack, and also to determine the amount of oxygen circulating in the arteries.

Treatment

If congestive heart failure results from a curable cause such as a lung infection, thyroid disease, or anemia, treatment is directed toward the causative condition. Unfortunately, curable causes are not common. The treatment plan is directed at assisting the heart to pump the blood supply effectively from the heart to the body. Eliminating excess fluids from the body is equally important.

Mild congestive heart failure may be treated by reducing physical activity, restricting the use of salt in the diet, and taking a diuretic to reduce the excess fluid in the body. *Digitalis* will also be prescribed, since it improves the contraction of the heart muscle.

Severe congestive heart failure requires hospitalization in order to administer more potent diuretics and other necessary medications to improve the work done by the heart. Close monitoring of the oxygen levels in the blood is also necessary.

Digitalis

Digitalis is an important medication in the treatment plan of an individual suffering from congestive heart failure. It improves the contraction of the heart muscle, thereby improving the output of blood from the heart and decreasing the amount of backflow congestion. Digitalis also acts on the electrical system of the heart, slowing the heart rate.

The most commonly used preparation of digitalis is Lanoxin (digoxin). The dosage used depends on the severity of the disease, although it is usually 0.25 milligrams. Sometimes a larger, initial "loading dose" is prescribed. Usually, the daily dose of digitalis is taken after breakfast, provided the pulse rate is normal. If symptoms that suggest digitalis sickness or toxicity develop, a physician should be consulted. Digitalis sickness is more common in older people, since the kidneys become less able to clear the medication from the body. A dosage of 0.125 milligrams four to five times a week may be effective in maintaining therapeutic results in older people. (See Chapter 25, *Common Medications.*)

Health Education

It is important for those who suffer from congestive heart failure to understand how the heart functions and what causes heart failure. This information may

Signs of Digitalis Toxicity

- lack of appetite
- vomiting
- abdominal discomfort
- disturbances in color vision
- nausea
- diarrhea
- changes in the heart rate and rhythm, especially low pulse rate (less than sixty)

help them understand the importance of modifying activities and diet as necessary. It is also important to learn possible symptoms of heart failure and when these symptoms indicate that medical attention is necessary. For instance, a weight gain of two to three pounds (0.9 to 1.35 kg) a day or an increase in the amount of swelling of the ankles may indicate impending heart failure.

Adherence to a low salt diet is very important. Depending on the severity of the condition, daily consumption of salt may be limited from 1 to 4 grams a day. It is important to review with a nutritionist or nurse foods that commonly have a high quantity of salt, keeping in mind that salt is used in processing and preserving many of our foods. The water supply in many communities is high in sodium. Baking soda and medications such as Maalox, Gelusil, prednisone, and Indocin also have a high concentration of sodium and should be avoided. (See also Chapter 8, *Nutrition.*)

Physical exertion and stressful situations should be avoided. An understanding of the types and amount of exercise and activities is important. Work schedules and household tasks may need to be reorganized. Rest periods during the day should be allowed for.

If medications are prescribed, one should know the name of the medication, what it does, and when to take it. Fluid pills or diuretics will increase the frequency and amount of urination. Sometimes a potassium supplement is necessary, since potassium is removed from the body through the urine. Weakness, faintness, leg cramps, or abdominal cramps may signify a decrease in blood potassium, and the need for a supplement.

Those taking a digitalis preparation should check their pulse daily for its rate and regularity. If the pulse rate is below 60 beats per minute or is irregular, a doctor should be notified. Digitalis is not for chest pain; it is for heart failure. If chest pain develops, an additional digoxin tablet should *not* be taken. Chest pains should be evaluated and specific treatment prescribed.

Disease of the Heart Valves

The valves of the heart maintain a one-way flow of blood from the *atria* to the *ventricles* and from the ventricles to the great vessels (*pulmonary artery, aorta*). During the resting phase (called *diastole*), the *tricuspid* and *mitral* valves open, allowing blood from the atria to enter the ventricles. During this phase the *pulmonic* and *aortic* valves are closed. Then both ventricles contract (called *systole*), closing the tricuspid and mitral valves, and pump blood out through the pulmonic and aortic valves to the lungs and the rest of the body. During this phase blood returns from the body and lungs, filling the right and left atrium respectively, preparing for the next cycle.

Abnormalities of the valves may exist because of congenital malformation or may be acquired as a result of inflammation from diseases such as rheumatic fever, syphilis, or lupus erythematosus. Damage to the valves as a result of inflammation does not necessarily end following treatment. Fibrosis and calcium deposits that continue because of normal aging further deform the valve and interfere with its functioning. With aging the normally occurring stress to all four valves will cause them to thicken and become more rigid. If a preexisting disease has damaged a valve, this normal aging process may be accelerated.

Valvular damage may interfere with the function of the valve in one or both of two ways. It may narrow the valve (*stenosis*), making it difficult for the blood to move forward; or it may interfere with closure of the valve, causing blood that has entered the chamber to flow backward (*regurgitation* or *insufficiency*).

Symptoms

The symptoms occurring as a result of valvular disease depend on the valve or valves affected. For instance, with mitral stenosis (narrowing of the mitral valve), symptoms might include shortness of breath during exertion or while lying flat and chest pain with exertion. The severity of the symptom will depend on the amount of damage to the valve.

Diagnosis

In the great majority of cases, the history and physical exam of the individual will establish the diagnosis. By listening carefully with a stethescope to the opening and closing sounds made by the heart valves, as well as to the sounds of the blood flow, your medical provider can obtain a great amount of information. A chest X ray and an EKG are useful for confirming the clinical diagnosis and identifying secondary problems. *Cardiac catheterization* and *angiography,* both highly specialized tests, may be required for proper evaluation of the valves if surgery is being considered.

Treatment

Valve Surgery

Heart valve replacement surgery began over twenty years age. A pig valve or a mechanical valve, both reliable and durable, is used to replace the diseased valve.

Surgery is not generally recommended for individuals who have a diseased heart valve but do not suffer from symptoms related to it. Selection of patients for the operation is usually limited to those whose condition cannot be controlled medically. Surgery should not be delayed, however, until serious incapacity or heart failure occurs.

Heart Transplants

In December, 1967, Dr. Christiaan Barnard received worldwide exposure after performing the first human cardiac transplant using the heart of another human being. Before that time unsuccessful transplants of a primate (monkey) heart into a man had been done by others. Today over two hundred people are referred each year to the Stanford Medical Center in California to be evaluated for this surgery; additional transplants are done at a few other medical centers in this country. Using stringent criteria, only 15 percent of the applicants are selected as appropriate candidates for a transplant. The majority of patients considered exhibit severe or end-stage heart disease caused by ischemic heart disease or disease of the heart muscles.

Surgery is performed on these individuals only if they are free from other major diseases or active infections. The candidates are generally younger than fifty-five, but this is not a fixed rule.

Infection, especially early in the postoperative period, and rejection of the transplanted heart remain problems interfering with survival. Furthermore, atherosclerosis may affect the transplanted heart.

Another difficulty associated with transplantation surgery relates to the donors. Guidelines for the pronouncement of brain death are not uniform in all states. The donor must also be in a location that allows transfer of the heart in a reasonable period of time to the hospital where the transplant surgery is to be done.

Eighty-five percent of these patients may return to their previous jobs after a three-month period. The expected five-year survival rate since 1974 is equal to approximately 45 percent.

Noninvasive Aids in Evaluating and Diagnosing Heart Disease

Electrocardiogram (EKG)

The electrocardiogram is the most commonly used diagnostic tool in the assessment of cardiac health. The machine records the electrical activity of the heart. It does not give an electrical shock. It records changes characteristic of a lack of oxygen to the heart muscle, injury (infarction) of the muscle, and enlargement of the heart. Effects of medications such as digoxin and quinidine may also be evaluated with this test. Signs of an increase or decrease in levels of calcium or potassium in the body may appear on the EKG tracing.

Phonocardiography

In phonocardiography, several small microphones are placed on the chest wall in order to graphically record the sounds made during various events in the heart cycle. This test can identify the normal heart sounds, as well as murmurs, gallops, and other abnormal sounds. The test is not uncomfortable and does not take a long period of time.

Echocardiography

Echocardiography utilizes ultrasonic beams to evaluate people with suspected disease of the heart valves, congenital heart disease, cardiomyopathy, and coronary disease. An ultransonic beam passes through the heart structure and echoes are returned. The echoes are converted into electricity, which then can be recorded as wave patterns on film. The various areas within the heart are identified by their characteristic patterns of motion. The procedure is harmless but tiresome, since it takes thirty to sixty minutes.

Ambulatory Electrocardiography (Holter Monitor)

The Holter Monitor electrocardiogram is essentially a portable EKG. A small machine is worn for twenty-four hours in order to assess the cardiac (heart) rhythm during normal activities. It is important to keep a diary of activities and any specific symptoms experienced, including time and duration of both. Activities that are important to record include exercise, climbing stairs, emotional upset, arguments, smoking, bowel movements, urination, meals, sexual intercourse, medication use, and sleep.

Exercise Tolerance Test (Exercise Stress Test)

The exercise tolerance test has several uses. It is commonly used to confirm the diagnosis of angina. It is also a useful tool in assessing the effect of exercise on a person who has had a heart attack in order to recommend an accurate and safe exercise program. It is also a noninvasive method of screening patients who may be candidates for coronary bypass surgery.

The treadmill test is the most common method of stress testing. The speed of the treadmill and the incline are adjusted at scheduled intervals until the predetermined heart rate is achieved. The blood pressure, pulse, and electrocardiogram are monitored during the test and for ten minutes following the test in order to document any abnormalities. The test is discontinued if the subject becomes short of breath or has extreme fatigue, dizziness, or angina. The test is also concluded if multiple abnormal heartbeats occur or signs of lack of oxygen to the heart muscle are recorded on the electrocardiogram.

Approximately 80 to 85 percent of those with angina will have a positive test, meaning that this study documents a lack of oxygen to the heart muscle. There is an appreciable number of negative tests that are false, especially when the individual is not able to achieve the required heart rate because of poor physical conditioning. There may also be false positive tests. Many drugs, valvular heart disease, and anemia may also interfere with the test results.

Treadmill exercise tests should not be performed on people who have had a recent onset of angina or who have had increasing episodes of angina within a four- to six-week period of time. This test is not usually done on the post–heart attack patient for at least four to eight weeks. If there are complications following the infarction, the test is delayed further.

A thirty- to sixty-minute rest is advised following the test. It is also wise not to take a hot shower for three to four hours following the test, since this added heat stress may cause the blood pressure to fall with position changes.

Noninvasive Stress Thallium Scan

The main purpose of this test is to detect a lack of oxygen to the heart muscle. This noninvasive test is indicated for:

- patients who have no symptoms but do have an equivocal or a positive exercise stress test
- patients who have atypical chest pain
- patients with abnormal resting EKG and suspected coronary artery disease
- symptomatic patients with a negative exercise tolerance test
- patients unable to achieve an adequate heart rate response on the exercise tolerance test
- patients who have had bypass surgery, in order to confirm the normal functioning of the graft

The thallium scan provides a safe method of visualizing the blood flow to the various regions of the left ventricular heart muscle. The study is performed on an outpatient basis. Perfusion scans with radioactive thallium (^{201}Tl) are taken at rest and during exercise and are then compared. "Cold spots" indicate regions of reduced or absent flow caused by a decrease in the amount of oxygen to the muscle or by an old injury to the heart muscle.

❀

The thought of heart disease understandably produces enormous fear and worry in all of us. Yet, in the last twenty-five years, major strides have been made in treating heart disease and improving the quality of life for individuals with cardiac problems. Moreover, we now know that improving diet, stopping smoking, controlling blood pressure, and instituting a regular exercise program can benefit almost everyone—regardless of age. Heart disease no longer needs to be considered an incurable problem, and no one should avoid medical care because they think their problem is hopeless. We can now say that it is possible to have a healthy, functioning heart for a lifetime.

Chapter 14
The Lungs

Christopher H. Fanta, MD

The respiratory system consists of the *mouth, pharynx, larynx* (voice box), *trachea* (windpipe), *airway* (bronchi and smaller passages), and *lungs* (composed of tiny air sacs called *alveoli capillaries,* and connecting tissues). It communicates directly with the external environment and exchanges at least 2,600 gallons (10,000 l) of air every day. Included with this continual flow of air are particles and gases that must be filtered.

It is therefore not surprising that the respiratory system is particularly prone to disease and that the incidence of respiratory illness increases as we age. That, combined with the cumulative effects of smoking and exposure to toxic substances in the air, means the lungs and airways are under continual onslaught from the external world.

Many of the infections that affect the chest are transmitted from person to person via fine droplets of moisture coughed, sneezed, and spoken into the air. The most common infection is the *common cold,* caused by one of many viruses that are in the environment throughout the year. *Pneumonia* is an infection of the lungs that, although less common and devastating than before the age of antibiotics, still represents a problem for older people. Combined with influenza, it is the fifth leading cause of death. *Tuberculosis,* once a major killer, has become rather uncommon. Most cases of TB now occur as reinfections from a dormant tuberculosis bacterium that was once an undetected illness. Possibly as result of lowered resistance, the infection reappears.

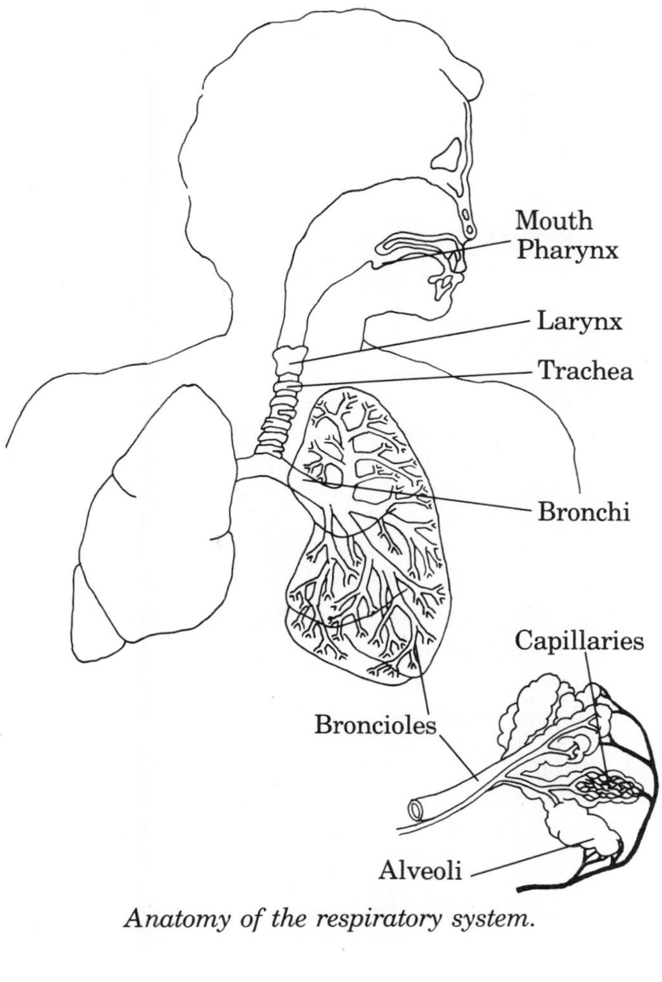

Anatomy of the respiratory system.

Chronic *bronchitis* affects as many as 20 percent of the adult American population. It results from long-term irritation to the lungs, usually from smoking cigarettes. Not only are chronic bronchitis and *emphysema* devastating in their own right, but they further increase the likelihood of acquiring serious infections in the lungs.

Lung cancer is still increasing dramatically in America. (It had a twenty-five-fold increase in men over the last forty-five years!) It has long been the most frequent cancer among men and is now rapidly becoming the number one cancer killer in both sexes because of increased smoking among women. Unfortunately, most of these cancers are discovered too late for a surgical cure. Since we do not have good medical therapy for advanced lung cancer, approximately 90 percent of patients are dead within five years. As in chronic bronchitis, smoking has been established as an important factor in the cause of lung cancer.

The respiratory system defends itself with the filtering function of the nose, with sneezing and coughing that clears the airway, and with a blanket of mucus that coats the airways. The mucus traps particles and dissolved gases and removes them in expectorated secretions during coughing and clearing the throat. A microscopic defense squad of scavenger cells also removes foreign particles and organisms that enter the respiratory system.

This protective system can be overcome, however, by overwhelming exposure, chronic irritation (cigarette smoke, industrial pollution), or weakening of defenses by certain medications or repeated illness. When this happens, cough and sputum production become a symptom of a disease process, not a defense.

Symptoms of Lung Disease

The symptoms of pulmonary (lung) disease are generally not subtle. Thanks to years of colds and flu, we are usually expert at recognizing the symptoms of upper respiratory tract (upper airway) infections. These symptoms include runny or stuffy nose, cough, and fever.

The symptoms of pneumonia, or infection within the lungs, are more dramatic. They include the production of large amounts of thick, discolored (purulent) sputum, high fever, shaking chills, prostration, and chest pain that worsens with each deep breath (called *pleuritic chest pain,* or pleurisy). There may also be a sensation of shortness of breath and a rapid breathing rate. These are all signs that more than a simple cold is brewing and should be investigated by a family physician or other trained medical person.

Coughing up blood (*hemoptysis*) may complicate an infection of the lungs, may result from a blood clot to the lungs (*pulmonary embolus*), or may be a sign of lung cancer. **It is a symptom that cannot be ignored** or explained away with excuses—"I thought that I had probably just ruptured a small blood vessel in the back of my throat from coughing so much." A thorough examination should be done immediately by a medical provider if blood is coughed up.

The sensation of chest congestion or tightness may result from increased bronchial secretions that narrow the airways. Wheezing, a musical sound during breathing that sometimes can be heard with the naked ear or with a stethescope, may accompany congestion. Wheezing is an indication of narrowing and spasm of the airway and may occur because of asthma, chronic bronchitis, a tumor, or other less common illnesses.

The distant cousin of the wheeze is the snore, which occurs when the back of the mouth becomes narrowed during inspiration. For most, snoring is an innocent, perhaps endearing (or annoying) idiosyncrasy. For a few it is associated with restless interrupted sleep, episodic blockage of the airway during sleep, and excessive daytime sleepiness. This is the newly described *sleep apnea syndrome,* which links the respiratory system with sleep disturbances. If you snore and find that you are fatigued during the day because of restless sleep, you should consult your medical provider about the possibility that you suffer from sleep apnea syndrome.

Examining the Lungs and Chest

In examining the chest, all physicians tap on the chest wall and listen to breath sounds with a stethescope. This is done to detect any alterations in the usual production and transmission of sounds through the chest that can indicate disease.

Normally the lungs are an air-filled container. If the normal resonant percussion note created by tapping with the fingers is dulled, there may be a mass; if crackles are heard in the stethescope, there may be fluid in the air sacs (alveoli); and if wheezing is noted, it may indicate air rushing through secretion-filled small airways. It is for these reasons that the medical provider will tap on the chest, feel with his/her hands, and listen with the stethescope.

Few of today's physicians are as skilled at these techniques as chest physicians in the tuberculosis sanitariums of old. The story goes that one TB specialist became so adept at chest percussion that, when going to visit at someone's house, he could simply knock on the door and tell how many people were home. If this is a lost art, the reason for the change is that the chest X ray often has a greater sensitivity than hands and ears. But the techniques of physical examination and chest X ray are complementary. Wheezes may be heard when the chest X ray looks normal, but on the other hand, small masses may be seen on the X ray when the physical examination is normal. Therefore, you should expect a thorough physical examination from your medical provider, as well as a chest X ray and other diagnostic tests.

Even in a world sensitized as ours is to the risks of unnecessary radiation exposure, the feeling among the vast majority of physicians is that chest X rays (even repeated X rays) are safe. The radiation dose from a single chest X ray is less than one ten-thousandth of a *rad* (a unit for measuring radiation), far below the recommended guidelines for safe yearly radiation exposure (0.5 rads). In fact, it is less than the background environmental exposure present all the time in certain parts of the country. You would need five thousand chest X rays in a year to total 0.5 rads. Although no one is in favor of unnecessary chest X rays, it seems highly prudent to have one or more if they are needed as part of your medical examination.

Common Tests of Lung Function

Two types of tests that one might encounter while having illnesses of the lungs investigated are pulmonary function tests and arterial blood gas tests. Pulmonary function tests are designed to measure the maximum amount of air the lungs can contain and the resistance to the flow of air in and out of the lungs. One of these tests, *spirometry,* involves taking the largest possible breath in (inhaling) and then blowing it out (exhaling) completely. Exhaling should be done as fast and as completely as possible so that the spirometer can measure the maximum lung function. Spirometry is useful in diagnosing obstruction to the exhalation of air, seen in asthma, chronic bronchitis, and emphysema.

Tests of arterial blood gases measure the concentration of oxygen and carbon dioxide in the blood after it has passed through the lungs. The measurement requires taking a blood sample from the artery for analysis. Since arteries are deep and surrounded by more nerve endings than veins, the sampling process may be quite painful. I suggest that, if you need such a test, you ask that the person drawing the blood anesthetize the skin and underlying tissues prior to drawing the blood. The anesthetic takes no more than a minute to inject and can convert a traumatic and painful experience into a nearly painless one.

Arterial blood gases are also useful in measuring the functioning of the lungs. Abnormalities found in this test can help to determine the nature and severity of many kinds of problems, including pneumonia, chronic bronchitis and emphysema, pulmonary embolism (blood clot in the lungs), and other disorders.

Chronic Bronchitis and Emphysema

Chronic bronchitis and emphysema are medical terms whose definitions have undergone transformation over the years. Consequently, they tend to be used loosely, interchangeably, and incorrectly by many physicians and nonphysicians. Correctly defined, chronic bronchitis means the presence of cough and sputum production for a minimum of three months of the year, for at least two years in a row. Emphysema, on the other hand, is a destructive process in the walls of the air sacs that causes the lungs to lose their elasticity and thus their ability to force air out during exhalation.

Chronic bronchitis results from overproduction of mucus by enlarged and excessively numerous mucous glands in the airways. This develops in reaction to irritations, such as cigarette smoking. The excess mucus plus swelling of the walls of the airways leads to obstruction to the flow of breathed air, especially during expiration.

Thus, chronic bronchitis is one of the *chronic obstructive pulmonary diseases,* sometimes referred to by medical professionals by the acronym COPD. When the disease becomes severe, breathing is limited, producing shortness of breath. At first this may occur only with strenuous activity, but as the disease progresses, even minimal exertion may be difficult.

You can see the obstruction to air flow by watching someone with COPD breathe. There will be a prolonged period of exhaling and sometimes the pursing of the lips. It can be measured more exactly with the spirometer, as described previously.

Emphysema is also a disease in which the flow of air is obstructed during breathing. The disease process involves destruction of the walls of the alveoli of the lungs. These air spaces become overdistended and lose their normal elasticity.

The person with emphysema experiences persistent breathlessness with little cough or sputum production. The lungs will probably be overinflated, so that the person appears to be barrel-chested, and they will look large and clear on a chest X ray. Expiration takes longer than normal. These changes can be accurately demonstrated with the pulmonary function tests mentioned earlier.

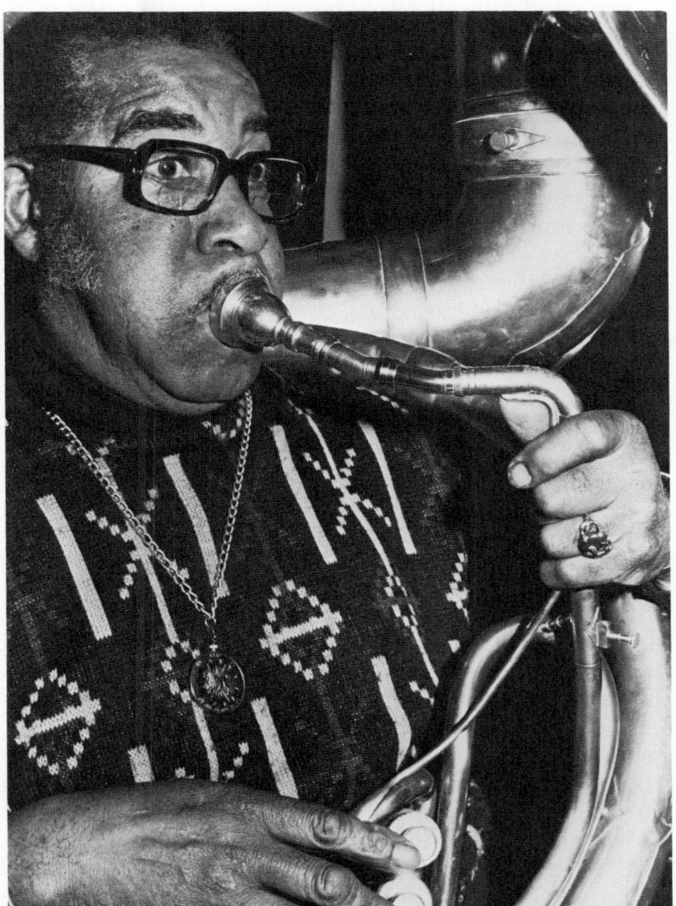

Both chronic bronchitis and emphysema (as well as cancer) are devastating responses of the lung to the ravages of continued cigarette smoking. We are what we breathe, and although not all cases of these diseases are the result of cigarette smoking, most are. Based on the comparisons of disease frequency among urban versus rural populations, it is clear that air pollution, though a contributing factor, plays a relatively minor role.

Unfortunately, we are not yet very knowledgeable in ways of treating the addiction of cigarette smoking. A local chapter of the American Cancer Society can direct smokers to smoke-ending clinics or workshops. Various systems of graduated filters, substituted oral gratifications, and even hypnosis can be tried. But by and large these only supplement the one necessary ingredient: willpower. Each smoker must decide to quit and have the fortitude to withstand the considerable (but transient) physical and psychological discomforts of withdrawal from nicotine.

Let no one who reads this ever say, "But my doctor never told me to quit." If you smoke: *quit. Now.*

Chronic bronchitis occasionally results from heavy occupational exposure to dust in mines, mills, and other factory settings. In some cases it may evolve from repeated childhood bronchial infections. In even rarer instances, emphysema may result from an inherited protein deficiency (alpha -1 antitrypsin deficiency). In the vast majority of cases, however, cigarettes are the underlying cause both in emphysema and chronic bronchitis. In fact, most cigarette smokers have a chronic cough, phlegm production, and shortness of breath that represents a mixture of both diseases.

Once established, these diseases do not go away with the cessation of smoking. But the accelerated rate of decline in lung function can be halted. Untreated, and with continued smoking, the person will suffer repeated chest infections, progressively debilitating shortness of breath, heart failure, and death.

Treatment

The medications prescribed for chronic bronchitis and emphysema are similar to those used in asthma. The mainstays are bronchodilators, which relax the muscles that ring the airway. This allows for a freer passage of air and easier breathing.

The medications can be taken in tablet, capsule, or liquid form, inhaled in a mist from small pressurized containers, or injected under the skin or into a vein in emergency situations. Although a myriad of different bronchodilator preparations exist, the medications within them fall into two different categories. One is a family of medicines related to aminophylline. These include Slo-Phyllin, Choledyl, Theo-Dur, Tedral, and Marax. The other clan of medicines includes relatives of epinephrine (adrenalin). These include Isuprel, Bronkosol, terbutaline, and metaproterenol. All of these bronchodilators may have stimulantlike side effects, including shaking, palpitations, nervousness, and nausea. Nausea and vomiting are particularly common with excessive amounts of the aminophylline group of medications.

Side effects should be reported to a medical provider so that the dosage may be adjusted to fit individual needs. A useful blood test is available to measure the level of aminophylline in the blood. It can indicate whether the appropriate amount of medication has been prescribed.

Steroid medicines such as prednisone, though not strictly speaking bronchodilators, are also sometimes used to treat chronic bronchitis. They are thought to act by reducing the inflammation in the bronchial walls, rather than by relaxing the muscles that surround the airways. Because these medications have potentially serious side effects when used for long periods of time (i.e., months to years), they should be used only when other measures fail. Some of these side effects include high blood pressure, diabetes, thinning and weakening of the bones, and cataracts.

Antibiotics play an important role in treating the chest infections that often complicate chronic bronchitis and emphysema. Because the consequences of pneumonia may be devastating, antibiotics such as ampicillin or tetracycline are often prescribed at the very first sign of infection, including symptoms like fever and discolored (yellow or gray) sputum. These symptoms should be promptly reported to a medical provider.

A number of other measures are often used to treat chronic bronchitis and emphysema, but they are of debatable value. They include humidification, expectorants (to help clear secretions), chest physiotherapy, and breathing retraining exercises.

Home oxygen use, however, has been shown to be of undisputed benefit for many people. If chronic obstructive pulmonary disease (emphysema or bronchitis) is severe, it may cause persistently reduced oxygen levels in the blood. This is much like living atop Mount Everest. Every little amount of effort causes shortness of breath. For these people home oxygen use for at least eight to twelve hours a day can increase the ability to tolerate exertion. It can help with dressing, walking, and doing simple things around the house. It will also decrease the stress that low oxygen levels in the blood put on the heart. Home oxygen systems have been designed to be portable, simple to use, and unobtrusive in the home. They can also be taken on trips outside of the house.

Finally, in the person free of heart disease, exercise will not harm the lungs and can generally be encouraged. It can strengthen the respiratory muscles, promote a more positive sense of well-being, and improve breathing.

Lung Cancer

Over 112,000 new cases of lung cancer will be diagnosed in the United States this year. Even among those of us who work daily with lung cancer patients, it continues to be an enormous tragedy. This is because the best hope for long-term survival is surgery, and at least three-fourths of people come to the physician with inoperable cases. In other words, by the time the patient sees the doctor, the cancer has spread and surgery is not feasible.

Untreated, fewer than 10 percent of those with lung cancer will survive for five years. Even with the best of medical therapy, the prognosis for most people with lung cancer remains grim. More Americans will die of lung cancer this year than died in the Vietnam War, yet as many as 18 to 23 percent of today's teenagers are already smoking cigarettes regularly. As in COPD, smoking is apparently a primary cause of lung cancer.

I would like to describe lung cancer in terms of a patient of mine. We will call him Mr. Jones. He gave the typical history: a cigarette smoker with a chronic cough, mild shortness of breath, increasing fatigue over the past few months, some lack of appetite, and weight loss. When he no longer could attribute these symptoms to a bad cold, he went to see a doctor.

After a physical examination, a chest X ray was taken. It showed a spot on the lungs, a shadow on the X ray where normally there is none. This indicated that there was an abnormal mass of tissue where air-filled lung ought to be. Suspecting that this might indicate a cancer, we collected some of Mr. Jones's expectorated sputum in a cup and sent it to the pathologist. Sputum contains cells that are sloughed from the airways and can be useful in diagnosing cancer of the lung. In Mr. Jones's case, it did not show malignant cells.

At this point it was decided to try to obtain a biopsy specimen from the lung mass. Years ago this would have required a major operation. With the development of modern fiber-optic equipment, however, it was possible for Mr. Jones to undergo a relatively minor procedure under local anesthesia called *fiber-optic bronchoscopy*.

In this procedure a pencil-thin tube is passed through the anesthetized nasal passages into the trachea and bronchi (airways), allowing the surface of these channels to be examined by direct visualization. A growth originating from the wall of one bronchus (one part of the wall of the airway) was seen. Through the bronchoscope was passed a fine wire, at the end of which a tiny biopsy forceps was employed to take a sample of the mass.

An alternative procedure, also requiring only local anesthesia, would have been to pass a long but thin needle through the chest wall and into the mass. This is accomplished with the aid of X rays to guide the placement of the needle. This technique is called *percutaneous aspiration* and is used for masses located in the perimeter of the lungs that cannot be reached with fiber-optic bronchoscopy.

Treatment

The biopsy sample was read by the pathologist as containing squamous cell carcinoma, one of the four principal types of lung cancer. The four types (squamous cell carcinoma, adenocarcinoma, large cell undifferentiated carcinoma, and small cell undifferentiated carcinoma) all behave differently. The first three seem to act most alike, whereas small cell carcinoma has long been the black sheep. It tends to grow most rapidly and to spread outside the lungs, *metastasize,* early and widely. Curiously, the same properties that have made it the most aggressive killer in the past have made it the most amenable to chemotherapy now. Although generally not amenable to surgical treatment, small cell carcinoma of the lung does respond to drug treatment with at least a temporary decrease in size and in some cases even complete cure.

For Mr. Jones the best hope for long-term survival was surgery. This meant removal of the tumor and repair of the involved lung. To be as certain as possible before surgery that all of the cancer could be removed, it was necessary to determine that it had not yet metastasized. In this case we needed sophisticated liver, bone, and brain scans that use safe, radioactively labeled dyes injected into a vein. Sometimes procedures are necessary to sample lymph nodes as well, although we did not need to do this for Mr. Jones. We also used pulmonary function tests to see that Mr. Jones had sufficient lung function to be able to stand surgery and the removal of a portion of his lung.

Ultimately Mr. Jones was found to have a cancer localized to one lung and amenable to surgery. The lung was removed, he made a trouble-free recovery over one week's time, and then returned home. Now, after three months, although shortness of breath prevents him from playing tennis, he remains generally active. His respiratory function is good, and he can do most light activity. We will see him periodically in clinic to make sure that his cancer is not recurring.

What if Mr. Jones had been less fortunate and his cancer had spread to his bones, causing great pain and obviating the possibility of surgical cure? In that situation radiation therapy offers effective relief of pain. A series of painless treatments during which high concentrations of radiation are focused on the cancerous bone (or lung, or lymph nodes, depending on the site of involvement) are generally highly successful in shrinking the tumor and relieving symptoms. Whether radiation treatments can actually *cure* a localized lung cancer is a subject of ongoing controversy in pulmonary medicine. It remains much debated whether the person unwilling or unable to undergo the pain and risk of major surgery can be effectively treated with ultra-high-dose radiation therapy for a localized cancer. Although generally free of serious symptomatic side effects, radiation treatments, especially in very high doses, may occasionally cause inflammation and scarring of the normal lung tissue caught in the radiation field.

Derivatives of apricot pits, such as laetrile, and other illicit "magic potion" drugs have no effect on the growth of lung cancer. They are born of alchemy, invested with the hopes of desperate people, and then falsely heralded as panaceas like the patent medicines of old. Progress in the treatment of lung cancer will come from the slow but inexorable advances of scientific research and experimentation, not from some remote clinic for profit promoting so-called drugs of unproven worth.

Pulmonary Embolism

All of the blood in the body passes through the blood vessels of the lungs on each circuit around the body. At rest about 4½ quarts of blood (about 4 l) circulate through the pulmonary vessels each minute. These blood vessels at their smallest are about 1/100 of a millimeter in diameter, little bigger than the red blood cells that pass through them single file, and so act as filters for the blood system. Particles in the blood that are larger than these tiny vessels will impact on the vessels and be removed from the circulation before they can reach such vital organs as the brain.

The lungs can filter minute particles from the blood without problem, but larger particles, trapped by larger blood vessels, stop the flow of blood through those vessels and leave a part of the lung without blood supply. The trouble might develop as follows. An older person has been bedridden for many days or has just been through a major operation or has bad varicose veins in the legs. Because the blood is passing relatively slowly through the veins of the legs, a blood clot forms and fills one of the veins in the calf. This clot, or *thrombus,* may manifest itself by redness, swelling, warmth, and pain in the lower leg or, in as many as half the cases, may give no indications of its presence at all.

Then suddenly a small portion of this clot of blood breaks loose and floats through the bloodstream, unimpeded until it reaches the lungs. In the blood vessels of the lungs, it lodges in the first vessel with a diameter smaller than itself, stopping up the flow of blood through that vessel and creating havoc in the lungs. The portion of lung tissue beyond the plugged vessel may or may not die, depending on the availability of alternate sources of blood from other, nonoccluded blood vessels, but in any case a disturbance in the ability of the lungs to oxygenate the blood results. Commonly, the person with this clot to the lungs (*pul-*

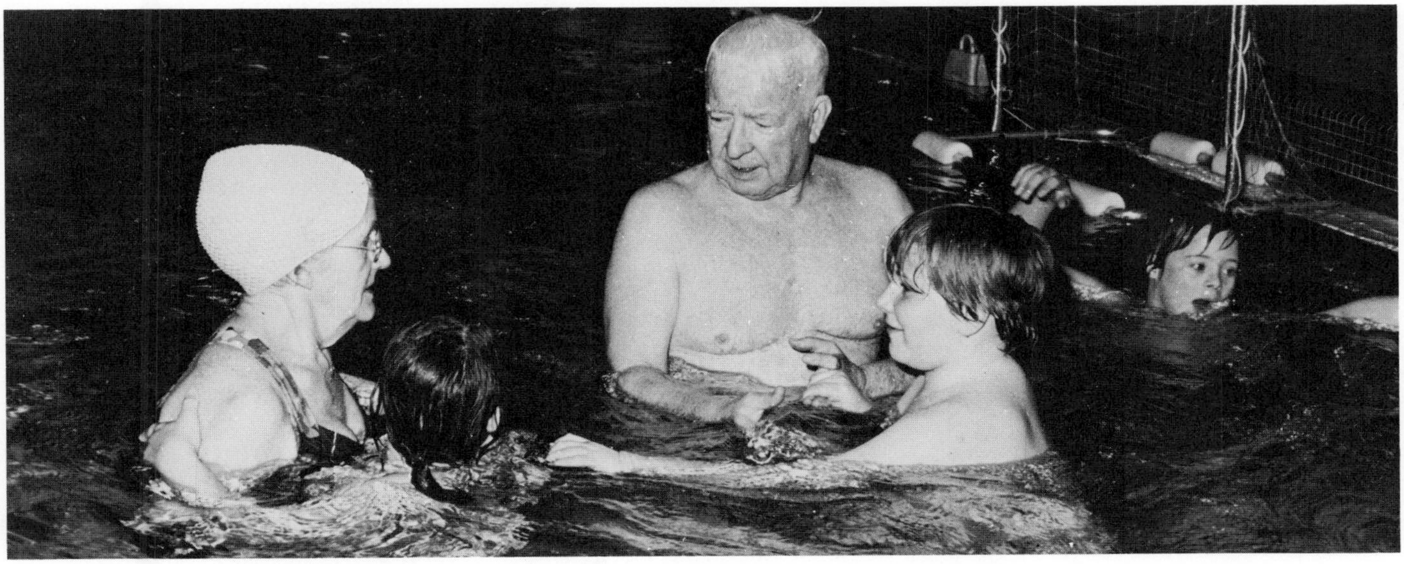

monary embolus) experiences the sudden onset of rapid breathing and hunger for air. A sharp "pleurisy-like" pain may develop, and blood may be coughed up. In other cases one may simply become suddenly short of breath, with no other clues as to the cause.

The standard treatment for pulmonary emboli is anticoagulation medication to impair the body's ability to clot blood and therefore to form new clots in the legs. This form of medication has often been called a "blood thinner." By interfering with the ability to make clots, anticoagulation increases the risk of serious bleeding, if the patient is injured. Thus, the treatment of pulmonary emboli, which is usually continued for about six months, carries with it certain dangers. A physician must therefore be very certain of the diagnosis before starting treatment: he or she does not want to subject the patient to an unnecessary risk of anticoagulation, yet does not want to allow a second and perhaps fatal clot to form in someone who has indeed had a pulmonary embolism.

Unfortunately, despite the importance of accurate diagnosis, this disorder remains one of the most difficult to diagnose. In older, hospitalized persons, many pulmonary emboli go undetected until after death, at autopsy. Physical examination, chest X ray, and analysis of blood gases may indicate only a rapidly breathing patient with low blood oxygen, nonspecific results found in numerous lung ailments. If pulmonary emboli are suspected (for instance, because there has been recent orthopedic surgery and one leg is painful and swollen), two tests of potential value may be performed.

One, called a *lung scan,* involves injection of minute quantities of radioactive protein molecules into a vein. This material circulates around to the lungs, or at least to those portions of the lungs to which blood is flowing. In a person with a pulmonary embolus, a scan over the lungs will reveal radioactivity in all portions except those where blood clots have prevented blood from passing. This test is painless, rapidly performed, and very sensitive to even quite small emboli. Unfortunately, it is also not very specific, in that a variety of different lung disorders can impair blood flow to one portion of the lungs and give an abnormal lung scan. The radiation exposure, though greater than that of a chest X ray, is not toxic and causes no side effects.

The other test, the definitive one for the diagnosis of pulmonary emboli, is called *pulmonary angiography* and involves X rays of blood vessels. This procedure is a more major undertaking. It consists of passing a thin, flexible tube through the veins, to the heart, and on into the blood vessels in the lungs. Dye is then injected through this tube, and multiple X-ray pictures are taken of the dye outlining the pulmonary vessels. If the flow of dye is suddenly cut off from one blood vessel, a blood clot is blocking that vessel. This method can detect the presence of pulmonary emboli with great certainty, but since it requires introduction of catheters into the heart and lungs, highly skilled personnel, and some discomfort to the patient, it is usually reserved for those situations in which no other means can resolve the question of whether or not a pulmonary embolus has occurred.

In recent years medicine has made progress in preventing blood clots from forming in the legs in the first place. Patients who must be confined to bed in the hospital for long periods are now often given small injections of the anticoagulant heparin. In these small doses, the medication prevents formation of new clots in the veins of the legs without causing any significant risk of bleeding. Other preventive measures that may help include having bedridden patients wear support stockings and encouraging them to periodically wiggle their feet up and down to keep the blood circulating briskly through the legs. The best way to deal with the difficult problem of pulmonary emboli is to prevent them.

Preventive Measures to Maintain a Healthy Respiratory System

I have heard it said that at one time in China physicians were paid to maintain health rather than to treat illness. Vaccination against infection has been a major advance in the maintenance of respiratory health. Influenza vaccine gives protection against the epidemic strains of influenza, a respiratory tract virus that causes unnecessary deaths, particularly in the older-age population and in those with underlying lung disease. The rare neurologic disease that followed some injections of the swine flu vaccine in 1976 has not been associated with the influenza vaccines since. Yearly vaccination is safe and is recommended for all those over the age of fifty or those with chronic pulmonary illnesses.

More recently a vaccine has been developed against the major bacterial cause of pneumonia, the pneumococcus. Pneumococcal pneumonia is not only the most common cause of pneumonia in adults, it also can be a serious and even fatal pneumonia, even in this age of penicillin and other powerful antibiotics. Effective prevention against most strains of the pneumococcus bacteria is provided by a single injection of the pneumococcal vaccine Pneumovax. The protection afforded by one injection lasts at least three years, so there is no need for a yearly injection, as with influenza vaccine. Again, persons over the age of fifty or with any form of chronic respiratory disease would be well advised to receive this preventive medicine. It is a treatment of which the "health maintenance" physicians of ancient China would have been proud.

Chapter 15
Breast Cancer

Marcia Bowling, MD; Mark Huberman, MD; and C. William Kaiser, MD

Every year more than 90,000 women in the United States and Canada are diagnosed as having breast cancer. More than 34,000 die from this disease. It is the most common cancer in women, and one's risk of developing it increases with age.

We do not know the cause of breast cancer. But early detection through self-examination and regular examinations by a family medical provider can help find breast malignancies early—before they have a chance to spread to other parts of the body. This is essential, because early detection vastly increases the chance of curing the disease. All women should know how to examine their own breasts and should do so at least once a month.

Signs

Breast cancer usually appears as a painless lump or thickening in the upper, outer portion of the breast, the area nearest the armpit. It may, however, appear in any portion of the breast, so it is essential to examine the entire breast each month. Discharge from the nipple or redness of the skin are other potential signs. If the cancer has spread to the lymph nodes under the arm, there may be swelling in the armpit.

Women who have any of these signs should see a medical provider immediately. They should get confirmation of their symptoms and should not hesitate or wait because of embarrassment. Breast cancer will not go away on its own.

Self Breast Examination

All women should examine their breasts for lumps, discharge, and change in the normal skin color and texture at least once each month.

A. Hands glide more easily over wet skin, so examine breasts during bath or shower. Move the flat part of your fingers over all portions of the breast. Feel in your armpit for lumps.

B. Standing in front of a mirror, look at your breasts with your arms over your head. Check for areas of swelling, dimpling of the skin, or changes in the contour of the nipple. Squeeze each nipple between thumb and forefinger and note any discharge. This should also be reported to your medical provider.

C. Repeat step B with your hands at your sides.

D. Lie down with a small pillow under your right shoulder and feel your right breast with the left hand. Keeping your fingers flat, move hand in a circular direction, gradually moving closer and closer to the nipple. Check as you did in step A for lumps or changes in skin texture or contour. Squeeze each nipple and look for discharge.

REMEMBER:

1. Most breast cancers are found by women examining their own breasts.
2. Most breast biopsies show noncancerous lumps.
3. Prompt diagnosis and treatment may vastly improve your chances of successful outcome. See your physician immediately if you find a lump or other suspicious change.

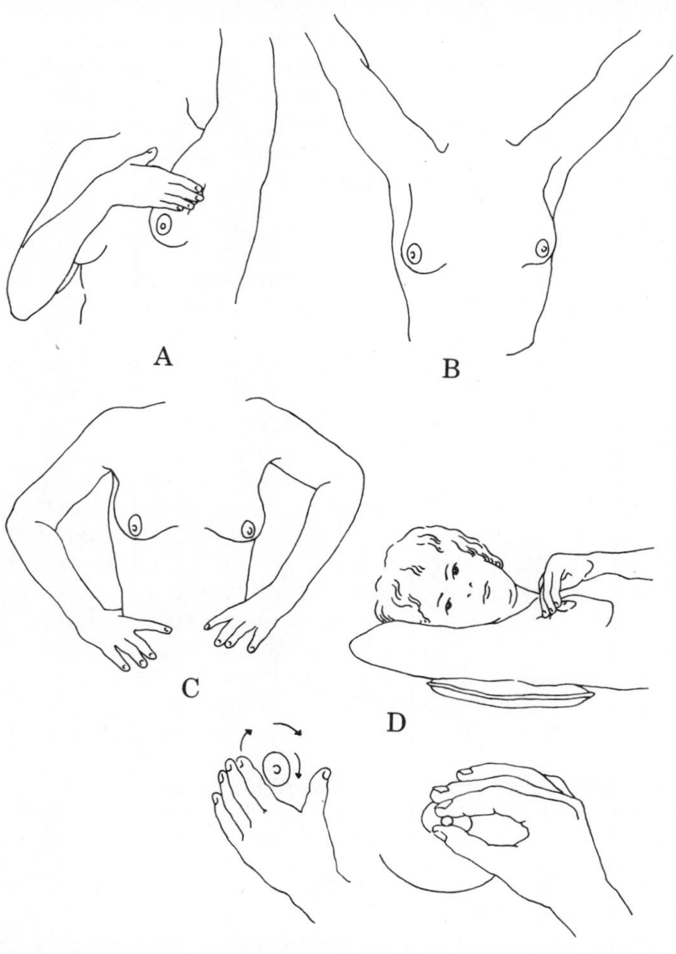

Diagnosis

The diagnosis of breast cancer begins with an examination by the medical care giver. If a suspicious lump or other sign is noted, the next step is one of a number of X-ray–type techniques. *Mammography* is an X-ray examination of the breast. *Xerography* is like mammography, but it uses a specially coated paper instead of X-ray film. *Thermography* detects changes in temperature that may indicate a breast malignancy. In recent years concern has grown over the safety of mammography. Although it is not recommended for every woman, it is considered safe and essential for women who have a suspicious lump or other potential sign of a malignancy.

If any of these exams are positive, the diagnosis is confirmed (or not) by obtaining a piece of breast tissue by a surgical procedure called a *biopsy*. This may be performed in a physician's office under local anesthesia. A tissue sample is taken either with a needle or through a small incision in the skin. The sample is then analyzed under the microscope by a pathologist. In a few days to a week the results will be in and a final diagnosis made. —M.B.

Treatment

The treatment of breast cancer has undergone some major changes in recent years. Old concepts are being reevaluated, and new treatment strategies and medicines are coming into use. There are two major aspects to the treatment of breast cancer. The first is the treatment of *primary* breast cancer, that is, breast cancer confined to the breast. The second is the treatment of *metastatic* and/or *recurrent* breast cancer: breast cancer that has spread beyond the breast and local lymph glands under the arm, or breast cancer that has come back after the primary therapy.

Surgery

The treatment of primary breast cancer is a good example of how medical practice has reevaluated old beliefs and made changes necessary for the improvement of medical care. In years past, the treatment of choice was *radical mastectomy,* removal of the entire breast and the major muscles of the chest that lie beneath it, as well as removal of the lymph glands under the arm. We now know that a *modified radical mastectomy,* also called *total* or *simple mastectomy,* is just as effective. With this operation the entire breast is removed, but the chest wall muscles are left intact. In addition, the underarm area, or *axilla,* is also explored to remove all accessible lymph nodes. This simpler surgery results in much less deformity of the chest and very little, if any, swelling of the arm on the side where the surgery was done. Studies are now underway to find out if even more limited surgery is equally effective in the treatment of primary breast cancer.

❝ I would like to share some experiences that I had concerning breast cancer. Although I am not quite fifty-five, I feel that my experiences are probably shared by almost every woman who has had a malignancy, especially of the breast.

Most of my life I have enjoyed excellent health. I have had a number of different careers, including teacher, mother of four, and investment counselor. I have always been active and found my illness to be a great shock. My mother had had breast cancer, and died when I was ten. My cancer was particularly frightening and emotionally painful because of that.

I discovered the lump in my breast myself. It was small, and I could push it around. My husband made me see a physician immediately. The doctor tried to aspirate it, but it would not aspirate. The following day the physician removed it, and in a few days the pathology report indicated that it was malignant.

I was offered two alternatives. The first was a modified radical mastectomy with examination of the lymph nodes under my arm. If the nodes were involved, I was to have chemotherapy. The second was a wide excision (removal) of the lump with nine weeks of radiation. Although the lump had been removed for the pathologist, a more complete procedure was thought to be needed to be certain that all the malignant tissue nearby had been excised. My immediate reaction was to try to save the breast and only have part of it removed. That meant choice number two, the wide excision of the lump. I did some reading and other investigation, and I then knew that I did not want to have radiation. I was more fearful of the radiation than the surgery. I also did not like the idea of chemotherapy, but I understood that that might be necessary in either case.

The matter-of-fact attitude of the surgeon who performed the initial procedure to biopsy the lump was very threatening to me. I asked for a referral for a second opinion. She said, "You don't need a second opinion. I can do this type of surgery on a kitchen table."

I began to get conflicting advice from friends and relatives. Everyone was well meaning, but no one was really helpful. I also continued to read about the controversy between different medical procedures and treatments for breast cancer. I investigated an interferon experiment but found that I would never know whether I received the treatment or a placebo.

I consulted the physician who pioneered mammography. He told me that I could live until ninety without anything more than having the lump removed. Before having the surgery, I had an extensive examination of the other breast, including a mammogram. A precancerous condition was found, and I felt that some form of treatment on the other breast was therefore necessary.

Finally, I chose to have a modified, bilateral mastectomy with immediate implants and reconstruction of the breasts and nipple grafts. In retrospect, I would have chosen the same set of procedures but would have postponed the implants and reconstruction until the healing of the mastectomy was complete. This is because I had a number of complications associated with the reconstructive surgery. Actually I have not healed completely yet, and it has been many months.

Immediately after the surgery, I felt that I was glad to be alive. I felt no pain, but there was tightness in the area of the operation. I also had a great deal of draining fluid from the surgical incision; it did not hurt but was very bothersome. I had to return to the hospital after my discharge because one complication occurred after another. The implant had to be removed, and still later additional reconstruction needed to be performed.

The recurrent postsurgical complications made me feel very depressed. I did a great deal of crying and felt that I had not been prepared for these

> events by my surgeon. I had been told that the healing would take two to three weeks, but instead it has taken months.
>
> Although there have been problems in my marriage, my husband was very supportive, helpful, and truly concerned for me throughout this. I am thankful that he was available to help me when I really needed him.
>
> Going back to work was truly exhilarating. I also returned eventually to my social activities, like playing bridge, and found this very important. Somewhere, perhaps in a marginally unconscious part of me, I always felt that with my heredity I would get cancer. Maybe it made me more conscious of my lump. It has been a long ordeal, but I am happy to be alive. I know now that I will stay in my marriage, and that I am proud of my career and my own financial success. And I am proud of my children. ❞
>
> —Elaine Kessler, 54

Radiation

X-ray or radiation therapy has also been used to treat primary breast cancer. When radiation therapy is to be used in this way, the tumor lump in the breast is removed, but the rest of the breast is retained. The lymph glands under the arm may also be removed. Following this rather minor surgery, the breast and underarm area are treated with X-ray beam. This approach is rather new, and it has not yet stood the test of time. It appears to be just as effective as surgery, however, particularly for women with small breast tumors. The appearance of the breast after such treatment is generally excellent. Radiation therapy may not, however, be suitable treatment for every woman with breast cancer.

Many women hesitate to go to their doctors for a biopsy of a breast lump because they are afraid they will wake up to find their breast has been removed. Immediate surgery of this sort is no longer standard practice. Each woman should discuss the possibilities of treatment with her physician prior to biopsy of a breast lump. If the breast lump is malignant, mastectomy need not be done right away. Some women prefer to wait and discuss the options of surgery or radiation therapy at a less stressful time. There is no evidence that waiting several days or even several weeks represents a further danger.

The evaluation of the lymph glands under the arm is an important part of the treatment of breast cancer because it helps predict if a woman's breast cancer is likely to recur after surgery. If the lymph nodes have cancer cells in them at the time of surgery, the risk of developing more cancer at some point in the future is high. If the lymph glands are not involved with tumor at the time of surgery, there is an 80 percent chance that primary treatment will cure the breast cancer. By evaluating the risk of recurrence, the doctor is able to choose whether *adjuvant therapy* will be beneficial after surgery or radiation.

Adjuvant Therapy

Adjuvant therapy, which has improved the survival rate of breast cancer patients, consists of powerful cancer-killing drugs, or chemotherapy, and sometimes hormones. The involvement of lymph glands is a signal that microscopic spread of cancer to other parts of the body may have occurred already. The purpose of adjuvant therapy, therefore, is to kill off the small numbers of remaining cancer cells that cannot be removed by surgery or killed by radiation. Adjuvant chemotherapy is given for one to two years in four- to six-week cycles. Unfortunately, chemotherapy may have severe side effects, which I will discuss later.

At the time of surgery, the surgeon will also send to the lab a piece of the breast tumor to measure estrogen receptor protein levels in the cancer tissue. This is a measurement of the capability of the tumor cells to bind hormones and grow in response to them and is important in evaluating the efficacy of hormonal therapy in each particular case. This information also may be of use in deciding whether adjuvant therapy is indicated. In addition, knowledge about the ability of a tumor to bind hormones will be useful in selecting therapies in the future if the tumor should recur. Finally, the presence or absence of estrogen receptor protein may give significant information about the risk of recurrence after primary therapy.

Proper treatment for primary breast cancer is essential. The ideal treatment is best individualized. The physician should explain fully to each patient what treatment options are available and explain the reasons for treatment recommendations. Including surgeons, radiotherapists, and oncologists (cancer specialists) in this discussion will help the patient in making a decision. It is, in addition, every patient's right to obtain a second opinion about treatment for breast cancer.

Treatment of Recurrent Cancer

Cancer that has recurred after the primary treatment is referred to as metastatic disease, or disease that has spread beyond the local area of the breast. It is very important for women to realize that even widespread breast cancer can be controlled or put in remission in the majority of cases. Remissions may last many months or years. The three major forms of treatment for metastatic cancer are chemotherapy, hormone therapy, and radiation therapy. These are used either by themselves or in combination, depending upon the situation.

The first step in the treatment of recurrent breast cancer is diagnosis. This may require sampling a piece of tissue (biopsy), especially if a long time has passed since the initial treatment for breast cancer. Other studies, such as X rays of the bones and chest, or scans of the bones, liver, or brain, help the physician understand the extent of the disease and evaluate the efficacy of the treatment. After the biopsy and tests have been done, the physician will choose the best type of treatment for the particular patient. This decision is based on many different pieces of information, including age, the period of time between the first diagnosis of breast cancer and its recurrence, previous treatment, the specific organs involved by the disease, the results of the estrogen receptor test done on the initial breast cancer and on the recurrent breast cancer if that is available, and the general medical condition of the patient.

Chemotherapy

Chemotherapy refers to the use of powerful drugs that kill cancer cells. Usually two or more different drugs are used in combination to maximize their effect. Most of these drugs are nonspecific, which means they may kill normal cells as well as cancer cells. Thus, side effects are associated with the use of chemotherapy. Generally these are mild and well tolerated by the patient, but serious side effects can occur.

Nausea and vomiting are common side effects. These occur only in the period when the drug is taken and usually disappear within a day of stopping the chemotherapy drug. In many patients the nausea and vomiting may be prevented or treated with pills. It is important to realize that not all patients have nausea and vomiting and that these symptoms vary in severity from patient to patient. Hair loss is a frequent and unfortunate side effect of many of these drugs. Most patients adapt to this by obtaining a wig, the cost of which will be covered by most insurance companies and Blue Cross/Blue Shield. A small number of patients will develop sores in their mouth. These will heal when the drugs are stopped, and often physicians can avoid their recurrence by changing the dose of medication.

The most serious side effects associated with these drugs relate to lowering of blood counts of the three types of blood cells that are manufactured by the bone marrow; red blood cells, which carry oxygen; white blood cells, which fight infection; and platelets, which stop bleeding when we cut ourselves. Most patients have mild or moderate suppression of the blood counts, which usually causes them no problems. Their blood counts return to normal within two to three weeks after chemotherapy is stopped. Some patients, however, experience a severe lowering of the blood counts. Although at these times they may feel no differently, they are susceptible to severe infection or bleeding. Patients on chemotherapy must report to their physicians immediately if they have a fever, chills, or other signs of infection, and if they observe any sign of bleeding. Even if these severe complications occur, they can be treated in most cases with prompt medical attention. Physicians will monitor the blood counts very carefully to minimize severe complications. These side effects may sound very frightening to the patient about to begin chemotherapy. Most patients manage very well on this treatment, however, and continue to live productive lives.

Hormone Therapy

Hormone therapy is another mainstay of the treatment of breast cancer. Based on the bits of information mentioned above, a cancer specialist can predict which patients are most likely to respond to a hormone therapy. Many types of hormone therapy are used in breast cancer, including some that add a hormone and others that block the effects of other hormones, either with medication or by removing the glands that produce them. In premenopausal women, removal of the ovaries is often a very effective form of treatment. In women who have had menopause, high doses of female hormones or estrogens are an effective form of therapy. A new type of hormone therapy, anti-estrogen pills, has become very useful recently. This may sound contradictory—and we do not fully understand the mechanism by which these therapies work—but it is related to the response of *abnormal* (cancer) cells to these chemicals. Other hormone drugs are progesterone, androgens or male hormones, and cortisonelike medications. These drugs have some side effects, but generally they are mild and well tolerated. Some side effects are nausea, vomiting, water retention with swelling of the ankles, and hot flashes. In addition, removal of the adrenal glands is often effective in patients who have responded to hormone therapies. In the past this required major surgery. We are now able to obtain the same result with a medicine, thus avoiding the need for surgery. Finally, some patients whose tumors are sensitive to hormones may respond to removal of their pituitary gland.

Radiation Therapy

Radiation therapy is a third form of treatment. This involves the use of invisible radioactive particles to kill cancer cells. Unlike chemotherapy and hormonal therapy, which affect the entire body, radiation therapy is a localized form of treatment. This means that the only cancer cells affected are those that lie in the path of the radiation beam. Generally, radiation therapy is used along with one of the other therapies to relieve severe symptoms, such as those from a painful bone affected by the cancer. Radiation is also useful in treating areas that chemotherapy and hormone therapy have difficulty reaching, such as the brain or the spinal cord. The specific side effects associated with radiation therapy depend on the area that is treated. Generally, radiation is well tolerated with only mild problems, if any at all.

Breast cancer is indeed a very serious and, unfortunately, very common disease. Many women are cured of this disease by their original therapy, however, be it surgery or radiation, with or without chemotherapy. For those women who are not cured by their primary therapy, effective therapy can control the breast cancer for periods of time varying from months to many years. Although these women often need to be under frequent medical care and on treatment, they are able to live relatively normal and productive lives.

—M.H.

Breast Reconstruction after Mastectomy

Breast reconstruction is a relatively new procedure that allows for creation of a breast mound after mastectomy. A nipple may also be constructed. This operation is becoming increasingly available because of advances in surgical technique by plastic surgeons and the decline in use of radical mastectomy. A number of surgical and nonsurgical options can be used for reconstruction. The choice should be based on individual needs, and the information provided by a physician. I will describe one of the more common approaches. It is important to emphasize that there now appears to be little justification for radical mastectomy, which removes the breast and the large pectoralis muscle that lies under the breast and covers the chest wall. The modified radical mastectomy, which most surgeons now perform for early breast cancer, preserves this muscle, enabling easier reconstruction of the breast.

The issue of reconstruction should be discussed with the surgeon before a mastectomy is performed. The type of incision and the amount of tissue removed may be influenced by the knowledge that further operations are planned.

The Breast Prosthesis

Women who do not wish to have reconstructive surgery may choose prosthetic devices that can be worn inside a brassiere. These can be fitted and purchased in corset shops in many large department stores or in smaller specialty shops. In many cases the fitting and prosthesis is covered by medical insurance.

Information on recovery after mastectomy, obtaining a prosthesis, and the many emotional issues involved in having a mastectomy is provided by volunteers from the Reach to Recovery Program of the American Cancer Society. Women who are interested in this information should consult their local telephone directory for the chapter of the American Cancer Society near them. The chapter should be contacted prior to the mastectomy procedure, so a volunteer can come to the hospital and discuss the issues before the surgery. The volunteer will also aid the patient in choosing and obtaining a prosthesis while she is in the hospital.

The National Cancer Institute publishes *Breast Cancer Digest,* a pamphlet that contains information concerning breast prostheses and answers many questions about breast cancer. It can be obtained by writing:

U.S. Department of Health and Human Services
Public Health Service
National Institutes of Health
Bethesda, MD 20205.

Refer to the *Breast Cancer Digest* by title and use "NIH Publication No. 80-1691" for further identification.

Additional information concerning breast cancer may be obtained from a local chapter of the American Cancer Society (listed in *Breast Cancer Digest* or the phone book) or through the national headquarters:

American Cancer Society, Inc.
777 Third Avenue
New York, NY 10017.

Exercises, bust developers, and hormone creams have not been proven effective in restoring a breast mound or normal chest wall shape after a mastectomy. Exercises to restore and maintain mobility and strength to the shoulder and arm on the side that has been operated on, however, are recommended. Most hospitals will give women a series of exercises and show them how to perform them daily at home.

Breast reconstruction is usually not undertaken if the patient has had an excessively large tumor removed, or if there is a high risk of recurrence in the area of the operation or in other parts of the body. Furthermore, most surgeons prefer to wait four to six months after the mastectomy before beginning the reconstruction process.

The technique of reconstruction usually involves two to three operations performed over a period of six months. First the plastic surgeon creates a breast mound by inserting a silicone-filled bag (prosthesis) under the skin or muscle on the mastectomy side of the breast. If the muscle has been removed by a prior radical mastectomy, a flap of muscle from the side may be brought up over the chest wall, under the skin surface, to cover the area. The prosthesis may then be inserted below the muscle flap in a later operation.

Many women are satisfied with a breast mound alone and do not wish further surgery. For those who desire a new nipple and areola on the breast mound skin, a thin skin graft from the nipple and the areola of the remaining breast may be applied.

The emotional impact of the surgery for breast reconstruction is usually far less devastating than the feelings of depression and loss associated with the removal of the breast. Women generally feel very positive about the reconstruction process because its goal is to restore what has been lost. Furthermore, since women are not offered the option of breast reconstruction unless there is little risk for redeveloping breast cancer, it is usually a promising sign. The atmosphere is one of hope because the cancer has been successfully treated.

Ideally, before leaving the hospital, both after the mastectomy and the reconstruction, doctor and patient should talk about caring for the wound and about sexuality. I feel that the physician should be the one to initiate this discussion, since many people are embarrassed to talk about sex with their doctor. If the physician does not bring up these issues, however, the patient should. I recommend that the patient's husband or sexual partner also be present.

Men may have anxieties about resuming sexual activity after mastectomy or the breast reconstruction operations. They may be concerned about hurting their partner, catching her cancer, or being exposed to radioactivity if radiotherapy has been part of the treatment. All of these fears are groundless, but men do have them. A discussion with the physician will help answer these questions and establish a common understanding.

❋

Those contemplating breast reconstruction might find it helpful to look at some articles on the subject available in medical journals. Several of these illustrate the technique used. The physician can obtain copies, or they may be found in the libary at a medical college. I suggest the following: *Resident and Staff Physician,* January, 1979, p. 58; *Annals of Surgery,* volume 187, 1978, p. 492; *American Journal of Surgery,* volume 138, 1979, p. 777.

—C.W.K.

Chapter 16
The Digestive System

Hank Pizer, PA-C

Unlike other parts of the body, the digestive system does not usually wear out with aging. The common medical problems that arise are more likely to be a result of dietary indiscretion (fatty foods, refined carbohydrates, alcohol, food additives) or stress than a function of advancing years. Ulcers, hemorrhoids, diverticuli, constipation, and gallstones, for instance, are usually partially or totally caused by life-style, eating habits, or nervous tension built up over many years.

Fortunately, it is never too late to change one's diet. Regular bowel movements should not be a problem for the average person. A small change in diet—for example, adding a few tablespoons of bran to food each day and avoiding white bread and other refined carbohydrates—can eliminate chronic constipation for many people. Hemorrhoids and gall bladder disease will also often respond to a change in diet. Ulcers may be controlled with diet, antacids, and techniques for reducing emotional stress.

In short, many of the problems of the digestive system can be controlled and minimized. Dietary changes will be necessary. Often this means changing patterns that have been established over an entire lifetime. But the rewards are enormous. The suggestions that were made in Chapter 8, *Nutrition*, will help most people to lose weight, have regular bowel movements, and prevent many common medical problems of the digestive system.

The digestive system, also called the gastrointestinal system, is a continuous tube that stretches from the mouth to the anus. It is about thirty-six feet (about 9 m) long and is connected to the liver, gall bladder, and pancreas, which produce chemicals that are essential to the digestion of food.

Digestion begins in the *mouth,* where food is chewed and mixed with saliva that begins the breakdown of starches. The *esophagus* carries the meal to the stomach, where the *cardiac sphincter* (or lower esophageal sphincter) acts as a gate, allowing food to pass into the stomach but not backward into the esophagus. The J-shaped *stomach* contains millions of glands that produce enzymes and hydrochloric acid essential for the breakdown of food. When food enters the digestive tract, a signal is sent to these glands to produce and secrete the digestive chemicals. At the lower end of the stomach is another gate, the *pylorus,* which prevents the backflow of food from the intestine into the stomach.

The *small intestine* is a long, convoluted tube, about 22 feet (6.6 m) long, where the balance of digestion takes place. It is composed of three sections: the 10-inch (25.4-cm) *duodenum,* the 9½-foot (2.85-m) *jejunum* and the 12½-foot (3.75-m) *ileum.* Attached to the small intestine are ducts that connect the liver, gall bladder, and pancreas to the duodenum. Digestion of food occurs as a result of mechanical churning of the food and chemical action by an array of essential enzymes. Fats are broken down by *bile,* produced in the liver and stored in the *gall bladder,* as well as by pancreatic juices. Proteins, already partially metabolized by *pepsin* in the stomach are further digested by *enzymes* from the pancreas and small intestine. Bacteria also act on food.

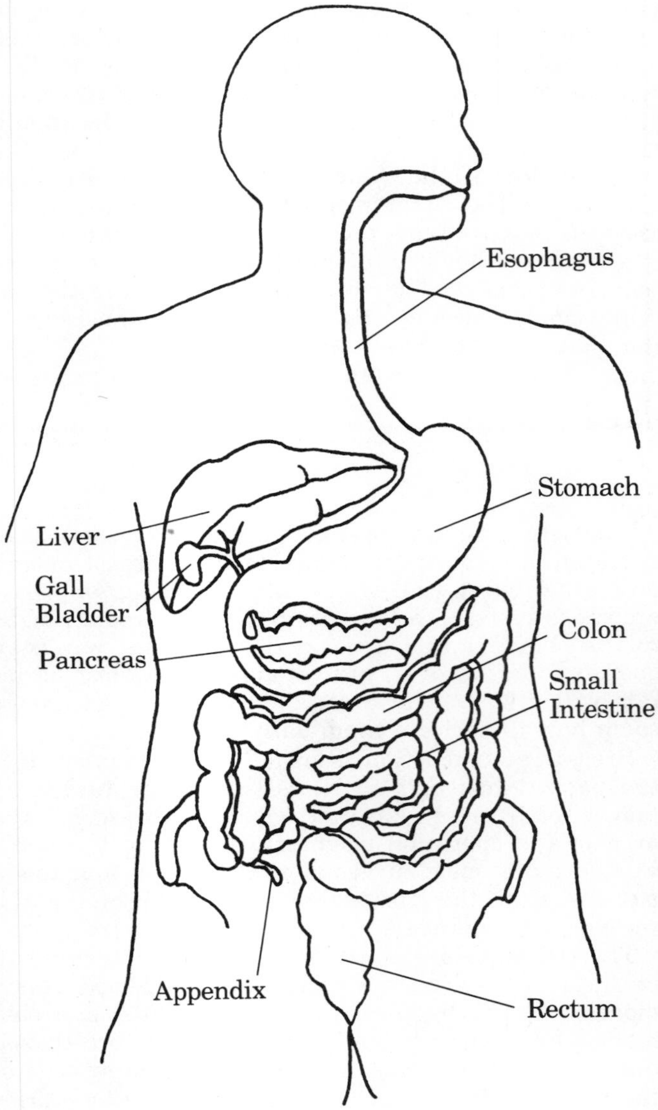

Anatomy of the digestive system.

The *liver* is the largest digestive organ of the body. It stores sugar, makes proteins, and converts unused sugar into fatty acids, which are a storehouse of energy. The *pancreas* is a straw-colored organ about six or seven inches (17 cm) long. It produces *insulin* and *pancreatic juices*. Insulin is needed for sugar metabolism, and pancreatic juice, a combination of chemicals, helps neutralize acid produced in the stomach.

The *colon,* or large intestine, is about 4½ feet (13.5 m) long. At the juncture of the small and large intestines is a valve that prevents the backflow of food. This is also the region where the *appendix* is located. In non-meat-eating animals this part of the body digests cellulose found in plants. In humans it has little importance, and normal digestion is possible after appendectomy. The large intestine absorbs fluid from the digested food and stores feces prior to excretion. Some digestion is performed by bacteria that inhabit the colon.

Common medical problems such as constipation, gas, diarrhea, and food poisoning are disorders of the digestive system that most people face at one time or another. Usually they are related to diet, nervousness, poor intake of fluid, or too little exercise. These are things that we can do something about ourselves. By changing our life-style, we can control or eliminate these unpleasant and altogether too common problems.

Constipation

Constipation refers not only to failure to pass stools; it also means difficulty in passing extremely hard stools. Millions of people suffer from chronic constipation, although most of them could avoid it with some simple changes in life-style. Constipation usually results from a combination of factors: emotional tension, diet lacking in bulk, poor intake of fluids, insufficient exercise. It only indicates serious illness when it marks a significant change in bowel habits or stool size.

People over fifty-five in Western countries have difficulty passing stools in large part because they exist on a diet high in refined foods and low in fiber. An apt comparison is to imagine a machine that is designed to chew up rocks, branches, and gravel but instead is fed only finely ground sand. Sooner or later that machine will get bound up. As was pointed out in Chapter 8, *Nutrition,* a few tablespoons of bran added to one's diet each day will be sufficient to provide the necessary bulk for the digestive system. The fiber provided by the bran, and also by fruits, vegetables and whole grains, will add bulk to the diet and help soften stools.

Self-treatment with enemas and laxatives is *not* an answer to chronic constipation. Eventually people get hooked on these preparations, just as others do on drugs, and find that they cannot move their bowels without them. Bowel movements are not necessary each day, but everyone should be able to move feces when they feel they must.

If a laxative is needed, understand that there are basically four different types. One type increases bulk. Examples are Metamucil and Serutan which are commercially formulated and work much the same way bran does, but are far more expensive. A second type is mineral oil, which acts as a lubricant by coating the inner lining of the digestive system with oil. Colace, a third type, softens the stool. Mineral oil and stool softeners may have some negative effects, such as reducing the intestinal absorption of nutrients and increasing the loss of oil-soluble vitamins A, D, E, and K. It is thought by some that they may be carcinogenic,

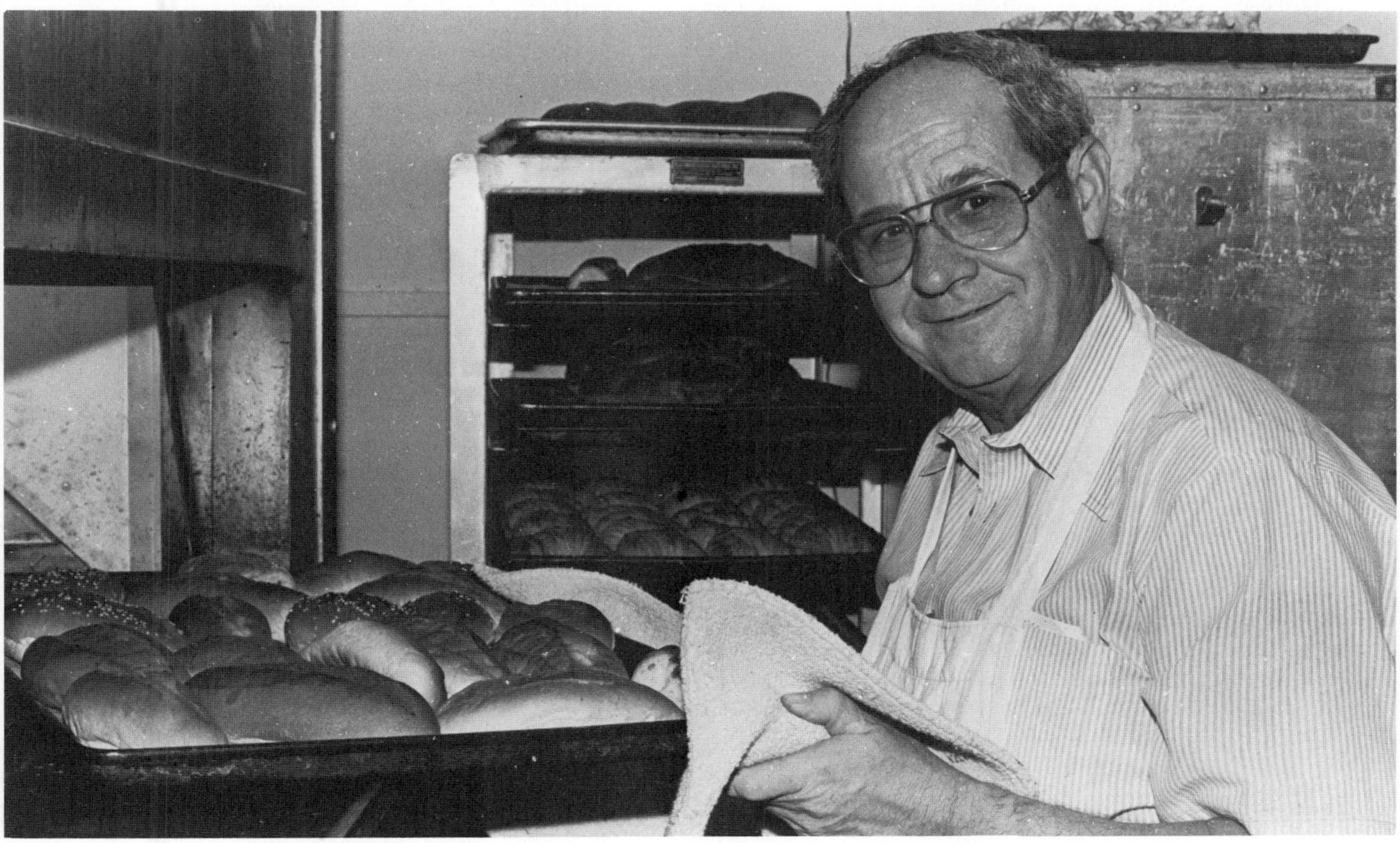

Avoiding Constipation

- Drink eight or more glasses of liquid a day, in the form of water, juices, teas (avoid excessive use of coffee and caffeine-containing teas).
- Eat high-fiber foods as often as possible. Try to have whole-grain breads, brown rice, or bran at most meals.
- Avoid all refined carbohydrates like white bread, rolls, and fast foods, which tend to be high in sugar (and fat).
- Exercise regularly.
- Allow regular and adequate time for bowel movements, so that you do not feel rushed.
- Do not use laxatives on a continual basis.

If constipation persists, get a full medical evaluation.

but this has not been proven. Some also feel that it is unwise to mix mineral oil and Colace. The fourth type, irritant purgatives, include milk of magnesia, cascara, and suppositories that stimulate the intestine to expel feces. They are usually highly effective but may bring on painful cramping.

Enemas wash out the colon. They should be used only under medical supervision. The effectiveness of coffee enemas and other naturopathic methods of cleansing the colon is largely unproven; they may even be dangerous. There are occasional reports of death resulting from coffee enemas. Like those who abuse laxatives, some people become addicted to enemas and cannot defecate without them.

If you have a problem with constipation, have a thorough medical evaluation. If an examination does not turn up any underlying disease, work out a change in diet and life-style with a medical provider. Realize that emotional as well as physical and dietary factors are related to defecation. Stress produces constipation. Individuals suffering from constipation may have to deal with the underlying problems that are affecting their digestive system.

Diarrhea

Diarrhea is the passing of frequent watery, unformed stools. An average person usually passes about 100 to 200 grams (3½–7 oz.) of stool a day. With diarrhea the volume may increase to 300 grams (10½ oz.) a day or more. Not only feces, but also water and salts that are essential for maintaining normal body balance are lost.

Persistent diarrhea can occur for many reasons. Loose, watery stools for more than a few days deserve a medical examination. Diarrhea may be a symptom of nervousness, an infection, or a more serious problem like colitis (and other inflammatory problems of the bowel), cancer, or an allergy. It may indicate intolerance to a drug being taken or a problem absorbing nutrients from the digestive system. Have the problem thoroughly investigated to rule out all of these possibilities.

Traveler's Diarrhea

Diarrhea is a common, but most unpleasant, symptom to have while traveling. It is usually produced by an organism (*E. coli*) normally found in the intestine, but of a type the traveler is not accustomed to. In most cases the symptoms of watery discharge and cramping pass in a few days to a week. During that time lost fluid and salts should be replaced with flat cola, ginger ale with a small amount of salt added, fruit juice, gelatin, or light pudding.

Most medical professionals advise against the use of Lomotil or opiate drugs to stop the diarrhea. It is thought that the bowel movements are necessary to purge the intestine of the pathogenic organisms. These drugs should be used only if ready access to a toilet is impossible or the lost fluid cannot be replaced with drinks.

There are no proven ways to prevent this problem with drugs. Some suggest Pepto-Bismol, one teaspoon three to five times daily, or antibiotics like tetracycline, streptomycin, or sulfa drugs. None, however, has been shown to be useful in experimental testing. The best strategy is still to exercise care in the food and water one ingests.

Food Poisoning

The symptoms of food poisoning are familiar to most of us: vomiting (often painful and explosive), diarrhea, nausea, cramps, and sometimes fever and chills. Pto-

Tips for Travelers

- Avoid tap water. Remember: ice in alcoholic and soft drinks may be made from impure water.
- Tea and coffee should be made from water that has been brought to a rolling boil.
- Carbonated drinks in their bottle or can, beer, wine, and distilled alcoholic beverages are usually safe. If you are uncertain, drink from the bottle, not a glass. The glass may have been washed in impure water.
- You can sterilize your own water by:

  Boiling vigorously for ten minutes.

  Adding ten drops of laundry bleach (1 percent chlorine) per quart or liter of water and letting stand for thirty minutes. If the water is cloudy, use twenty drops.

  Adding five drops of tincture of iodine (available at most drugstores) per quart or liter and letting stand for thirty minutes. Use ten drops if water is cloudy.

  Let the water stand in an uncovered container overnight to remove the iodine or chlorine taste.
- Brush your teeth in purified water only.
- Peel skins off fruits and vegetables before eating.

maine poisoning (its medical term is *salmonellosis*) is one type of food poisoning. There are, however, many other types. Aside from microorganisms, even chemicals like lead, arsenic, cadmium, and strychnine may contaminate food and produce these symptoms. Chemical poisoning usually presents other symptoms like convulsions, or bluing of the lips or fingers, along with the intestinal ones.

Food poisoning, like traveler's diarrhea, commonly passes on its own. The poisoning from staphylococcus found in spoiled milk or cream, for example, usually comes on within one to seven hours after ingestion and passes in a day or two. Sufferers may, however, feel weak for many days afterward and may find it difficult to eat a normal diet.

As with diarrhea, it is important to replace the fluid, salts, and nutrients lost through the watery stools. Gelatin, sodas, juices, water with some sugar and/or salt added will all be helpful. Keep food simple and bland, and *gradually* return to the usual diet. Avoid coffee, alcohol, spicy food, and drugs.

In warm regions with inadequate refrigeration, some foods should be eaten only with extreme caution. Seafood, dairy products, and meats may all become contaminated if they have not been refrigerated or preserved adequately. The food should smell and taste fresh and should be thoroughly cooked. Avoid street vendors that keep unrefrigerated food out in the sun.

Gas

Gas production is a normal part of the activity of digestion. Although people worry about this problem, it rarely has to do with the condition of the digestive system; rather, it is usually related to what we eat or how we eat it (too hot, too cold, or too fast). Whether we are conscious of it or not, we pass about 1,000 to 1,500 cc's (1 to 1½ qts.) of intestinal gas daily. Nitrogen, oxygen, methane, hydrogen, and carbon dioxide are produced in the intestine by the action of normal resident bacteria on the food we eat. Some foods, like beans and other legumes, are well-known gas producers. Bacteria act on the sugars (carbohydrates) these foods contain. Other foods such as milk products and wheat may produce gas in those who are allergic to them.

In addition, some of the gas comes from air that is swallowed during eating and drinking. Nervousness also produces gas, just as it may cause constipation, diarrhea, and other symptoms in the digestive tract. Even highly spiced foods can cause gas and gas pains.

Belching is not the release of gas produced by the action of bacteria on the food we eat. It comes largely from air that is swallowed and trapped in the lower portion of the esophagus. After a meal a carbonated drink may release a belch by freeing this trapped air.

Repeated belching, especially when not associated with meals, is not normal. It can be a sign of nervousness, an ulcer, disease of the pancreas or gall bladder, or aerophagia (excessive swallowing of air). Persistent belching merits a medical investigation.

Gas pains and bloating may be related to posture. Sitting hunched over allows gas to accumulate and distend the abdomen. If you are uncomfortable at work or after a meal, try getting up and walking around. This will help gas move out and through the digestive system. At home and at work, try to be as active as possible. Body motion helps to move food and gas through the system.

Hemorrhoids

Hemorrhoids are dilated blood vessels in the anal area. There are two types: *internal* and *external*. External hemorrhoids are obvious tags of skin that represent dilated veins. They look like small, rounded, purplish swellings and become more prominent when the sufferer strains. They are covered with a protective layer of muscle and so are not very likely to bleed. Internal hemorrhoids are usually more serious and more painful. Located inside the anus, they may protrude to the outside and look like an external hemorrhoid, except that they are not covered by muscle. Because of this they can bleed when the sufferer strains.

Hemorrhoids are an almost universal phenomenon with increasing age. Part of this common ailment, however, has nothing to do with aging, but with a diet poor in fiber, and with tension and straining to have bowel movements. It is believed by some that hemorrhoids are an inevitable result of walking upright, which places pressure on the rectum. Studies of people in primitive cultures, where a high fiber diet is common, point instead to diet as an important cause. In these regions hemorrhoids are far less common than in our society.

For most people hemorrhoids can be kept in check by one of a number of strategies, thus avoiding the need for surgical removal. Begin with increasing the bulk in the diet, as was described in Chapter 8, *Nutrition*, and in the section on constipation. This eliminates the need to strain during bowel movements. Sitz baths (soaking in a warm tub) twice a day will reduce pain and itching.

Creams may also help. Creams containing steroids reduce inflammation but should be used for only short periods of time. Applying lubricating cream, petroleum jelly, or mineral oil to the anus on a daily basis will be soothing and will ease bowel movements. For times of flare-up, instead of using toilet paper after bowel movements, use a wet washcloth and soap for cleansing. Apply a small amount of cream to the rectal area after cleansing.

Many steroidal and nonsteroidal creams and suppositories are available for relief of hemorrhoid symptoms. The nonsteroidal forms (for example, Anusol, Preparation H, Nupercainal) may be purchased without a prescription, whereas the steroids require one. The steroid forms are more effective for reducing pain, itching, and inflammation but should not be used for more than a few weeks at a time. Moreover, they should be employed in conjunction with a complete program that includes dietary change, sitz baths and stress reduction. If continued use of creams or suppositories is desired, a *non*steroidal antiinflammatory cream should be used. Persistent pain, bleeding, or discharge from the rectum deserves a prompt and thorough medical examination.

Some hemorrhoids will recede with the change in diet and life-style that has been described. Those that continue to be painful or bleed profusely should be removed by a surgeon. A number of different kinds of surgical procedures can be performed. The type that will be used depends on the preference of the surgeon, the size of the hemorrhoids, and individual needs.

Gastritis and Peptic Ulcer

Gastritis is a general term for inflammation of the stomach. Sometimes laypeople call this heartburn because of the sensation of burning and pain in the upper abdomen (where the heart is). Gastritis may be caused by a number of things (e.g., alcohol, aspirin, and tobacco), but most common is irritation caused by excess acid production. Tension is often a major factor in causing gastritis.

Peptic ulcer is the medical term for an ulcer (open sore) in either the duodenum (first part of the small intestine) or stomach. Ulcers are produced by excess stomach acid and enzymes that damage the lining of the stomach or duodenum. Usually these sores are about ¼ to ¾ inch (0.6 to 1.8 cm) in diameter and most often are found in the duodenum. They are uncomfortable and dangerous, principally because they can bleed. Sometimes this bleeding is severe enough to cause life-threatening hemorrhage.

Gastritis and peptic ulcer disease are often linked. After months or years of persistent gastritis, an ulcer develops. Moreover, both problems are often caused by the same set of factors: emotional stress, drinking too much alcohol, smoking, and less commonly, diseases of the stomach. The direct cause of all ulcers is acid and enzymes that corrode the stomach. Controlling, preventing, and healing an ulcer (as well as controlling most gastritis) therefore involves controlling acid production.

The signs of an ulcer are "gnawing" in the upper portion of the abdomen, pain in that region, weight loss and thirst. These symptoms may also indicate a hiatus hernia (see page 108), but much of the time they indicate excess stomach acid irritating the duodenum or stomach. In addition, darker than normal stools, a sign of active bleeding from the ulcer, may appear.

Most people who have ulcers or irritation in the duodenum find that food relieves their symptoms. Ulcers in the stomach, however, although less common, seem to provoke the opposite reaction—food often makes the symptoms worse.

Life-Style and Ulcers

Much has been said, some of it unfairly, about the role of life-style and personality in the development of ulcers. There does appear to be some relationship between ulcers and the need to succeed, anxiety, compulsiveness, perfectionism, and impatience. Nonetheless, people who are outwardly calm also get ulcers.

Ulcers also come in times of social and political unrest, for instance, during war and famine. Malnutrition and deficiencies of vitamins A, B, C, and protein can produce ulcers. The ulcer in this case seems to arise partially because of the emotional stress and partially because of the stress of poor diet.

In other words, although personality and life-style patterns are associated with ulcers, as well as many other medical problems, the entire story is more complex than that. It is difficult to know whether the personality traits precede the ulcer or vice versa. Possibly some underlying emotional conflict creates both the ulcer and the general personality traits of compulsiveness and drive.

Whatever the individual dynamics, it is a good idea for ulcer sufferers to seek some emotional counseling along with medical therapy. Many methods, including individual and group therapy, relaxation exercises, and meditation may be helpful.

Substances to Avoid If You Have an Ulcer

Caffeine: coffee, tea (nonherbal), cocoa, chocolate, cola drinks, No Doz
Spices: black pepper, cayenne, white pepper, chili powder, curry powder
Drugs: aspirin, Indocin, Butazolidin, cold tablets with aspirin, pain medicines with aspirin, Alka-Seltzer
Tobacco: cigarettes, pipe tobacco, cigars, snuff, chewing tobacco
Alcoholic beverages

Drugs, Diet, and Ulcer

Since dietary indiscretion can cause ulcer, it is not surprising that improving the diet can promote healing of an existing ulcer. Some substances increase the stomach's production of acid and should be avoided by those who have or have had an ulcer. The chart above lists them.

Most carbonated drinks and fruit juices are less acid than the stomach fluids and usually do not irritate the digestive system. If the ulcer is actively bleeding, however, their use may be restricted. In general, they are safe.

In planning a diet, think about food as both a pleasure and a potential ulcer producer. In other words, it is impractical for most people to completely abstain from caffeine, alcohol, spices, and the other foods listed in the chart. Find out what foods cause symptoms, and then take them only in moderation. There is no point in trying to stick to a diet that restricts desirable foods. Instead, the diet should be balanced to individual tastes.

Diet in the Treatment of Ulcers

Food is one of the tools for treating ulcers. As mentioned earlier, most people with duodenal ulcers find that food relieves their symptoms of heartburn and gnawing.

In the past, ulcer patients were encouraged to eat a diet high in milk products and other alkaline foods. This diet was called the Sippy diet, named after the physician who designed it. The Sippy diet is no longer used very often. It is too high in cholesterol to be recommended for most people over fifty-five, since the risk of heart disease is also high in these years. Moreover, diet can be manipulated in other ways to produce the same effect. The accompanying chart describes some of the principles of an ulcer diet. The most important point is to have *something* in the stomach to buffer the acid. Although this should not be taken literally, eating a pepperoni pizza is probably better

Principles of an Ulcer Diet

1. Eat enough to maintain your normal weight. Neither binge nor starve yourself.
2. Try to maintain a bland diet without caffeine, tobacco, alcohol, or spicy food. Allow yourself to enjoy these substances sometimes, but only in moderation. Avoid them if you have any symptoms, such as pain, heartburn, or gnawing.
3. Eat ample amounts of roughage and fiber foods. They are not harmful.
4. Restrict carbonated drinks only during acute attacks.
5. Under most circumstances, there is no need to avoid citrus juices. They do not increase acid production and are usually less acidic than stomach juices.
6. Eat small, frequent meals and exercise regularly to reduce stress.
7. Take an antacid about an hour after eating, since an ordinary meal neutralizes acid production for less than an hour and then increases it.

Meal and Antacid Schedule for Active Duodenal Ulcers

8:00 A.M.: breakfast
9:00 A.M.: antacid
10:00 A.M.: snack
11:00 A.M.: antacid
Noon: lunch
1:00 P.M.: antacid
3:00 P.M.: antacid
4:00 P.M.: snack
5:00 P.M.: antacid
6:00 P.M.: antacid
7:00 P.M.: dinner
8:00 P.M.: antacid
10:00 P.M.: antacid
11:00 P.M.: snack and two tablespoons of antacid

If you do not have symptoms, you may skip the 11 A.M. and 6 P.M. antacid doses. Be aware, however, that when you have symptoms, you may be doing damage to the lining of your stomach or duodenum, so that the idea is to prevent the gnawing and burning. If you feel hungry or nervous, take your antacid at these times.

than having an empty stomach. Remember: small, frequent meals and antacids form the basic diet plan for ulcer disease.

Medical Treatment

Treating ulcer disease begins with *preventing* ulcer formation. Since "no acid, no ulcer" is a fairly valid concept, diminishing acid production and neutralizing what acid is produced are the goals of treatment.

Antacids and food are the best initial forms of therapy. Both are effective for a maximum of about twenty to forty minutes, because the stomach regularly empties itself. Antacids relieve symptoms for a somewhat longer time than food, however, because acid takes some time to build up. Antacids should be taken on a regular basis, usually about every two hours. Taken at four-hour intervals, they appear to be only about half as effective.

There are many kinds of antacids on the market, those containing *aluminum* and *magnesium* being the most commonly recommended. *Baking soda* (sodium bicarbonate—found in such preparations as Rolaids and Alka-Seltzer) will neutralize stomach acid, but it sometimes produces a rebound effect of greater acid production. Its use is also not advised because it contains sodium, which can aggravate high blood pressure. *Calcium carbonate* (Titralac, Tums, Di-O-Gest) also works to neutralize acid but can be very constipating and may create abnormally high levels of calcium in the body, which can damage vital organs. Like baking soda, calcium carbonate may have a rebound effect. For these reasons aluminum- and magnesium-containing antacids are generally the best alternative.

Even these preferred antacids, however, produce some undesirable side effects. The antacids that contain only magnesium (milk of magnesia) produce loose stools, whereas those that contain aluminum (Basaljel, Amphojel) tend to constipate. Mylanta, Gelusil, Maalox, and Trisogel are combinations of aluminum and magnesium. Some people find it best to alternate two types of antacids, for instance, Mylanta and Basaljel. Antacids may also produce gas (flatulence); some of them contain simethicone to counteract that. Simethicone can also be taken by itself (as in Mylicon) to relieve gas symptoms.

Antacids should be taken after meals, usually an hour after eating and then two hours later. See the above chart for a sample meal and antacid schedule. They should not be taken with tetracycline medications, since they inhibit absorption of the antibiotic from the stomach. If you are watching your sodium intake, be aware that certain antacids contain sodium. Read the label of any antacid you are considering for sodium content and discuss this with your medical provider.

Certain other medications—antispasmodics (Donnatel, Pro-Banthine), sedatives, and tranquilizers—have been used to help with peptic ulcers. The antispasmodics inhibit the transmission of messages from the nerves to the stomach, which reduces both acid production and the ability of the stomach to empty. They have a number of potential side effects, including blurred vision, difficult urination, and reduced perspiration (which may interfere with temperature regulation). They also affect many other parts of the body and should be used only with an understanding of their diverse side effects. Discuss this with a medical provider. They are often prescribed for nighttime use. Tranquilizers and sedatives also have been used in controlling ulcers, but they can be both physically and emotionally addictive and may interfere with driving, working, and other necessary activities. In general, these medications are used in conjunction with antacids, never by themselves.

Cimetidine (Tagamet) is a relatively new medication for people with active duodenal ulcers. Because of potential side effects, it should be taken only for short periods (usually up to eight weeks) for acute ulcer attacks. It is not for daily prevention of symptoms. Among its possible side effects is an increased susceptibility to bleeding among those taking Coumadin as an anticoagulant. It can and probably should be taken along with antacids to relieve pain.

Surgery

Ulcers that do not respond to the conservative medical treatment described may require surgery. There are many possible surgical procedures. Some remove the ulcer (if it is in the duodenum); others remove part of the stomach and cut some of the nerve supply to the part of the stomach where acid and enzymes are produced. The type of operation performed depends on where the ulcer is located, its size, and the preferences of the surgeon.

Endoscopy is a safe, relatively painless procedure for looking directly into the stomach and first portion of the small intestine. It involves passing a fiber-optic instrument via the mouth. The procedure usually takes less than thirty minutes and is performed without general anesthesia.

Hiatus Hernia

Sometimes the symptoms of a hiatus hernia mimic those of ulcer disease. A hiatus hernia occurs when a portion of the stomach slides, rolls, or protrudes upwards through the diaphragm into the chest cavity, and stomach juice (which is acid) can flow back into the lower portion of the esophagus. Sometimes one gets a bitter or foul taste in the mouth, especially after lying down. The cause of a hiatus hernia is unknown.

Differentiating hiatus hernia from ulcer disease should be the job of a medical provider. Since the symptoms are often similar, it may be necessary to swallow some barium contrast liquid and have X-ray pictures taken as it courses down the esophagus and into the stomach.

Often the symptoms of hiatus hernia can be controlled with diet, much like those of ulcer disease. Sitting upright after meals will also help. If these conservative methods do not provide relief, however, surgery can be performed to correct the hernia. Because these operations are not always successful, they are considered only after medical therapy has proven unsuccessful.

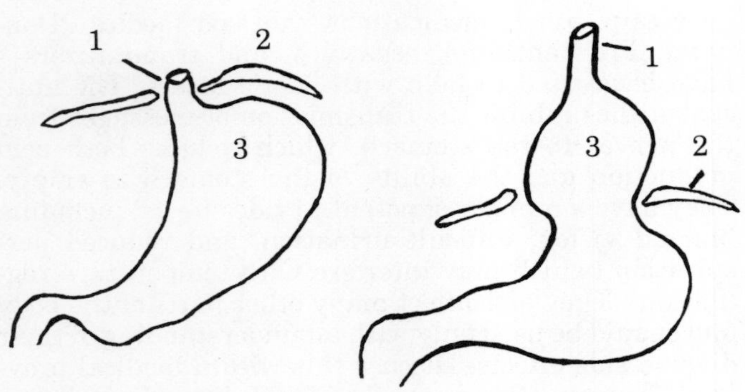

Hiatus hernia. Left: *normal esophagus (1), diaphragm (2), and stomach (3).* Right: *sliding hiatus hernia—stomach (3) passes through diaphragm (2), altering the angle between the stomach and the esophagus (1).*

Cancer of the Colon

Cancer of the colon is the most common tumor-producing death in people over seventy-five. It is an extremely common type of cancer in all people over fifty-five, and one of great concern to both the public and to medical practitioners. This is because effective drugs do not exist for treating cancer of the colon, and lesions are often discovered too late for surgery to be curative.

Screening

Increasing survival from cancer of the colon and limiting its devastating effects on the overall population depends on early detection of the disease. The most effective method of screening oneself for colon cancer is the inexpensive and simple *stool guaiac test,* which reveals small amounts of blood in feces, an early potential sign of a tumor. The test kit, available from a medical provider, consists of a card on which small samples of bowel movements are placed. The specimens should be obtained after a few days of eating a high-fiber diet and avoiding red meat, horseradish, turnips, and vitamin C, all of which might make the test falsely positive.

Physicians differ on exactly how the specimen should be taken. A commonly used approach is to take a small amount of stool from each of two parts of the bowel movement for three days. All six cards should be mailed to a physician for analysis. Follow the directions of a medical provider, even if they are somewhat different from these, so that he or she is aware of how the specimen is being collected. What is most important is that this test is performed regularly, at least once a year, so that potentially cancerous lesions can be discovered.

Physical examination by a medical professional is another part of screening for cancer of the colon. Since many of these cancers can be felt in the course of a rectal examination, this simple procedure is basic to early detection. Sigmoidoscopy, using a lighted instrument to look into the colon, is also an extremely valuable tool in diagnosing cancer of the colon. It is often not practical to do this as a screening test in a regular physical examination, however. Although not actually painful, it is uncomfortable and too expensive for most people to have it performed annually.

Unfortunately, in most situations there are few, if any, symptoms of cancer of the colon. Sometimes there may be a change in the normal bowel patterns such as a feeling that one has not completely evacuated the colon. Weight loss, generally not feeling up to par, and an increasing abdominal mass are other signs. Cancer of the colon is often a silent disease until it is far advanced. For this reason the stool guaiac test is very important.

Treatment

Surgical removal of small lesions found in the intestine is the basic goal of treatment for colon cancer. This can provide a cure, but only if the tumor is found early.

Once it has spread, the chance of survival longer than five years becomes small.

❝ I was in good health until a few years ago, when a number of things started happening to me. I had retired with a good income and enjoyed having less pressure. I had felt that I tended to become anxious when I felt pressure, and figured, "So, why continue?"

My health remained excellent until just after my wife's death. That was six years after I retired. I had been under the care of a physician for a prostate condition, when I began to feel thirsty. The doctor referred me to another physician, who found an extremely high sugar level in my blood. I had diabetes. I was hospitalized for one week until the sugar content came down to within a normal range. I took insulin for four months and then started on an oral medication. I watched myself to see that I didn't get bruises or infections which are potentially serious for diabetics, and was able to accept the medical regimen that I had to observe. I slept well and, for the most part, ate everything.

Yet there remained a nagging worry about my health. I remained under a doctor's care for about four years and then noticed an itchy feeling in my stomach. The doctor recommended X rays. Two days later he called me to say that I had cancer of the colon. He felt that the disease was just at its outset. I had no other symptoms—no bleeding, no weight loss.

He recommended surgery, and I had the operation to remove the cancer two weeks later. Before the operation I became very nervous and feared death. I couldn't sleep, my appetite was reduced. After retirement I often visited the men I worked with while they were in the hospital. I was very aware of the effect of serious illness. I felt that even if I survived the surgery, I would have only a short time to live. This depressed me even more. I did feel that if I did die, I had had a wonderful life. I had enjoyed my experiences. If I had to die, that would simply be it for me.

I emerged from the operation feeling well almost immediately. I felt relieved of anxiety, because my doctor informed me that everything was fine. I had nothing to worry about. I picked up my old activities very quickly.

About a year later I got a new interest in my life. I met a woman I cared a great deal about, and I wanted very much to be well and active.

I should also mention something about my wife's death. She died very suddenly from heart failure. I was there when she died. I tried to revive her with mouth-to-mouth resuscitation but was not successful. She was just sixty-two and had retired about fifteen days before.

I was very depressed by these circumstances. My son tried to help by sending me to Europe. I was supposed to stay five weeks, but I returned in three weeks. Nothing helped. I didn't sleep. I couldn't deal with the vision of her lying on the floor dead. That depressed feeling remained with me until the other events that I mentioned came into my life.

Now, as to the future, I want to live as I do now. I want to enjoy my family, my friends, and my activities. There is still with me the feeling that I might have a recurrence of the malignancy. If I don't feel well now, there is always the nagging suspicion that I might be having a recurrence. If I'm alone, I'm particularly vulnerable. If I'm involved in something I like, the anxiety is dissipated. ❞

—Frank Amodeo, 73

There is an ongoing effort to find new chemotherapeutic drugs to treat colon cancer. To date, this has been a rather frustrating endeavor. New drugs in various combinations are being tested in clinical trials in cancer centers. This kind of therapy should be supervised by oncologists who participate in these studies. Usually the surgeon who performs the operation will recommend an oncologist or treatment center where follow-up care can be obtained.

Radiation therapy in most cases of cancer of the colon is not curative. It remains an important additional form of treatment, however, because radiation can shrink the tumor mass. This is useful for relieving intestinal obstruction or pain created by the tumor.

Colostomy

Removing all or part of the large intestine is often necessary when treating cancer of the colon. A colostomy will then be created, through which evacuation of feces can occur. The hole through which the feces evacuates is called the *stoma*. Its size, placement, and configuration will depend on the type of operation and the preference of the surgeon.

Care of the colostomy has been simplified by the development of different types of bags that fit comfortably under clothing and irrigating equipment that is compact and easy to use. One can work, travel, swim, and participate in social activities with little inconvenience. Only contact sports, which may dislodge the appliance or injure the stoma, may be ill-advised.

Colostomy care does require emotional adjustment and some practice. Instruction in daily care begins in the hospital, after the surgery. The nursing staff will demonstrate all aspects of the process, and as one recovers from the surgery, there will be time to become proficient. The emotional adjustment inevitably takes more time. There is uncertainty about how one will function in the day-to-day world, and how others will react to the colostomy. Most areas have ostomy societies in which people meet and discuss problems related to colostomy care. They are an extremely valuable resource.

A useful booklet, prepared by people who have colostomies, is called "All About Colostomies." It can be obtained for fifteen cents from:

American Cancer Society
Connecticut Division, Inc.
270 Amity Road, Suite 217
Woodbridge, CT 06525.

Other useful resources are *The Ostomy Handbook,* by Edith S. Lenneberg and Miriam Weiner of the Stoma Rehabilitation Clinic, New England Deaconess Hospital, Boston, MA 02215; and *Colostomies: A Guide,* by Edith S. Lenneberg and Alan Mendelssohn, MD, of Wayne State University Medical School, Detroit. You can obtain these booklets from:

United Ostomy Association, Inc.
2001 West Beverly Boulevard
Los Angeles, CA 90057.

Information concerning an ostomy association near you can be obtained by writing the United Ostomy Association.

Diverticulosis and Diverticulitis

Diverticuli are sacs or outpouchings that occur in the intestinal wall, usually in places where arteries pass through the muscle. They are related to years of eating a diet poor in fiber, which causes the bowel muscle to strain to move the feces through the gut. In countries where the diet is rich in fiber, and among vegetarians, the incidence of diverticulosis is far less than that in Western countries, where about half the people over seventy have diverticuli.

Diverticulitis is the inflammation of these saccular pouches. About 10 percent of people with diverticuli suffer acute attacks, which are probably the result of small perforations in the bowel that become infected. Signs of diverticulitis are pain in the abdomen (usually the lower left portion) and a change in normal bowel habits, such as frequent loose stools, constipation, or bleeding. If the inflammation progresses so that there is fever, it must be treated with antibiotics. If it does not, then a soft or liquid diet, along with mineral oil or a stool softener like Colace until bowel movements are painless will be helpful.

After the period of inflammation has passed a diet *rich* in fiber will help prevent future attacks. This will not eliminate the small outpouchings already formed, but it may help prevent new ones from forming. The fiber will aid normal strain-free movement of feces through the intestine.

Gall Bladder Disease

Gallstones and inflammation of the gall bladder and its drainage ducts are extremely common, especially in overweight people. The exact connection between gall bladder disease and aging, weight, and diet is not known, but the incidence is so high in Western countries that diet and life-style must play some role.

It is widely believed that diets rich in meat and fat contribute to gall bladder disease. As evidence of this, after World War II the incidence of gall bladder disease increased in the Japanese as they began to adopt a Western-style diet. Diets low in fiber also probably play a causative role since fiber aids in the absorption and metabolism of bile and cholesterol which make up gall stones.

Bile is an acid produced in the liver for the metabolism and absorption of fats. Between meals the bile is stored and concentrated in the gall bladder and then released when food enters the first portion of the intestine.

Gallstones are made up of bile salts and cholesterol. We do not know exactly why they form but they may result from excess ingestion of fats, along with incomplete emptying of an overworked gall bladder. For whatever the reason, aging brings an increased likelihood of forming large, painful, and potentially dangerous stones in the gall bladder or the ducts that lead from the gall bladder to the intestine.

Once stones form and obstruct the flow of bile, infection, pain, and jaundice can occur. Pain may or may not come with fatty meals. When it does occur, it is usually felt under the right portion of the rib cage, but this is also somewhat variable. In about one-fourth of those suffering from gallstones, some jaundice, visible as yellowing of the skin and the white of the eyes, may appear. In many people, however, the stones produce neither pain nor jaundice.

The presence of gallstones can be diagnosed in a number of ways. Two of the most common are X rays with a tracer dye and the use of fiber-optic instruments passed via the mouth and into the intestine to look into the gall bladder region.

The prevention of gall bladder disease is perhaps more relevant than its detection. Many people can accomplish this with dietary change, particularly reducing the amount of fat ingested. For most people this means eating red meat only in small amounts and not on a daily basis. Increasing the dietary fiber also helps, as does losing weight.

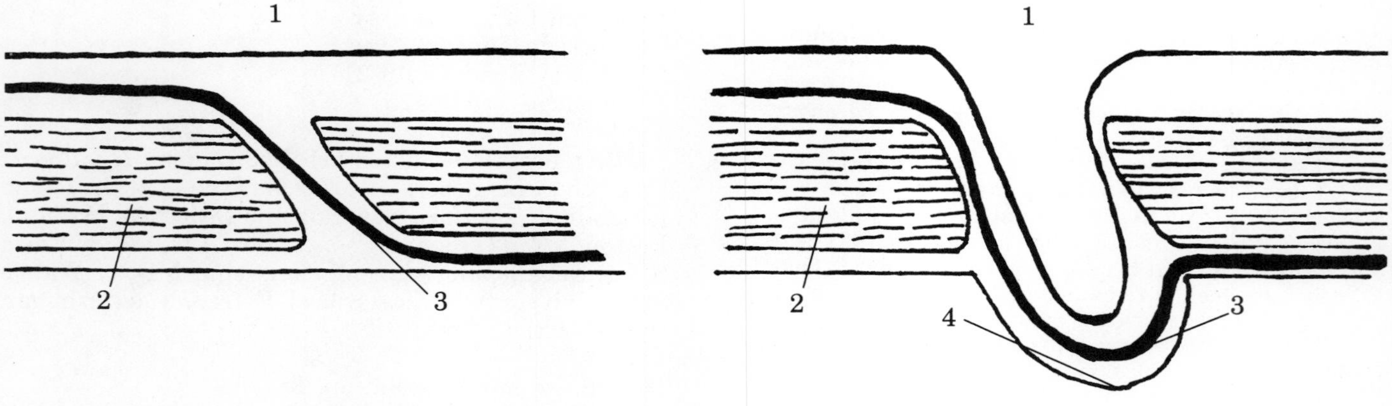

Diverticulosis. Left: *cross section of normal colon, showing inside colon (1), muscle in colon wall (2), and blood vessels that pierce muscle wall (3).* Right: *colon with diverticulum—pressure inside colon (1) causes the weaker blood vessel area (3) in the muscular wall (2) to bulge, resulting in a diverticulum (4).*

Some stones may cause no symptoms. There is no fixed rule about whether and when small stones that do not produce pain or inflammation should be removed. Some physicians prefer doing this before an acute attack, because emergency surgery is potentially more dangerous than elective surgery. This is particularly true in people over sixty, who have a higher risk than average when having an operation.

When gallstones cause pain, fever, jaundice, and inflammation, most physicians encourage removal of the gall bladder. This is done in the operating room, under general anesthesia. If there are only very small stones, the surgeon may choose to remove only the stones; but in most cases the entire gall bladder is removed. It is possible to live a normal life, eat a normal diet, and remain entirely healthy without the gall bladder. Leaving it in may increase the likelihood of stone formation in the future and the need for another operation.

Disease of the digestive system is probably not an inevitable outcome of normal aging. We have been endowed with a complex system that can satisfy our metabolic needs throughout life if we take care of it with some relatively simple dietary and life-style measures. At the same time, the signs and symptoms of illness cannot be ignored. A healthy digestive system is absolutely essential for the metabolism of food, upon which all life is based.

Chapter 17
The Genitourinary System

Hank Pizer, PA-C; and Marcia Bowling, MD

The genitourinary system is composed of the kidneys, ureters, bladder, urethra, and genitalia. The kidney is an essential organ of body regulation and waste elimination. The genitalia are organs of reproduction.

The physiological changes in the genitalia of women that are associated with menopause were discussed in Chapter 3 by Dr. Alice Rothchild. Further discussion of these changes and their relationship to certain medical problems will be found in the discussion in this chapter by Dr. Marcia Bowling.

The Urinary System

The *kidney,* along with the lungs, skin, and intestine, is an organ for waste elimination and for regulation of the body's balance of fluid, salts, acidity, and other products of body metabolism. It also filters drugs, toxic substances, protein, and sugar. The bulk of this process occurs in the *cortex,* or outer portion of the kidney.

We have two kidneys that sit behind the intestines, above the waistline at the level of the twelfth rib. Each kidney is about 4½ inches (11.5 cm) long, 2 to 3 inches (5.08 to 7.62 cm) wide, and a little more than 1 inch (2.54 cm) thick. Both kidneys touch the diaphragm and move up and down with breathing.

The kidney is highly vascular: about one-fifth of the body's blood volume is located in the kidneys at all times. Blood is filtered continuously, and waste products pass in the urine into the ureters and bladder. About 99 percent of the fluid is reabsorbed into the bloodstream. In addition to regulating body fluid and waste removal, the kidney is an essential organ in the control of blood pressure.

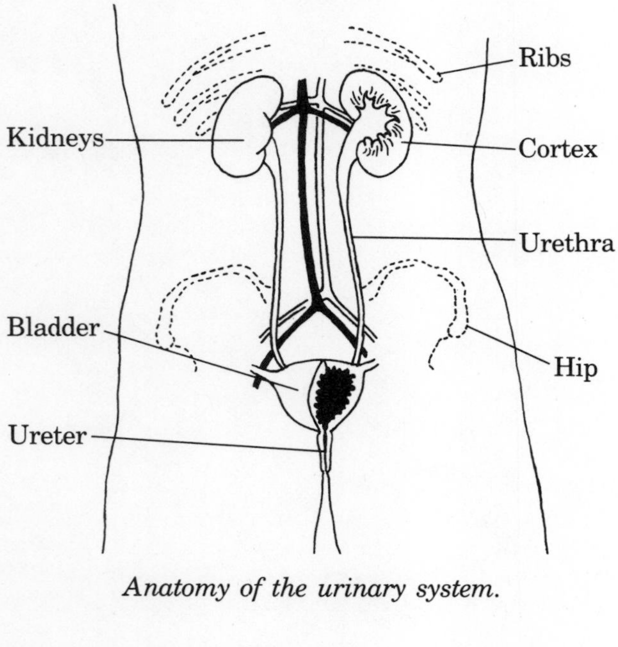

Anatomy of the urinary system.

The *ureters* connect the *bladder* to the *kidney.* Urine is forced into the bladder, a muscular organ, by rhythmic contraction of each ureter, and a set of flaps at the entrance to the bladder prevents the urine from flowing backward. In men the bladder is found behind the pubic bone. In women, it lies between the uterus and the pubic bone.

The *urethra* is the tube that drains the bladder. In men it is about 8 inches (20 cm) long and carries both urine and semen. The first inch or so of the urethra (nearest the bladder) is surrounded by the prostate gland, which will be described more fully later. In women the urethra is approximately 1½ inches (4 cm) long and opens into an area between the clitoris and the vagina. The increased incidence of bladder infections in women is in part caused by the proximity of the urethra to bacteria that reside in the vagina and to the shortness of the tube.

Normal Aging

The aging of the kidney has been studied in great detail by physiologists. It has been observed that the kidneys shrink in size and lose up to 50 percent of their overall filtering capacity. The kidney contains many blood vessels, and these decrease in number with aging. Some researchers hypothesize that the diminution of kidney function results from the decrease in blood flow through the kidney.

Despite these changes it would be false to conclude that the aging of the kidney inhibits activity or diminishes longevity for most people. Kidney disease is not one of the top ten causes of death in people over fifty-five. Perhaps this is because the kidney contains an enormous extra reserve of filtering capacity. In some situations changes in kidney function are a factor in the type and quantity of prescribed medication. This is something that the professional need be concerned with and not part of the day-to-day life of people over fifty-five.

With advancing years it is increasingly common to feel the need to urinate during the night. The feeling that one needs to void suddenly, even with relatively little in the bladder, is also common. The reason for these changes in bladder function is not well understood. Since the bladder muscle remains relatively intact with aging, it is felt that changes in the nerve supply are most likely to be a factor.

It is *not* normal to feel pain, burning, hesitancy, or a sudden increase in the frequency of urination. The likelihood of having an infection in the bladder increases greatly with advancing years. *Incontinence,* or the inability to control one's need to void, is also not normal. Any of these symptoms are signals to have a complete medical evaluation of the urinary system.

Medical Problems

There are many diseases of the *genitourinary* system. Bladder infections (*cystitis*) can usually be treated by a family medical provider. More complicated illnesses demand the care of a specialist.

Genitourinary problems in men are usually treated by a urologist, a surgical specialist. Women are more often seen by a gynecologist, also a surgeon; but they too should see a urologist if the problem affects the kidney or bladder. Nephrologists are medical specialists in the care of kidney disease. They manage dialysis care, as well as treating nonsurgical diseases of the urinary system.

Urinary Tract Infection

Urinary infections affect both men and women but are more common in women. Usually they are localized in the bladder but, if left untreated, can ascend into the kidney. This type of infection, called *pyelonephritis*, is particularly dangerous. It can cause an extremely serious infection throughout the body and may produce permanent scarring of the kidney. Thus, bladder infections should be promptly treated by a medical professional.

The signs of a bladder infection are:

- feeling the need to urinate more often (urgency)
- urinating more often (frequency)
- pain or burning while urinating (dysuria)
- sensation of pressure in the lower abdomen
- blood in the urine (hematuria)

Kidney Stones

Kidney stones form from excessive concentration of particles normally found in urine. The formation of these stones usually occurs suddenly and without warning, although infection, disorders of calcium metabolism, gout, dehydration, and injury may cause stone formation. Occasionally excessive milk or vitamin D ingestion may produce stones. The diagnosis of the problem will depend on an evaluation by a trained medical provider.

The signs of a kidney stone attack are pain in the side, blood in the urine, difficulty urinating, and pain in the groin or lower abdomen. If you suspect a stone, you should get emergency medical care. Usually the pain is so severe that people proceed immediately to their nearest hospital, but if you have any doubts be aware that kidney stones are potentially serious and should be treated as soon as possible.

If you have pain and feel that you need to urinate, save your urine and take it to the hospital. Better yet, strain it and bring the residue for analysis. Knowing the chemical content of the stone is an important part of treatment as it will help your medical provider decide on ways to prevent further stone formation.

Preventing the recurrence of kidney stones depends on the type of stone formed. As a general rule, increasing daily fluid intake to at least four glasses of water will be beneficial. In addition, those who tend to form stones should seek treatment of urinary infections early. These infections increase the risk of stone formation.

Incontinence

Incontinence is the inability to retain urine. This may result from injury to the spinal cord, stroke, multiple sclerosis, senility, or with relaxation of the pelvic organs after menopause. Any change in the normal pattern of urination warrants a complete medical evaluation. Usually a thorough investigation involves an examination by a urologist (see also *Relaxation of the Pelvic Organs* in the next section).

Hernia

A hernia occurs when the muscles and ligaments that make up the abdominal wall weaken and allow a portion of the intestine to come through. It is more common in men, although it happens to women as well. A hernia is usually quite obvious in people over fifty-five. It may be situated in the groin, umbilical region (belly button), or other portion of the abdominal wall. The protruding portion of bowel is usually soft and can be pushed back into the abdominal cavity with one's finger.

In the groin area, two types of hernia can occur: *direct* and *indirect*. Direct hernias are more common in men over fifty-five and are seen in the area above the scrotal sac. The indirect hernia allows bowel to enter the scrotum and usually occurs in children. *Femoral* hernias occur in the crease where the upper thigh and abdomen meet. They are more common in women.

The hernia is *reducible* when you can push the bowel back into the abdominal cavity. It is *incarcerated* when you cannot do this. If the blood supply to the bowel is interrupted, the hernia is *strangulated*. This may cause death of the affected bowel tissue and serious illness.

Hernias should be repaired by surgery. If they are caught early and are reducible, they may be treated as an elective operation. If they are incarcerated or strangulated, surgical repair should be performed promptly. The surgery involves removing the sac containing the intestine and repairing the muscles and ligaments. If the hernia is large, a piece of metal or plastic may be inserted to cover the defect.

Trusses and binders are not considered effective therapy; nor do they protect one from getting a hernia during lifting or athletic activity. After surgical repair, men may use an athletic supporter if there is pain in the scrotal area during the healing period.

Postoperative recovery from the surgery is usually rapid. One should avoid any heavy lifting or straining for a fairly prolonged period, because closing the defect does not make a strong abdominal wall. Once the muscles have healed, normal activity can be resumed. Ask a medical provider or surgeon when strenuous work can be resumed. Individuals who are recovering should eat a high-fiber diet, drink ample fluids, and take a stool softener if prone to constipation since straining during bowel movements can retard healing or possibly reopen the hernia. Bathing with soap and water is permissible, and rubbing a bland lubricating cream on the scar area may reduce pain and itching.

Fever, redness in the scar area, pain, or a change in bowel patterns are signs of possible infection or damage to the bowel. Report these symptoms to the surgeon or family medical provider. —H.P.

Genitourinary Problems in Women

Since the turn of the century the definition of "older woman" has changed considerably. In 1900 a woman of fifty-one would have been considered old. Since that time, over twenty years has been added to the life span

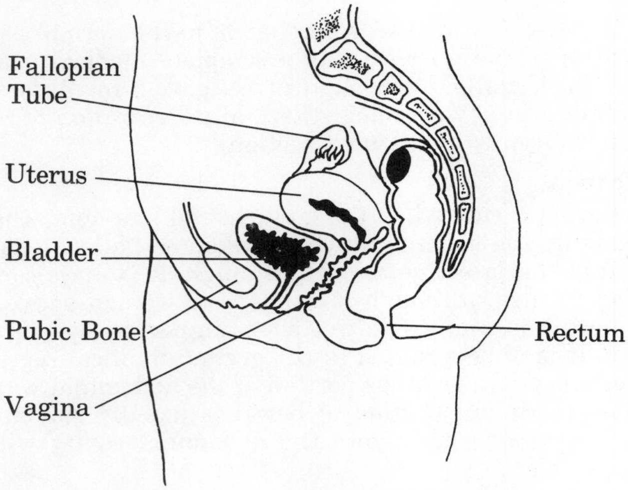

Anatomy of the female pelvis.

of the average woman, and few consider women in their fifties or sixties to be old.

Many of the medical problems that affect the genitourinary system of women have to do with anatomical and physiological changes associated with menopause. These are discussed by Dr. Alice Rothchild in Chapter 3, *Menopause and After*. I am going to present some additional information concerning the medical problems associated with changing estrogen levels.

To review, changes occur in the breasts, vagina, and internal pelvic organs during and after menopause. The breasts lose some of their glandular tissue, the supporting elastic tissue weakens somewhat, and they become more pendulous. Pubic hair tends to thin, and the vaginal opening may become narrowed. The vagina itself may shorten slightly, and its mucosal lining may thin. Vaginal secretions may diminish as well, which often produces a change in the kinds of microorganisms that inhabit the vagina.

The internal pelvic organs undergo similar changes. The uterus shrinks to approximately half its previous size, as do the ovaries. Normally these changes go unnoticed, except during a pelvic examination by a medical provider.

Interestingly, advancing years also offer protection from some gynecological problems, among them fibroids (benign muscle tumors of the uterus), endometriosis (displaced uterine tissue that may cause pain and/or bleeding), ovarian cysts, and acute and chronic inflammatory cysts of the breasts (mastitis).

Relaxation of the Pelvic Organs

Relaxation of the pelvic organs is a term used to describe the loss of elasticity of the ligaments and fibrous tissues that support the organs in the pelvis: the bladder, uterus, rectum, and urethra. The degree of change varies greatly among women. It may be related to numbers of pregnancies or a traumatic birth that may have occurred.

Sometimes medical care givers call this condition *pelvic insecurity,* an unfortunate term since it carries negative social connotations. It, of course, has nothing to do with emotional insecurity. It is a relatively common consequence of aging, but it may bring with it certain medical problems.

Many women say that they can remember when they first noted the displacement (prolapse) of one of the anatomical structures. They may relate it to a fall or to a bout of sneezing or coughing. But, like most problems associated with aging, the change actually occurs gradually over time. The first symptoms may be a subtle heaviness in the pelvis, back pain, constipation, urinary retention, or urinary frequency.

Sometimes urine may leak when one coughs, strains, laughs, exercises, or moves from a sitting to a standing position. This is called *urinary stress incontinence.* It should be differentiated from a second type of incontinence, *overflow incontinence,* which occurs when there is loss of sensation of a full bladder. Overflow incontinence may be a result of drugs, anesthetics, tumors, being bedridden, a change in mental status (Chapter 19, *The Nervous System*); it is not caused by relaxation of the pelvic anatomy.

If you have difficulty holding your urine, see a gynecologist for an examination. This problem can be alleviated with Kegel exercises. To perform these exercises, begin by practicing during urination by attempting to tighten the muscles to interrupt the urinary flow. Once you can do this, you can perform the exercise any time during the day. Repeating this maneuver ten to twenty times, three to four times daily, may enable better urinary control. If unsuccessful, surgery is an alternative. There is usually no need for women to suffer the social inconvenience of incontinence.

Relaxation of the back of the vagina may produce a *rectocoele,* a pressing-forward of the large bowel and accompanying constipation. Often women with a rectocoele find that they can produce bowel movements by inserting a finger into the vagina and pressing toward the rectum while straining. As with urinary problems, rectocoeles can be repaired successfully with surgery. It is unnecessary to suffer with this unpleasant and uncomfortable problem.

Prolapse of the uterus occurs when the supporting ligaments stretch and relax and the uterus drops into the vaginal cavity. The cervix may appear just inside the outer lips of the vagina, or it may protrude slightly. This is usually not painful, but it may be quite uncomfortable.

Although advanced prolapse of the uterus usually requires *hysterectomy* (removal of the uterus), many times it can be treated less radically with a *pessary*, a device inserted into the vagina to support the uterus and prevent it from descending. Because the upper portion of the vagina is relatively insensitive to pain, most women are able to tolerate a pessary quite easily. Interestingly, pessaries have been employed for centuries.

Relaxation of the pelvic organs does not present a problem for the majority of women over fifty-five. Some degree of relaxation is commonplace. If you have symptoms of prolapse, back pain, or urinary irregularity, be certain to have an examination by a gynecologist. There is little reason to live compromised by these relatively normal aging changes.

Vaginitis

Vaginitis in women over fifty-five may result from decreased estrogen production. This produces increased fragility and thinning of the vaginal tissues and most frequently is felt as itching in the vaginal area. Cracks in the delicate vaginal mucous membranes may be produced by sexual intercourse or by irritation and chafing not related to sexual activity. Sometimes bleeding may result, which contrasts this type of vaginitis from that seen in premenopausal women. Before menopause, bacteria, or bacterialike microorganisms, often sexually transmitted, produce itching, irritation, discharge, and pain. The decreased vascularity (blood supply) of the postmenopausal vagina usually does not provide as welcome an environment for these organisms.

A standard treatment for *atrophic vaginitis* (the unfortunate term for the postmenopausal form) is topical application of estrogen replacement creams placed in the vagina. Some medical providers will try other alternatives before resorting to estrogen creams. It is sometimes necessary to perform a biopsy of the vaginal or vulval tissues to rule out the possible presence of cancer. This can be performed as an office procedure, using local anesthesia. As has been noted previously, although vaginal spotting or bleeding in a postmenopausal woman is often caused by small cracks in the tissues, it deserves a thorough medical investigation.

Although less common than prior to menopause, women over fifty-five may get symptoms of vaginitis from yeast infections. Also called *moniliasis,* this form of vaginitis is caused by a species of *Candida,* a fungal organism that normally resides in the vagina. It produces a whitish, often "cheesey" discharge, which may itch and burn in the vaginal area. When the normal balance of yeast and other organisms is disrupted, these organisms may proliferate and produce the unpleasant symptoms of vaginitis. This may also occur as a result of menopausal hormonal change, diabetes, or antibiotic therapy and may be aggravated by wearing tight-fitting nylon underwear that impairs ventilation, excessive cleaning of the vaginal cavity, or sexual contact. Yeast infections, however, are usually not considered sexually transmitted diseases, because *Candida* is not only normally present in the vagina, but is a ubiquitous organism in the environment.

Yeast infections are usually treated with a prescription vaginal cream or suppositories. Some women are also successful with vaginal douching, using an iodine preparation (such as Betadine) that can be purchased over-the-counter. Usually one douche a day for about a week to ten days is effective. Another method is to douche with one to two teaspoons (5 to 10 cc's) of white vinegar in a quart (1 l) of warm water. Self-administered douching should not be considered a substitute for good medical care.

Vaginitis may also be caused by the bacteria *Gardnerella vaginalis.* Often the discharge is yellowish and malodorous, but it may mimic a yeast infection. Since the causative organism is different, the therapy is usually different. Metronidazole (Flagyl), taken three times a day for ten days is generally employed.

Cancer of the Cervix

Although cancer of the cervix is most common in women in their forties, it can occur at any age. The number of cases of this type of cancer has been declining in recent years, possibly because of early detection with Pap smears. This appears to be another situation in which early detection of cancer brings positive results.

Vaginal bleeding is an important warning sign of cervical cancer. Cervical cancer is currently believed to be more common in women who have had multiple sexual partners, genital herpes infections, and venereal warts (condylomata accuminata).

When cervical cancer is detected early the superficial premalignant cells can be removed as an outpatient procedure. More advanced cell changes may necessitate a brief hospital stay for a very extensive cervical biopsy called a *conization.* This defines the extent of the abnormal cells. Treatment may also entail radiation and chemotherapy.

Pap Smears

A Pap smear is a screening examination for cervical cancer. It involves taking a sample of cells from the cervix and examining it under the microscope for abnormalities in growth and configuration.

There has been considerable controversy recently about Pap smears, particularly about how frequently they should be obtained. Although a yearly pelvic examination and Pap smear are routine among younger, premenopausal women, postmenopausal women may not need these as often.

The American Cancer Society has recommended, based on a study performed in Canada, that women between forty-five and sixty-five with negative smears in two consecutive years have a Pap test every three years. After age sixty-five the guidelines are less clear, and women should decide on the frequency of pelvic and Pap exams with their medical providers.

Gynecologists who disagree with these recommendations cite cases of women who have had a normal Pap smear one year, skipped a year, and then were found to have invasive and widespread cancer of the cervix. Many gynecologists therefore recommend a yearly Pap smear regardless of age. Since blood pressure, weight measurement, blood tests, urinalysis, stool and rectal examination, electrocardiogram, and other screening tests may be performed during this yearly visit, physicians cite this as another reason to go for a yearly Pap test.

Even if a woman has had her uterus, cervix, or both ovaries removed, she still should have regular Pap smears. For instance, if a woman has had a hysterectomy and an ovary is left (to preserve normal hormone levels), a Pap smear may help detect cancer in the vagina or ovary. Although the smear is less accurate in such cases than in detecting cancer of the cervix, it is a low-cost and safe test that can be of help.

Cancer of the Uterus

Cancer of the uterus most often affects women during and after menopause. Although it is one of the more curable types of cancer, it is the cause of death of approximately 11,000 women each year. This is because it is too often not detected and treated early.

The cardinal sign of uterine cancer is vaginal bleeding, spotting, or staining not associated with a menstrual period. Although this bleeding does not necessarily mean cancer, it is an important sign that *must* be evaluated by a physician. He or she will perform a *dilatation and curettage* (D and C) to obtain tissue for microscopic analysis. Be aware that taking oral estrogen replacement for menopausal symptoms increases one's risk of uterine cancer (see Chapter 3, *Menopause and After*). Obesity, hypertension, and diabetes may also increase one's risk.

The treatment of cancer of the uterus depends on the stage in which it is discovered. Surgical removal of the uterus (hysterectomy), radiation, chemotherapy, and hormone manipulation with drugs have been used alone or in combination.

Much has been written in the popular press about the abuse of hysterectomy, and many misconceptions about it exist. As a treatment for most cancers of the uterus, hysterectomy or hysterectomy plus radiation therapy is frequently the most desirable form of therapy if the cancer is localized in the uterus. In postmenopausal women, *oophorectomy* (removal of the ovaries) is almost always indicated. They are largely nonfunctional, and removing them frees women from fear of ovarian cancer, which is often most difficult to diagnose in its early stage. Also, it is possible for a tumor to spread from the uterus to the ovaries. Hysterectomy does not impair sexuality, and the operation is extremely safe.

Women with a malignant tumor of the uterus almost always have vaginal bleeding. It is therefore essential that any vaginal bleeding in a postmenopausal woman be promptly investigated by a physician. Although a Pap smear can be helpful in pointing out abnormalities associated with uterine cancer, it does not detect this disorder as effectively as it does cervical cancer.

Cancer of the Ovary

Ovarian cancer is generally a disease of women over fifty (average age at diagnosis is fifty-two). It is the fourth leading cause of death from cancer in women (exceeded only by breast, colon, and lung cancer). Each year 14,000 women die of the disease.

Some studies indicate that women who have never conceived are at greater risk than women who have had children. This finding is based on statistical analysis; the underlying reason is not known.

Unfortunately, cancer of the ovary is difficult to diagnose, and it is often not detected until the disease is far advanced. There is no screening test as yet to detect the disease, and the early signs may be extremely subtle. Nausea, difficulty moving one's bowels or passing gas, increasing waistline without weight gain, bone pain, or a vague feeling of abdominal pressure or fullness are potential symptoms. But often these are signs of ovarian cancer that is fairly widespread throughout the pelvic region.

The goal of treatment is surgical removal of the tumor mass, followed by chemotherapy, radiation treatments, or both. Although ovarian cancer can be a very aggressive type of tumor, it is also one for which chemotherapy and radiation are successful treatments. Many drugs have been shown to be active in arresting the cancer for various lengths of time, and new combinations are being tested to maximize the effectiveness of treatment. Since these treatments need to be evaluated in clinical studies to determine which ones are best, it is worthwhile for women to be treated as part of a study. There are many institutions where this can be done under the care of a gynecologic oncologist, a physician with specialized training in cancer care, who can follow the response to the medications and monitor their side effects.

Cancer of the Vulva and Vagina

These cancers are rare, accounting for only 1 to 2 percent of cancer in women. Unfortunately, many women do not report the sign of an abnormal lesion promptly to a physician and seek treatment only when the cancer is widespread. Denial seems to be a central factor in this. Any unusual lesion on the vagina or vulva requires immediate medical therapy, so that disfigurement or death does not result. Depending on the size and extent of the lesion, treatment may involve chemotherapeutic creams or surgery.

—M.B.

Genitourinary Problems in Men

There is no physiological menopause for men as there is for women. Without medical illness men can retain their capacity for reproduction until death. In fact, there are numerous reports of men who have fathered normal children in their nineties. Although the number of sperm and the amount of fluid ejaculated diminishes with age, the capacity to produce children is not lost.

Impotence is the inability to maintain an erection for the purpose of sexual intercourse. It is of great concern to men as they advance in years, often being associated with an inevitable decline in strength and social stature. There is nothing normal or inevitable about impotence, so any change in sexual functioning should be investigated by a physician.

With advancing age certain changes take place in the anatomy of the prostate gland that often result in difficulty urinating or obstruction of the flow of urine from the bladder. *Prostatism* is the general term used for difficult urination caused by enlargement of the prostate. Confusion sometimes exists between prostatism and *benign prostatic hypertrophy*. The latter is the *noncancerous* enlargement of the prostate gland, quite common in men over fifty-five, that gives rise to prostatism.

The Prostate Gland

The *prostate* is a cone-shaped, three-lobed glandular structure that lies in front of the rectum at the base of the bladder in men only. It covers the first inch or so of the male urethra as it leaves the bladder. The gland is covered by a tough, fibrous capsule, which does not stretch easily in response to enlargement of the glandular tissue inside the prostate. Because of this inelasticity, enlargement of the prostate may compress the urethra and inhibit the outflow of urine. This common and very unpleasant problem affects about 10 percent of men over fifty.

The cause of the enlargement is not well understood. In most men it is a noncancerous process, called benign prostatic hypertrophy, felt to be related to changing levels of estrogen and testosterone as men age. Whatever the cause, it is not uncommon for the gland to triple in size over the course of a lifetime.

The principal function of the prostate is to secrete fluid that enriches and transports sperm during ejaculation. It regularly produces about ½ to 2 cc's (1/10 to 4/5 of a teaspoon) of fluid each day. This is excreted

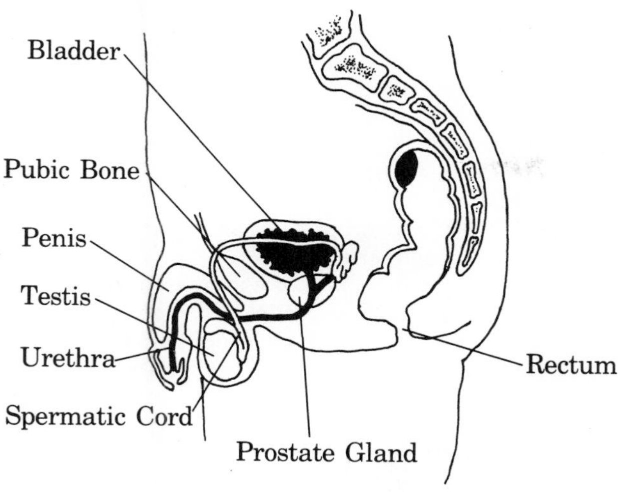

Anatomy of the male pelvis.

in the urine. During ejaculation about 3 to 5 cc's, 6/10 to 1 teaspoon, of fluid is produced. It comprises about 80 percent of the ejaculatory fluid called semen (sperm is only a small fraction).

The prostate enlarges and becomes functional at the time of puberty. It continues to grow slowly, so that by age forty most men demonstrate some enlargement, which may result in prostatism, but only 10 percent of all men actually will have problems with prostatism. Three diseases are usually associated with this enlargement: benign prostatic hypertrophy (BPH), carcinoma of the prostate (cancer), and prostatitis (infection). Unless caused by gonorrhea, prostatitis is not common in men over fifty-five. Carcinoma, however, is fairly common. It is the third leading cancer in men. Benign prostatic hypertrophy is by far the most common of the three conditions.

Prostatism

Prostatism is a general term for obstruction of the flow of urine from the bladder through the penis caused by enlargement of the prostate gland. The symptoms of prostatism most commonly include: difficulty starting a stream of urine; dribbling urine or having a reduced stream; urinating at night while in bed; dribbling slightly during the day onto the undergarments; decreased force of the stream; feeling that one has to urinate more often; sensation of a full or partially full bladder after urinating; or occasionally blood-tinged urine. Sometimes the symptoms are extremely subtle and are uncovered only in a routine physical examination. In other situations an attack may be precipitated by antihistamine drugs, tranquilizers or anticholinergics (for Parkinson's disease), or by cold weather

Besides the discomfort and social incapacity, prostatism can lead to damage of the kidneys and continued infections of the entire urinary system. Stagnation of urine provides bacteria with a place to grow and thrive. Obstruction may lead to back-pressure, which can damage the kidneys.

Evaluation of the prostate by a medical provider should begin with rectal examination. The two lateral lobes of the gland can be felt in this manner, and enlargement or suspicious growths (called *nodules*) can be uncovered. If there appears to be an irregularity, an *IVP* (injection of a dye into the arm and subsequent X-ray study to trace the excretion of urine from kidney to bladder and out) may be helpful in evaluating the problem. If there is still question after the IVP, further examination by *cystoscopy* may be needed. This involves inserting an instrument into the bladder, via the urethra, to visualize the urinary outlet. A *cystourethrogram* is an X-ray evaluation that provides similar results.

Benign Prostatic Hypertrophy

Many misconceptions exist about benign prostatic hypertrophy. I would like, instead, to present some facts. First, it is not cancer. Second, its surgical treatment does not usually lead to impotence or a diminution of sexual drive. Surgical treatment generally does result in ejaculation into the bladder (retrograde ejaculation) and sterility, but not impotence.

There are three types of surgery for BPH. The most commonly employed is the *transurethral resection* (TUR), in which the enlarged portions of the gland surrounding the urethra are "snagged" with an instrument inserted through the penis. Tissue that does not impede urinary flow is left in place. This procedure is relatively safe and easy, and it can be performed under spinal anesthesia with the patient awake. This procedure should produce neither impotence nor incontinence. After the operation a tube, called an *indwelling catheter,* will be left in the urethra and bladder to allow for the outflow of urine. It usually stays in for about three days after the surgery. When the urine is clear of blood, the catheter is removed and normal urination will gradually be restored.

When the tissue to be removed is too large to be drawn through the penis, surgery must be performed through an incision in the lower abdomen (*suprapubic* and *retropubic prostatectomy*) or just forward of the anus (*perineal prostatectomy*). Because these procedures invole an incision through the skin surface and general anesthesia, they involve some added risk. Unfortunately, prostatectomy usually produces impotence, and 10 to 15 percent of those so treated are incontinent of urine as well.

Some men cannot tolerate surgery either because of advanced years or a medical condition that greatly increases the risk of having an operation. In this situation a permanent indwelling urinary catheter may be necessary. The catheter will drain urine from the bladder into a bag that is strapped to the leg. Unfortunately the presence of the catheter is likely to produce infections. Although these can be controlled with antibiotics, often resistant organisms grow that are difficult to control.

Cancer of the Prostate

Cancer of the prostate generally occurs in men in their sixties, seventies, and eighties. It may not give rise to symptoms of prostatism and is thus unfortunately often discovered only after it has spread to the bones.

Sometimes small areas of cancer are discovered in the tissue removed to treat prostatism caused by benign prostatic hypertrophy. When this occurs, many physicians wait before attempting additional therapy to see if the entire cancer has been removed. During this waiting period, regular rectal examinations, at least twice a year, should be performed. During the digital exam, the medical provider will be feeling for suspicious lumps or signs of enlargement on the remaining portions of the prostate. Treatment for cancer of the prostate that is found to be localized to the gland is a prostatectomy, surgical removal of the prostate.

The alternative may also be local radiation, either implanted into the prostate or given by external beam. In cases where the cancer has spread to distant lymph nodes or bone, radiation therapy is usually employed. This treatment is palliative in that it reduces the painful symptoms, but it is not curative. If the cancer has spread to only small areas within the pelvis, radiation may be curative. Many ongoing studies are trying to find effective chemotherapeutic drugs for the treatment of prostatic cancer. Men who wish to be treated as part of one of these studies should contact the oncology department in their nearest large hospital.

Orchiectomy is the surgical removal of the testes. It is a common method of treatment of advanced prostatic cancer. It may be helpful in reducing bone pain and in slowing the spread of the disease. The surgery is relatively safe and simple. It involves, however, a serious emotional adjustment for many men. Surgical implantation of prosthetic testes is available for men who are concerned about appearance after the operation.

Impotence

As is true with sexuality and menopause in older women, many myths exist about sexual activity for older men. Impotence, or at least a lack of interest in sex, was once considered normal for older men. Conversely, continuing to want to have sexual relations was considered to be lecherous, dirty, deviant, or in some other way wrong. As medical attitudes about sexuality for older men and women began to change, it became apparent that doctors knew very little about what was a normal amount of sex for older people. In reality there is probably no general rule that applies. One thing is certain: impotence should neither be ignored nor considered normal. If you have a change in your ability to obtain or maintain an erection, have it investigated thoroughly by someone trained in this area of medicine. This generally means a urologist.

Men differ from women in that there is no set time for cessation of fertility. Nowadays one hears much talk about male menopause, but there is actually no point in a man's life when a significant decrease in testosterone (male hormone) production occurs. Most men may experience a change in the frequency of desire to have sexual relations, but this does not necessarily correlate with changes in levels of hormones in the body. In the absence of any particular medical problem that causes changes in the testes, brain, or other parts of the hormone-producing system, men remain capable of bearing children throughout life.

Myths about Male Erections

Males are capable of having erections from infancy, even though they are not capable of reproduction until puberty. Men have erections during sleep, generally approximately every ninety minutes. This is called *nocturnal penile tumescence*.

Myths about potency and the size of the penis are as common as they are false. Most men see flaccid penises in locker rooms or public men's rooms, which gives the impression that penis size varies greatly among men. In fact, regardless of size when flaccid, erect penises are usually about the same size. Furthermore, size has little to do with satisfying a partner during intercourse. This is because the vagina conforms to the penis during sex, and the inside is relatively insensitive anyway. It is the outer portion and the clitoris (which is completely external) that become stimulated and lead to orgasm.

Yet another myth is that sex is stressful to the heart (see also Chapter 13, *The Heart*). In fact, the average heart rate during intercourse is about 117 beats per minute, less than that during a brisk walk or a heated argument. There is little to support the popular myth that many men die during sex. The heart is taxed less during intercourse than during a cardiac stress test, and death associated with this test occurs about 1 out of every 10,000 times. Regrettably, sex is not a good way to get exercise, either for losing weight or building up the heart and lungs. It burns only about 150 calories on the average, far less than does a moderate exercise routine.

Finally, lowered hormone levels generally *do not* cause impotence in men, and injections of testosterone are not a cure for impotence.

What Is Impotence?

Masters and Johnson have defined impotence as "an inability to achieve or maintain an erection of quality sufficient to accomplish successful coital [sexual intercourse] connection." This does not mean that you are impotent if you have occasional failures caused by drinking too much, not being aroused, being nervous, or not being able to ejaculate. Impotence also does not have anything to do with how well you satisfy your partner.

If you can get an erection with masturbation, or if you wake up in the morning or at night with an erection, you are not impotent. These are signs that any difficulty in achieving an erection during intercourse has to do with how you feel about sex or your partner.

Causes of Impotence

Like other medical problems, there is no single underlying cause for all impotence. For most people it seems related to emotional factors like depression or anxiety. Yet certain medical problems can produce impotence. They may be related to the nervous system, such as a herniated spinal disc or a disease of the nerves that supply the pelvis. Impotence can also be caused by diseases of the blood vessels that supply blood to the pelvic area. Probably the single most common medical cause is diabetes, which probably affects both the nerves and the blood vessels that are involved in the erection mechanism.

Because there are many possible reasons for impotence, the problem should be fully investigated by a urologist. This specialist often works with other professionals, including psychiatrists or psychologists, to understand fully the emotional reasons for the problem.

Erection and ejaculation are physical processes under the control of two different branches of the nervous system. Ejaculation is stimulated by the *sympathetic nervous system,* the adrenalin-controlled system that we also use for "flight and fight" responses. Erection, on the other hand, is under the influence of the *autonomic nervous system,* which controls those body functions like digestion that we perform without thinking. Some medical problems, such as multiple sclerosis, alcoholism, and removal of the prostate, are more likely to produce impotence by interfering with the autonomic nervous system and the ability to achieve erection, whereas diabetes probably affects the sympathetic nervous system (and the blood vessels) and therefore the ability to ejaculate. Because the problems can be diverse and complex, it is important to undergo a complete medical, as well as psychological, investigation.

Evaluating Impotence

Depending on general health, personal medical history, and symptoms, a number of tests may be useful in establishing the cause of an impotence problem. Usually this means blood tests to screen for diabetes, thyroid disease, certain hormones produced in the pituitary gland (located in the brain), and some other substances located in the blood that may point to specific diseases. A rectal examination of the prostate, cystometrograms to evaluate the bladder, and tests of the blood flow through the penis may all be useful. The particular tests that are suggested by a medical provider should be discussed with each individual so he knows their use and significance for his personal history.

A fairly recent type of test is for NPT, or nocturnal penile tumescence, which records the frequency and intensity of erections during sleep. This tests the function of the autonomic nervous system, which controls erection, and can help tell whether the problem is primarily psychological or physical.

The test is performed by placing a pressure-sensitive gauge on the base and the tip of the penis. This device is painless and does not require any invasive medical procedure. It is left on during the night, and erections are recorded on a polygraph machine. It is probably best performed in the sleep lab and is usually used in medical centers before a surgical operation is contemplated in the treatment of impotence.

Penile Prosthesis

A relatively new approach to the treatment of impotence is the surgical implantation of a device for making the penis erect. There are two kinds of devices (prostheses). One is a pair of padded rods implanted along the shaft of the penis; the other is a pump that puts fluid into two reservoirs surgically implanted along the shaft.

Although some success has been reported with the rod-type prosthesis, it also has drawbacks. The first is that the penis remains permanently erect. Second, partners report that it may feel too hard or painful and may bend in the vagina during intercourse. The firm rods also may injure the soft tissue of the penis.

The pump-type device involves placing a pump in the scrotum, a reservoir that holds the fluid under the muscles of the abdomen, and inserting two inflatable cylinders along the penis. Pumping fluid into the cyl-

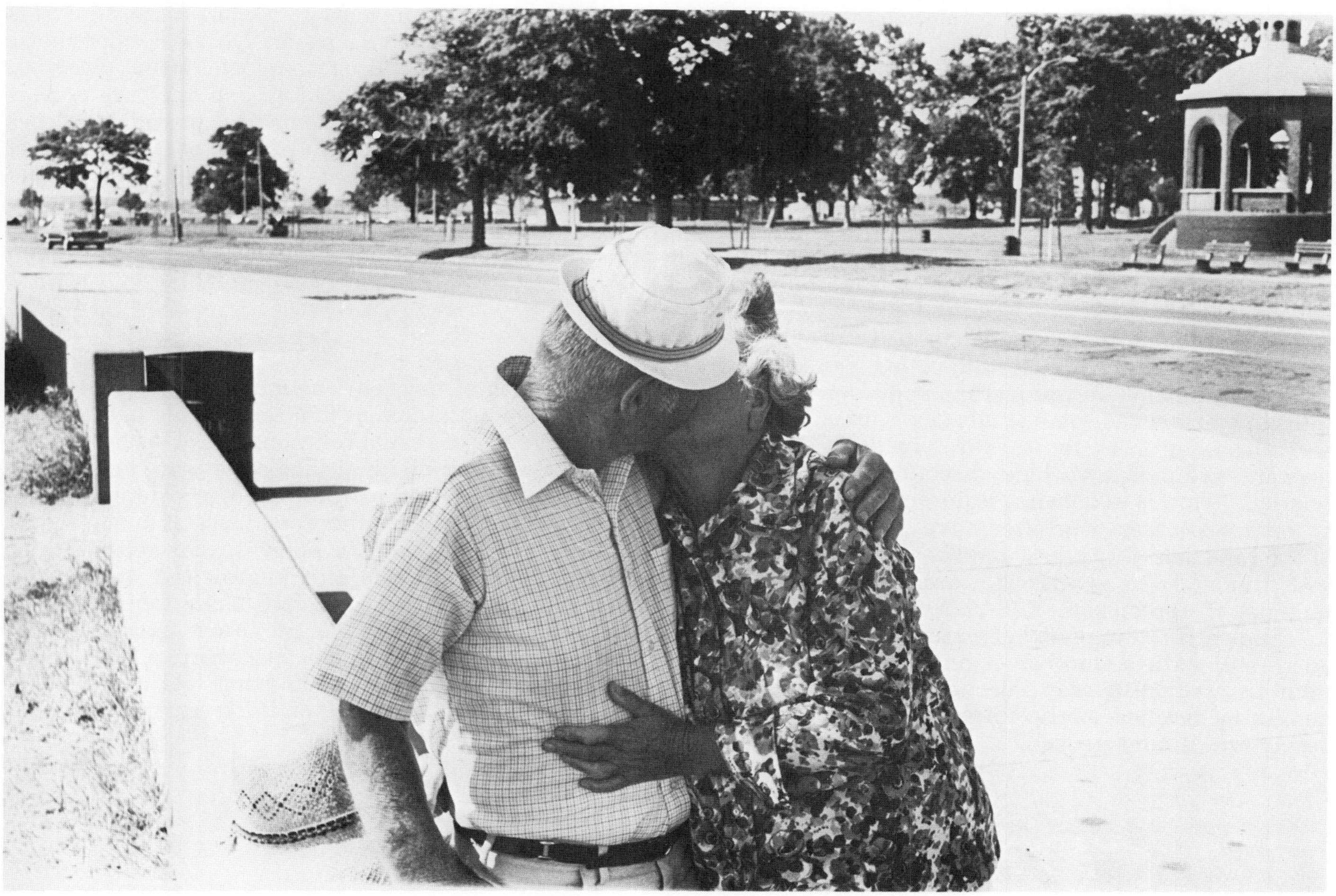

inders produces an erection, and the prosthesis can be deflated after sex by pushing a button that can be felt through the scrotum.

This device can produce an erection but not orgasm and ejaculation if they were not possible prior to the operation. It also may not be satisfying to one's partner if she is not accepting of the prosthesis. Since sexual relationships involve two people, it is helpful to undergo the entire process of medical evaluation with one's sexual partner, if at all possible.

The issue of implants for men raises the question of the role of the penis in confirming masculinity. Since the prosthesis does not ensure orgasm for either party, it may not in any way resolve sexual difficulties that exist. There are other forms of lovemaking and of loving that may be satisfying without sexual intercourse. This is a new area of medical intervention, and one that should be considered within the context of our social expectations. Many factors comprise maleness, and erection is only one of them.

—H.P.

Venereal Diseases

Sexually transmitted diseases in older people are often neglected by medical practitioners and not included in textbooks, reflecting a commonly held set of prejudices that assumes people in this age group are not sexually active with more than one person. Because this is not necessarily so, it seems appropriate to include a discussion of venereal diseases in this chapter as well.

Trichomoniasis, an infection produced by the organism *Trichomonas vaginalis,* is a form of vaginitis that is known to be sexually transmitted. Male partners do not get symptoms of this infection but act as carriers; they should therefore also be treated for it. The symptoms in women are similar to those of the other forms of vaginitis but may also include burning or discomfort with urination. Trichomoniasis can be diagnosed by a medical practitioner by finding the protozoan in a sample of vaginal fluid. The usual form of treatment is metronidazole (Flagyl), given in either a single large dose (eight pills) or as three pills daily for ten days.

Although somewhat unusual in older people, *gonorrhea,* produced by a bacterium called *Neisseria gonorrhea,* is epidemic in younger men and women. Symptoms in men are the same at all ages: pain on urination and discharge from the urethra. In postmenopausal women, symptoms include discharge, itching, and burning. This is somewhat different than gonorrhea in younger women, who often have no overt symptoms of the infection. Cultures should be taken by a medical practitioner from all possible areas of infection, including, if appropriate, the pharynx (from oral sex) and the rectum (anal sex). Treatment of gonorrhea is successful with a number of antibiotics that can be administered orally or by injection. All sexual partners should be notified of the infection, so that they can receive treatment as well.

Those over fifty-five can also contract *syphilis* or *herpes* through sexual activity. Syphilis is caused by the spirochete bacterium *Treponemum pallidum,* whereas herpes is produced by a virus.

Symptoms for both infections are similar in men and women. Both produce lesions in the area of sexual contact. Syphilis typically first appears as a red, raised firm lesion that is not painful. This *chancre* appears in the area of contact and then disappears after a few weeks without treatment. The next stage of syphilis appears as general malaise, possibly a low fever, and a skin rash that can cover any part of the body. This, too, disappears without treatment. These two stages of syphilis are the contagious stages. After the rash disappears, syphilis remains in the body without symptoms, only to reappear years later, after it has spread throughout the body and done damage to an organ. If syphilis progresses to this stage without treatment, it can cause blindness, mental incapacity, and death. Syphilis has been called "the great masquerader," because its symptoms mimic those of many other diseases. For this reason it is important to have a blood test that can reveal the infection. Once found, it can be completely cured by antibiotic therapy.

As with other viruses, however, herpes cannot be eradicated by any antibiotic treatment. The virus lies dormant in the nerves of the area of contact and may reappear at almost any time. The skin lesions of herpes are filled with fluid and have reddened borders. They are usually painful, last for about seven to ten days, and then disappear. If the history and appearance of the lesion is not readily diagnostic, viral cultures may be obtained for confirmation. Unfortunately, at this time there is no known cure for herpes. Symptomatic relief may be obtained by using cool soaks, avoiding contact with irritating clothing, and applying creams that can be suggested by a medical provider. Herpes is highly contagious, and 50 percent of those initially infected will have recurrent episodes. One should avoid sexual contact during the period when lesions are evident. (For additional information on herpes, see also the discussions in Chapter 11, *The Ears, Nose, and Throat,* and Chapter 22, *The Skin, Hair, and Nails.*)

—M.B., H.P.

✽

The health of the genitourinary organs is essential for both the maintenance of internal body balance and the enjoyment of sexual relationships. This latter area is one in which individuals and society are undergoing dramatic changes in attitude in regard to aging. We now know that, unless there is illness, it is normal for both men and women to enjoy sexual relationships throughout life. Sex is an integral part of our self-image and well-being. Therefore, changes in sexuality should not be considered an inevitable part of the aging process. Problems in this area require a thorough medical evaluation. We should not feel that our capacity to enjoy this facet of life ever wears out or completely wanes.

—H.P.

Chapter 18
The Skeleton

John Coblyn, MD; and Donald Abrams, RPA

The skeleton is composed of bones, ligaments, and cartilage. Together these structures give shape, strength, and protection to the body. Along with the activity of the many muscles, the skeleton provides the basis for movement, essential to life.

There are 206 bones in the body. They manufacture blood cells and store calcium. Ligaments hold bones together in the joints. Cartilage is the elastic tissue that supports and protects bones from damage caused by shock and movement. It also gives the skeleton the flexibility to bend. Tendons connect muscle to bone.

Rheumatologists are medical specialists who treat problems of the joints and soft tissues. *Orthopedists* are surgeons who treat problems affecting the skeleton that require surgery. Although these two specialties overlap somewhat, the sections of this chapter are divided along lines commonly associated with the work these physicians perform.

The Joints

Over 16 million people in the United States (at least 15 percent of all people over forty-five) think that they have *arthritis*. It is the most common crippler in America, Canada, and the other Westernized nations, and a multibillion dollar industry has arisen from its treatment. In spite of how common arthritis is, there is a fundamental misconception among physicians and the public about what it is, and what can be done about it.

In fact, there are over one hundred different kinds of arthritis. It is not just a disease of older people, nor does getting older mean that you will get arthritis. Its medical and surgical treatment has undergone vast improvements in recent years, yet many physicians still leave their patients with the depressing feeling that nothing can be done to alleviate their pain and improve their ability to function.

I have two principal goals in this discussion: to clarify what arthritis is and to explain what can be done for it with conventional medical and surgical therapy. In general, there is no reason for anyone to feel that he or she has to live with that pain and disability.

Not everything that hurts is joint pain or arthritis. Many people have pain caused by *tendonitis, bursitis* (inflammation of the padlike sac or cavity found in the area of joints), or *capsulitis* (inflammation of the covering of the joints). I will discuss these problems separately under the heading soft tissue rheumatism. The most common forms of arthritis are *osteoarthritis* (also known as degenerative joint disease), *rheumatoid arthritis, ankylosing spondylitis,* and *gout* and other "crystal" diseases. They all involve inflammation and degeneration of the joint; their differences will be explained in this chapter.

In additon to arthritis, bone diseases such as *osteoporosis* and *osteomalacia* affect older people. Many misconceptions exist about these diseases, so it is worth looking at them to identify what they are and what can be done about them.

The Structure of Joints

The joints of the body bear the great weight and stress of our movements. They act as shock absorbers and, with our strong muscles, provide support for the skeleton. The strength of the joint and its muscles protects it from wear and tear—but not forever. It is not surprising that arthritis is so common if we remember that few machines remain problem-free under constant use for fifty or sixty years.

To understand what arthritis is, we need to have an idea of the anatomy and workings of a typical joint. Most joints of the arms and legs work like a hinge. Adjoining bones are connected by *ligaments* and separated by *cartilage,* which reduces friction. They are also surrounded by *tendons,* which connect the muscle to the bone, and by *bursa,* a padlike sac that cushions the joint. All of these anatomic structures are covered by a *capsule,* which is fibrous on the outside and lined with cells on the inside.

Pain in the tendons, bursa, ligaments, or the joint capsule is not true arthritis, although it is often mistakenly called that. Arthritis is specifically inflammation of the inner lining of the capsule (called the *synovium*) or degeneration of the cartilage or bones within the joint. This occurs for nonspecific reasons in osteoarthritis or as a result of prolonged inflammation of the lining cells in rheumatoid arthritis.

Osteoarthritis (Degenerative Joint Disease, or DJD)

Osteoarthritis is the most common form of arthritis. It may occur in a number of different forms. It generally tends to run in families and affects the small joints of the hands most often. What is most reassuring about this problem is that it does not imply disease elsewhere in the body.

Osteoarthritis is "wear-and-tear" arthritis. We do not know why most degenerative joint disease occurs. In addition to the hands, the most commonly affected joints are those that do the work of carrying us around. That means the hips, knees, and less commonly, the ankle.

Previous injury to the cartilage of the joint seems to make development of degenerative joint disease more likely. This is because the normal padding and protection is worn away, and bone begins to rub on bone, producing pain. Because the padding between the bones

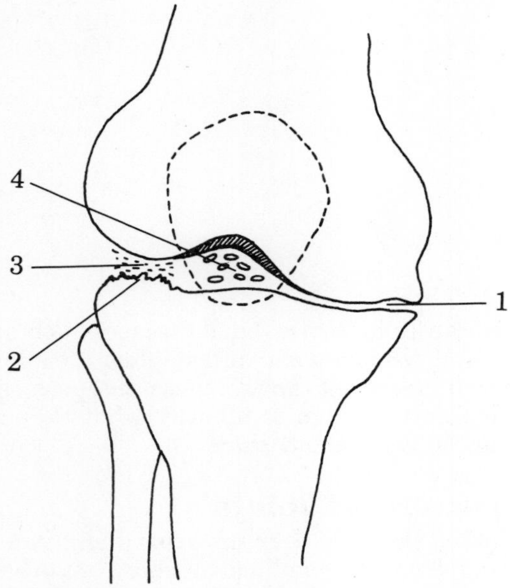

Typical arthritic changes in the knee joint: narrowing of the joint space (1); irregularities in the bony surface (2); inflammation (3); small pieces of bone eroded into the joint space (4). Any joint can be affected by degenerative joint disease.

has been eroded, this form of arthritis feels worse with exercise or walking and usually feels better with rest. Unfortunately, if the disease progresses and the normal space between the bones within the joint is lost, pain may also occur at rest.

A common sign of osteoarthritis is bumps, or nodules, on the joints of the fingers. These nodules, like the joints themselves, may be painful. The bumps will not go away with time, but the pain can be controlled with medication, local treatments, and rest.

Treatment of osteoarthritis is directed toward relieving the painful and limiting symptoms, not toward cure. Antiinflammatory medications are used. *Aspirin,* if it can be tolerated, *is still the best and most economical form of treatment.* Judicious use of canes and splints may also be helpful to rest and relieve the stress on painful joints. Local treatments applying heat to the skin overlying the joint (and creams like Ben-Gay or aspirin-containing preparations like Myoflex) may temporarily relieve pain as well.

Joint replacement surgery has revolutionized the treatment of severe osteoarthritis. Before this surgery was developed only twenty years ago, people with severe disease of the hips and knees were doomed to a life of severe pain and often were unable to walk. With the surgery people can walk without pain. In over 95 percent of cases, people come out of the surgery pain-free.

Whether this operation is needed depends on the symptoms. People who cannot control their pain with medication and who find that their lives are severely limited by pain will benefit from the surgery. Although it is a major surgery, it is one that most people tolerate well. Therefore, there is no reason for people to be crippled by this form of arthritis when it affects the knees or hips. Unfortunately, successful replacement of other joints, like the shoulder, ankle, or wrist, has not yet been developed.

Rheumatoid Arthritis

These forms of arthritis are different from osteoarthritis in several ways. Not only do they affect the joints in a different manner, but they also affect other parts of the body. The cause of rheumatoid arthritis (RA) is not well understood, but the current theory is that people are genetically susceptible to it and this inherent predisposition arises in reaction to some unknown environmental factor—perhaps a virus. After a virus infection, the theory goes, a chain reaction occurs in the body in which substances called *antibodies* are formed. Instead of fighting the infection, they attack the body's normal tissues. Rheumatoid arthritis is sometimes therefore referred to as an autoimmune disease: the immune system responsible for defense against infection attacks normal body tissues.

Rheumatoid arthritis is not only a disease of people over fifty-five, although it does affect people in this age group. More often women are affected earlier, but with advancing years this changes, so that men are equally affected by late middle age.

Rheumatoid arthritis may start suddenly with many swollen and warm joints, or it may develop insidiously

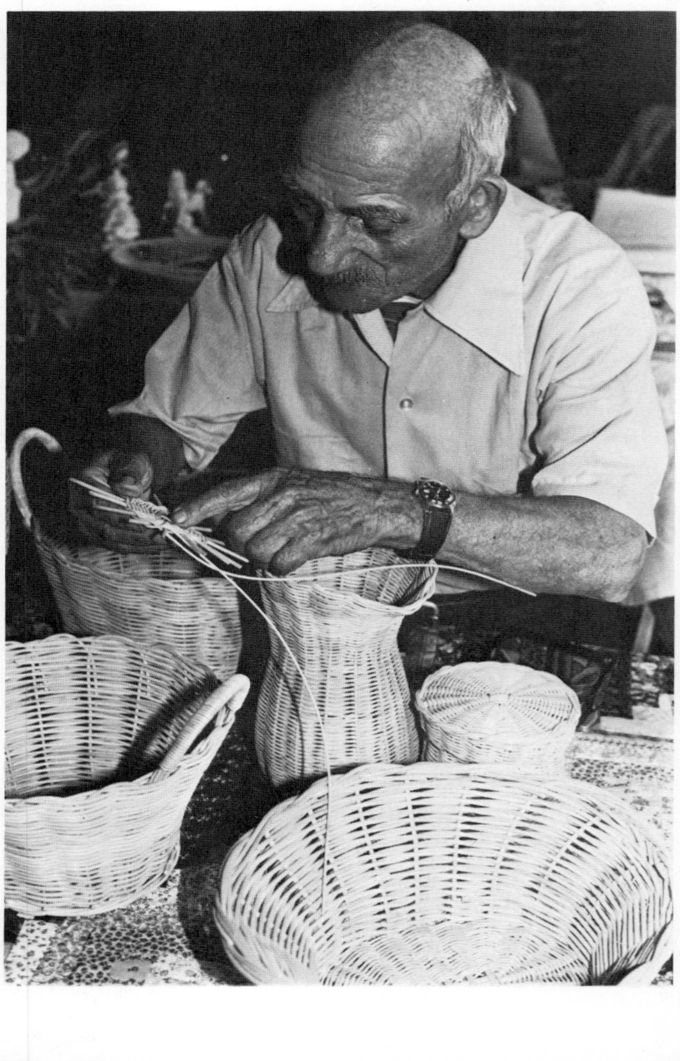

over many years, with one joint after another becoming involved. Or it may affect only one joint, like a knee or hip. It may affect other parts of the body like the skin (producing rashes and nodules), the lungs (producing nodules, fibrosis, or fluid in the lung cavity), kidneys, and other vital organs. People with rheumatoid arthritis may become anemic and tire easily.

The stiffness of RA differs from osteoarthritis in that it does not improve with rest. People commonly feel worse after a night's sleep, and this stiffness improves with movement. Symptoms of malaise and weakness similar to the flu may also be felt.

The treatment of RA involves time and usually two types of medications. Time is useful because some people (less than 5 percent) get better spontaneously, without treatment. The medicines either suppress symptoms of pain and inflammation or induce remission.

The suppressive medications like aspirin and the more expensive alternatives such as Motrin, Naprosyn, Clinoril, and Tolectin make one feel better but do not cure the disease. The symptoms tend to recur once the medication is stopped. Steroids, like prednisone, act in this fashion as well. The remission-inducing agents act differently. They are designed to promote a cure by arresting the autoimmune process. If they are employed early in the disease and if they are effective for a given individual, they should eliminate or reduce the necessity of taking suppressive medications.

Only three drugs have been proven effective as remission-inducing drugs: Plaquenil (hydroxychloroquine), gold salts, and penicillamine. Plaquenil has an interesting history. A derivative of quinine, it was first used to treat malaria. It is taken as a pill, and as with other remission-inducing drugs, must be taken for three to six months before results may be seen. The principal side effects are skin rash, stomach upset, and occasionally visual problems. Because the drug affects the eyes, it is important to have regular examinations by an ophthalmologist while undergoing the treatment.

Gold salts are given in a series of at least twenty consecutive injections. They have potentially toxic side effects; urine and blood tests must be taken periodically to follow the effects of the medications. Gold salts also may produce skin rash, kidney problems, and less commonly, blood and bone marrow toxicity. Usually when the gold treatments are discontinued, these side effects go away. Despite the potential side effects, gold salts have been extremely helpful for some people. Overall, about one-third of arthritic sufferers treated with gold salts get better, one-third get somewhat better, and one-third are not improved or have side effects that make further treatment impossible.

The latest drug that is useful in producing remission is penicillamine. Taken as a pill, it has similar side effects to the gold salts, but may not be as effective. In general, most rheumatologists treat first with Plaquenil, then gold, and finally penicillamine. There is a good chance that one of these medications will be successful, and I therefore encourage people to seek medical treatment. There is no reason to assume that these diseases are hopeless.

Since the remission-inducing drugs take a number of months to be effective, a suppressive medication will frequently be used during the initial period of treatment. For instance, it is common to use aspirin in combination with gold to reduce the painful inflammation and improve mobility.

The popular press is filled with nutritional approaches to treating arthritis. Often there is no attempt to differentiate the type of arthritis that is to be treated with a particular diet, nor to give the underlying rationale for the kinds of foods prohibited or eaten. There is no dietary therapy that has been proven to be effective in either rheumatoid or osteoarthritis. Overweight individuals may, however, benefit from weight reduction. This will help relieve some of the stress placed upon the joints of the hips, knees, and ankles when you are walking.

Finally, despite popular myth, wearing copper bracelets has never proven to be of any value in the treatment of arthritis.

> “ I have had arthritis for about twenty years. I remember when I first realized that I had it. I was sitting at a friend's house and could not get up. I went to a chiropractor, and she did me a world of good. I exercised, but then it gradually got worse. Later I went to an osteopath, and then to a doctor at a big local hospital,
>
> I saw the doctor, who asked me, "What do you do for it?" I said, "What can I do for it?" He said that the only thing was aspirin, buffered if you can't take it straight. I said, "That's what I take." I have never taken any of the fancy pills that cost a lot of money and are not any better.
>
> I was never laid up with my arthritis. I walk and take Bufferin a couple of times a day when it is bad. I crochet, I read, socialize with others, get around. Sometimes it affects my crocheting. You know some days are better then others. Crocheting is good exercise for moving my hands. You have to keep moving, keep exercising, unless the doctor tells you not to. I do all kinds of exercises, and it loosens me up, especially my hands.
>
> I write a lot, and walk. I walk around the block, around the grounds here, walk wherever I can. When I sit in my chair, I say my beads, which helps my hands. Then maybe I'll get up and write a letter. If there is any advice I can give, it is to keep going. Don't give up to arthritis. It may come with age, but you can't let yourself be idle or another four or five things may become a problem. I am eighty-eight now. When I was a kid, sixty years was a long life. You gotta keep going. ”
>
> —Margaret O'Mara, 88

Spondylitis

Spondylitis consists of a great number of diseases that can cause arthritis but are not as common as osteoarthritis or rheumatoid arthritis. The treatment of this group of arthritis is quite different than the ones already discussed. Spondylitis, and specifically *ankylosing spondylitis* (AS), a very common disorder, usually begins in young people, specifically young males, but occasionally it is undetected until later life. The true incidence of AS is unknown, but it may affect as many as 1 to 2 percent of the population. If a male has prominent low back pain that begins before age 30, AS should be a diagnostic consideration. Often these patients are ignored by physicians because their complaints are only of low back pain and often no signs appear on either X-ray or laboratory testing to support the symptoms. This type of low back pain can be differentiated from the type that one gets after heavy muscular work or from a slipped disc by its relation to rest and exercise. The back pain classically feels worse after a period of rest and there is the characteristic morning stiffness as in rheumatoid arthritis. Spondylitis is basically an inflammation of those areas that connect one disc to another in the back. In addition, there can be a large amount of inflammation in the sacroiliac joints.

The treatment of spondylitis is not nearly as successful as is that for rheumatoid arthritis. Medications such as aspirin and the nonsteroidal antiinflammatory agents are as effective as any agents we know. Different trials of Plaquenil, as well as gold, have been attempted, but the results of these agents are inconclusive. Exercises of the low back help maintain the tone, but their true role is unproven.

Gout and Other Crystal Diseases

Gout attacks are produced when uric acid crystals are shed from the bloodstream into the joints, where they produce painful inflammation. The uric acid crystals act as a foreign body, causing not only pain, but destruction of the inside of the joint.

Uric acid is a product of normal body metabolism. It is excreted in the urine and, for most people, never becomes a problem. Although we do not know why the majority of gout cases occur, certain drugs (such as diuretics used to treat hypertension), diabetes, alcoholism, and some cancers can increase the body's level of uric acid. When this occurs, gouty arthritis, kidney stones, and deposits in the ear or skin (called *tophi*) may develop. If left untreated for a long time, crystals may be deposited in the kidneys, causing serious disease.

If you have a warm, red, swollen joint, your physician may want to test you for gout by taking a blood test. A higher-than-normal level of uric acid in the blood indicates possible gouty arthritis. To be sure that uric acid has accumulated in the joint, it may also be necessary to remove fluid from the joint space and look under the microscope for crystals. This test is done as an outpatient procedure, takes only a few minutes, and is not painful.

Gout is not generally treated with aspirin. Indocin or other nonsteroidal antiinflammatory drugs are far more effective for the acute attack. Colchicine is a drug that is often used, but it can produce nausea and diarrhea. Cortisone is effective but should only be used for a short period of time, since it has many side effects.

After the acute attack has subsided, long-term drugs to prevent other attacks should be discussed. If the blood test shows only minimal uric acid elevation, treatment may be postponed until and if there are further painful attacks. In general, once daily medications are begun to treat gout, one is committed to this course for life.

Despite a huge volume of literature, diet has few if any *proven* effects on the course of arthritis. Gout can be affected by diet, however. Any food that changes the kidney's handling of uric acid (such as alcohol) or contains a high content of protein (liver, red meats, shellfish) may precipitate a gouty attack. With the advent of the modern drug treatment of gout, however, diet plays a relatively minor role.

Soft-Tissue Rheumatism

Not all that aches is arthritis. The bursa, tendons, and other parts of the anatomy in and around the joints may become inflamed and injured. In general, the reason for this is not well understood, nor is it solely a problem of people over fifty-five. Pain and inflammation in one or more of these areas near the joint is, however, quite common. It can occur with heavy exercise or with normal activity.

Most *tendonitis* occurs in the elbow, where it is commonly called tennis elbow, or in the thumb; but it can occur in other actively moving parts of the body. *Bursitis* is common in the side of the hip, shoulder, and knee. Correct diagnosis of these conditions usually rests with the physician or other medical provider, who will perform a physical examination, take X rays, and ask questions about symptoms.

Treatment of all types of soft-tissue rheumatism involves rest, sometimes immobilization with a sling or other support, and aspirin or other nonsteroidal antiinflammatory medications. If the pain and inflammation are particularly severe or prolonged, injecting steroids into the painful area may be helpful. Although the exact reasons why these areas of the body become inflamed are usually not known, successful treatment may frequently be expected.

Vascular Disease

In addition to problems in and around the joints, rheumatologists often see people who have trouble with their circulation. They usually complain of pain in their feet, legs, or hands, and this pain worsens with movement and improves with rest. When the disease is far advanced, they may experience pain at rest.

Usually these symptoms are caused by poor circulation as a result of a narrowing and stiffening of the arteries, which limits the flow of blood to the muscles in the extremities. The effects of the limited blood supply are evident in coldness in the extremity and lack of a pulse, especially in the feet. Various X-ray and sounding techniques can further substantiate the diagnosis of peripheral vascular disease.

No medical therapies have yet been proven to be helpful for peripheral vascular disease. Surgery to replace or repair the vessels is the treatment of choice. It is usually successful in restoring circulation and improving one's ability to move without pain.

Drugs and Their Side Effects

The public spends approximately one billion dollars a year on different cures for arthritis, many of which have no proven scientific or medical basis. In some cases people improve spontaneously and attribute their relief to these unproven methods. Only in the treatment of cancer have more dubious medications been tried and touted. This includes vitamin C, dimethylsulfoxide (DMSO), and certain other vitamins and diets that have all received publicity but have yet to be found effective in tests with large numbers of patients.

The cornerstone of treatment for most of the arthritis and arthritis-like problems discussed in this chapter is *aspirin*. Although it has toxic side effects in the large doses necessary for many people with arthritis (twelve to sixteen tablets a day or more), it is still the least expensive and most effective of the readily available medications. It is an excellent anti-inflammatory agent, as well as a pain reliever.

All aspirin is the same. It does not matter whether it is purchased in a pharmacy or a supermarket, nor does it matter whether it is "arthritis strength" or not. The preparations that are labeled as such merely contain more aspirin, so you can get the same effect by taking an extra tablet or two of regular aspirin to make a comparable dose. In general you will still pay less.

Aspirin has side effects that make taking it in large doses difficult for some people. It can cause stomach upset, gastritis (inflammation of the stomach lining), or ulcers. It can also cause loss of hearing or a sensation of buzzing in the ears. Less commonly, it may produce asthma, and virtually all people who take large amounts of it will show a small amount of blood loss in the stools, an indication of irritation and bleeding in the stomach lining. For these reasons it is wise to make regular visits to a physician if taking the amounts of aspirin usually prescribed for arthritis. Although aspirin is the most commonly used medication in America and can be purchased without a prescription, it is not harmless. If it were discovered today, it would not be an over-the-counter drug.

Aspirin substitutes are available for arthritis sufferers who cannot tolerate aspirin. Indocin, phenylbutazone, Motrin, Naprosyn, Tolectin, Clinoril, Meclomen, Ponstel, and choline magnesium salicylate are all aspirin substitutes. They should be reserved only for those patients who are intolerant to aspirin because of bleeding or stomach upset. Each of these agents can cause the *same* side effects of aspirin (although some less often) and unique side effects of their own, such as headaches and depression with Indocin, aplastic anemia from phenylbutazone, decreased renal function from Motrin, Naprosyn, and Tolectin, liver disease from Clinoril, and diarrhea from Meclomen. Of course, the list can go on—only to highlight the side effects of all drugs. Which agent to use after aspirin is totally dependent upon patient tolerance and the physician's experience; none have been proven to be better than aspirin. Moreover, using these products may cost fifteen to twenty times more per month than taking simple aspirin. Thus, although a wide variety of aspirin substitutes are effective, they have their own side effects and only sequential trials will determine which agent is tolerated and effective for an individual. They should be prescribed with caution, only after aspirin fails.

Hydrocortisone and other steroid drugs are the most effective antiinflammatory drugs known. They are useful for *short* courses of therapy (rarely for more than a few months) but are extremely dangerous for long periods of time. Their side effects include ulcers, weight gain, osteoporosis, redistribution of body weight, hair growth in undesirable places, thinning of the skin, and an increased risk of infection. Cortisone can also be injected into painful areas of bursitis and tendonitis, but again this should not be repeated over long periods of time. Individuals taking steroids should discuss their side effects and the goals of treatment with a medical provider. These medications should be used only with extreme caution.

—J.C.

Living with Arthritis

A helpful pamphlet for people with arthritis is called *Living with Arthritis*. It provides basic information on the major types of arthritis and their treatment, as well as a guide to many of the appliances that may be useful in adapting to the needs of daily living. It includes pictures of these aids and information on where and how they can be obtained. To obtain this pamphlet, write to:

Merck Sharp & Dohme
Division of Merck & Co., Inc.
West Point, PA 19486

Total Joint Replacement

In the last fifteen years, remarkable advances have been made in the replacement of worn out and seriously injured joints. The majority of the operations are on hips and knees that have been affected by arthritis, but the procedures are employed for injury or illness of other kinds as well. Replacement of joints other than the hip and knee has been less successful, but further investigation is actively under way for these joints as well.

The replacement of the hip joint involves insertion of artificial parts for both the long bone of the leg and the hip socket. The head of the prosthesis (the part that fits into the leg bone) is made of a strong, smooth metal. The socket portion is plastic, and they glide over each other, held together by the pull of the hip muscles. The materials are extremely tough and smooth, and there is little friction between the two parts of the prosthesis.

Recovery from hip replacement surgery is usually quite rapid. Usually one is able to walk with the assistance of a walker or crutches three to four days after the operation. Walking with full weight-bearing generally is possible in four to six weeks. The miracle of total hip replacement surgery is that movement becomes pain-free.

Recovery from total knee replacement surgery may take somewhat longer because there is more movement in the knee joint and a tendency for it to be stiff continues for up to three months after the operation. A total knee replacement prosthesis involves insertion of parts for both the bones of the thigh and calf, as well as the kneecap.

In about ten days to two weeks after the operation, it should be possible to walk in an immobilizing brace that supports the knee joint and limits its motion. In another week or two, the brace usually can be removed, and one can walk with crutches or canes. Stiffness may continue for up to three weeks, but walking should eventually be without pain, with a full range of motion.

—D.A.

Many alternative forms of medical and surgical therapy are available for people with the various kinds of arthritis. I find it disheartening to see people who have been told nothing can be done for them or that their only hope lies in an unproven wonder drug. It is possible to have a full, pain-free life with the judicious use of the treatments we now have available. If treatment has been unsuccessful I suggest consulting a rheumatologist who can work with you. Aging does not mean that suffering with the pain or limitation associated with arthritis is inevitable.

— J.C.

The Bones and Muscles

The skeleton, like other parts of the body, undergoes certain characteristic changes with aging. In general, height is lost because the spaces between the bones of the spine narrow. The bones also thin, a condition known as osteoporosis. This latter factor is responsible, in part, for the increased number of fractures that occur in people as they age. For the majority of people, however, osteoporosis is not a reason to be inactive or afraid of vigorous physical activity.

In spite of the physiological changes that occur in bones, the skeleton remains remarkably strong and viable throughout life. A prevailing myth claims that our bones heal more slowly as we age. Unless one suffers from other medical problems not necessarily related to the skeletal system, like diabetes or atherosclerosis, which impair blood supply to healing bone, normal healing can occur at any age.

A healthy skeleton can be maintained by regular exercise and good nutrition, as discussed in Chapters 7 and 8. In terms of our bones, this means taking in adequate amounts of vitamin D and calcium, as well as staying active. The strength of the skeleton is maintained by the constant stress and traction of our muscles exerting force upon the bones during exercise. It is therefore important for individuals who have had strokes or other medical problems to find ways to be active even with their limitation.

Minor injuries to muscles are extremely common in daily life and have become more common now that many people who were once sedentary are beginning to exercise vigorously. We all use the terms *sprains* and *strains,* even *myalgia,* interchangeably, although they have different meanings. *Bunions* and *calluses* are also common. To be more accurate, and to have a better understanding of how to treat these common problems, it is useful to learn their more exact meanings.

Myalgias, Strains, and Sprains

Myalgia is a nonspecific term for muscle pain. *Muscle strains* are mildly painful injuries to the muscle-tendon unit (the tendon attaches muscle to bone). Muscle strain is usually accompanied by swelling and some accumulation of lactic acid in the muscle. Lactic acid is produced when we burn complex sugars to provide energy for the muscle. Excess acid produces the *cramp* of overstressed muscles, usually most severe when out-of-shape people exercise. *Charley horse* is the lay term for small tears in the muscle fibers of the thigh or calf. This may occur along with excess lactic acid accumulation.

Muscle sprains are more severe injuries that occur when a ligament is torn (ligaments attach bone to bone). These injuries also produce pain and swelling.

Muscles are covered by a thin membrane called *fascia* (pronounced *fah-shuh*). At the end of the muscle, the fascia comes together to form the tendon. *Tendonitis* is a general term for inflammation of the tendon.

Common muscle strains are felt twelve to twenty-four hours after strenuous exercise or physical work. Unlike sprains, which usually are felt immediately after an overly forceful stretching of the muscle fibers, strains are often more generalized and slower to appear.

The treatment of strains is something that we all can become familiar with and use in our daily lives. First, all activity must be stopped when pain is felt. Second, ice packs should be applied for the first twenty-four to seventy-two hours. (Warm soaks can be applied later.) Cold reduces the pain, inflammation, and swelling. Third, the injury should be protected from further damage with a soft "ace"-type wrap bandage and elevated above the level of the heart to minimize swelling. Be careful that circulation in the fingers or toes of the injured extremity is adequate: they should feel warm and should be able to feel the light touch of someone pressing or stroking. If these sensations are impaired, a nerve or blood vessel may have been injured or the bandage may be wrapped too tightly. This is a sign to seek immediate medical attention. A full description of how to apply the wrap, heat, and cold is described in Part 4, *Emergency and First-Aid Guide.*

The rule therefore is: *rest; ice; wrap; elevate.*

If an injury is very painful, or there are signs of bleeding or rupture of the tendon or ligaments (if, for instance, there is an area of darkened discoloration or the extremity cannot be moved) it should be professionally examined and possibly X-rayed. These kinds of injuries may create fractures, since great force is applied to the bones. In the case of a fracture or other serious injury, application of ice and protection of the injury with a wrap will be helpful. Keep weight and stress off the injured area and get medical attention.

Preventing muscle injuries is the most useful strategy to adopt when starting to exercise. The detailed flexibility exercises presented in Chapter 7, *Physical Fitness,* help prevent strains, sprains, and other injuries. Do a warm-up and cool-down period of stretching. Do not use pain medications to cover up pain so that you can exercise more. Pain is a signal to rest. Injections of drugs and oral pain medications are a questionable practice in professional sports and have no place in the exercise routine of the average person.

Bunions

A bunion is the enlargement and protrusion of the ball of the foot (metatarsal bone). It occurs when the big toe has moved laterally, toward the outside of the foot, or when the metatarsal bone has moved towards the center. Probably the single most common cause, especially among women, is poorly fitting footwear. Sometimes bunions run in families.

Poorly fitting footwear, as well as the movement of the toes that exposes the ball of the foot, produces friction, which in turn stimulates enlargement of the covering of the bone. This occurs more often in people over fifty-five because of years of misuse and the gradual change in alignment of the bones of the feet. The rubbing also makes the area of the bunion red, swollen, thickened, and painful. Sometimes the toes curl and turn, making walking more difficult.

Bunions can be prevented by wearing shoes that provide room for the toes. Even if a bunion already exists, properly fitted shoes will avoid further aggravation of the problem. The toes should be able to point forward when you walk. There are also products that can be purchased commercially that help keep a space between the first and second toes. This keeps the big toe pointing forward, reducing the friction on the ball of the foot. An orthopedist or podiatrist can help with the purchase of this appliance.

You can also do some exercises to help straighten out the big toe. Gently stretch your big toe toward the midline, or inner side, of your foot for a few minutes, a few times each day. If you do this regularly, you can prevent bunion formation or reduce additional friction that will enlarge an already existing bunion.

If the bunion is extremely painful and restricts activity, it can be surgically removed by an orthopedist. There are many kinds of operations; the one the surgeon chooses will depend on the extent of the problem and the physician's personal preference. After the operation the same principles of foot care are essential to prevent new bunions—properly fitting shoes, exercises to move the big toe, and less friction on the ball of the foot.

Calluses

A callus is thickened skin. Like a bunion, calluses on the feet are produced through constant rubbing of improperly fitting shoes. Sometimes they occur because of poor posture while walking. Calluses on the elbow or hands usually result from friction during repetitive work.

Calluses that are painful or that restrict movement can be removed with one of many nonprescription preparations available in the drug store. They usually contain salicylic acid to dissolve the thickened dead skin. A family medical provider, podiatrist, or orthopedist can remove them as well. The important point is to prevent their formation to avoid the discomfort and potential restriction of movement. This means avoiding the continual rubbing that produced them. Calluses on the feet are a signal that shoes do not fit correctly or that the gait is abnormal. Calluses on the hands and elbows indicate that a change in posture during work is necessary. Protective padding on the elbows and heavy clothing on the arms can also help.

Low Back Pain

Pain in the lower back is an extremely common problem of people both before and after age fifty-five. Often this is a result of man's upright posture, which sets a highly movable upper spine upon a fixed lower spine, or *sacrum.* The twisting and moving of the upper portion against the lower creates strain on the *lumbar* region that lies in between. Tension and sitting for long periods at work also create low back pain.

Any sudden stress, or chronic stress created by muscular weakness, can produce an attack of low back pain. Obesity and poor posture, which place further stress on the muscles of the lumbar region, aggravate the pain.

The pain may be confined to the lumbar region of the back or it may travel (radiate) down the legs, in which case it is called *sciatica,* because the sciatic nerve supplies the legs and buttocks with stimulation. In general, sciatic pain appears a few days after pain is felt in the lower back, although it may appear immediately after a sudden twisting, lifting, or straining injury.

The symptoms of low back pain are usually aggravated by bending, twisting, lifting, sneezing, coughing, or straining during bowel movements. Because the pain is often extremely intense with movement, sufferers tend to stand and move stiffly in an attempt to keep themselves bent away from the injured area. Unfortunately, this usually creates added back strain and worsens the condition.

Although very incapacitating, most low back pain is only muscle strain. Because of this, the usual form of treatment is rest, augmented with local heat (like a hot pad, warm baths, and a hot water bottle applied to the lower back), pain medications, muscle-relaxing drugs, and massage. After the pain has subsided, it is a good idea to begin or continue a program of exercises like the Williams back exercises described in Chapter 7, *Physical Fitness*. It is also essential to learn strategies for lifting, working, and living that prevent back pain. Sufferers must learn what helps the pain, what brings it on, and what can be done individually to help.

The first strategy involves relearning how to move the body in relation to the back. Remember that the normal upright anatomy is based on a movable upper spine sitting on an immovable lower sacrum. Any object lifted at a distance from the sacrum will produce strain along that point. This occurs when objects are lifted with the back bent and the arms outstretched. Performing the same lift with the back *straight* and the arms at the sides will reduce this strain. The accompanying figure shows the correct way to lift, so as to minimize back strain. The strain in this method is on the legs, which are very strong compared to the back, not on the back. Bending, as well as lifting, should be performed in this fashion.

Williams exercises are useful for strengthening the abdominal and buttocks muscles. They also help to straighten out the exaggerated curvature of the lower back called *lumbar lordosis,* that most people develop. Further, they increase flexibility and help reduce weight along the waistline, additional aids in controlling back pain. These exercises do not cure back pain, but they do help strengthen the muscles that support the spine.

Other useful strategies include sitting upright in straight-backed chairs, avoiding slouching, sleeping on a firm surface (place a piece of plywood under the mattress to increase its firmness), and being certain to stretch before and after exercise and strenuous physical work. In general, most orthopedists find back braces, if they use them at all, helpful only during periods of muscle pain and spasm. After these symptoms subside, the brace should be removed so that the muscles are strengthened, thereby reducing the chance of future injury.

Disc Disease

In a relatively small percentage of people, low back pain is caused by herniation and dislocation of the disc that sits between the bones that make up the spine. This is often called a *slipped disc,* and the pain that

Helpful hints for a healthy back

Standing and walking

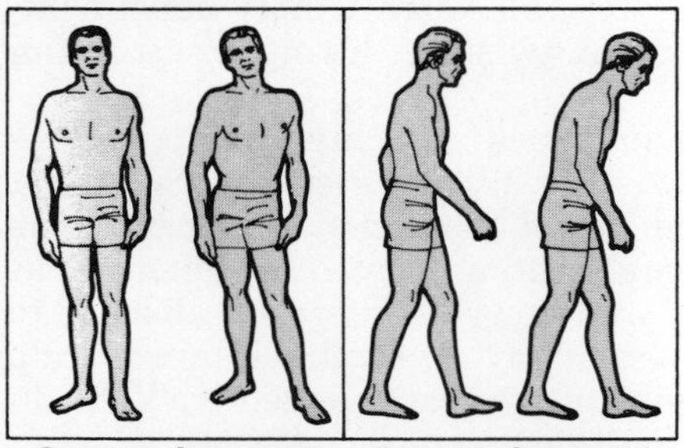

Correct Incorrect Correct Incorrect

Try to toe straight ahead when walking; put most of your weight on your heels; hold your chest forward and elevate the front of the pelvis as if walking up an incline. Avoid wearing high heels. Stand as if you are trying to touch the ceiling with the top of your head, eyes straight ahead. All the elements of good posture will flow from these simple maneuvers.

Sitting

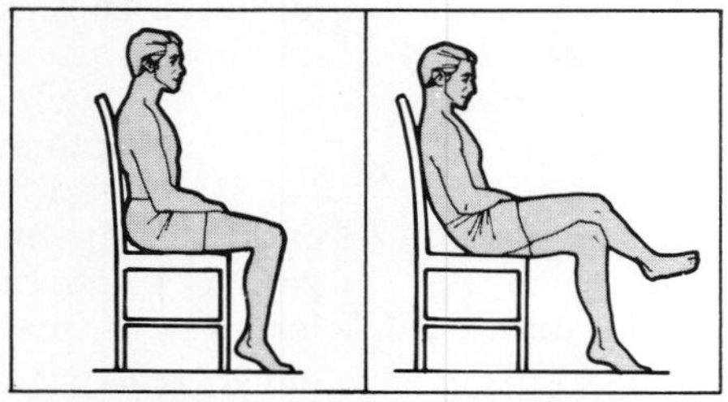

Correct Incorrect

Sit in a hard-back chair with spine pushed back; try to eliminate the hollow in the lower back. If possible, elevate the knees higher than hips while sitting in an automobile. Secretaries should adjust posture chairs accordingly. Sit all the way back in the chair with your back erect.

Lifting

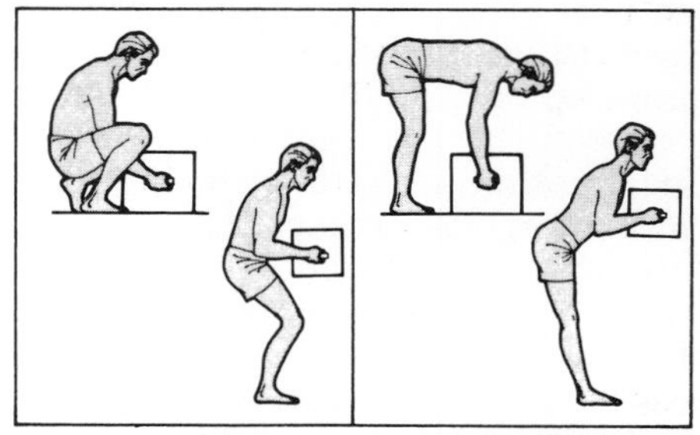

Correct Incorrect

Bend your knees; squat and lift with your thigh muscles, not your back. Never bend over with your knees straight and lift with the upper torso. Move slowly and avoid sudden movements. Try to avoid lifting loads in front of you above the waist line. Avoid bending over to lift heavy objects from car trunks, as this places a strain on low back muscles.

Sleeping

Correct

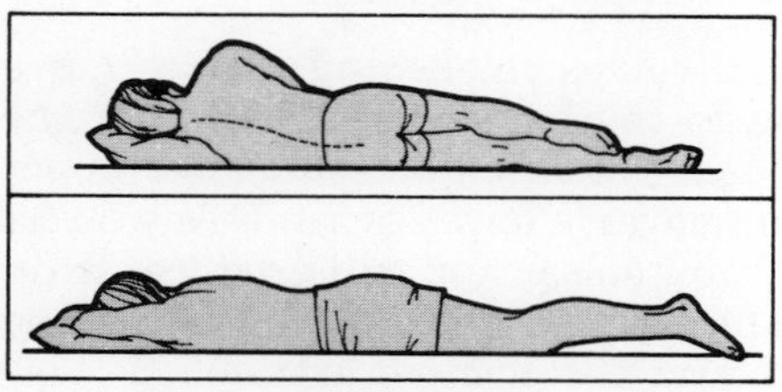

Incorrect

Sleep on a firm mattress; a ¾ inch plywood bed board is helpful and should be used with all but a very firm orthopedic mattress. With acute back pain, sleep with a pillow or blanket rolled under the knees and a pillow under the head. Keep your knees and hips bent when sleeping on your side.

Working

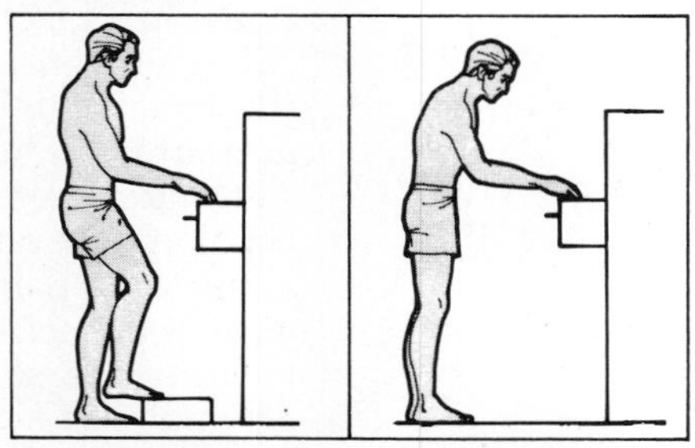

Correct Incorrect

Try to avoid fatigue caused by work requiring long standing. Flex hips and knees by occasionally placing a foot on a stool or bench. Take exercise breaks from desk work by getting up, moving around and performing a few back exercises in the standing position.

Driving

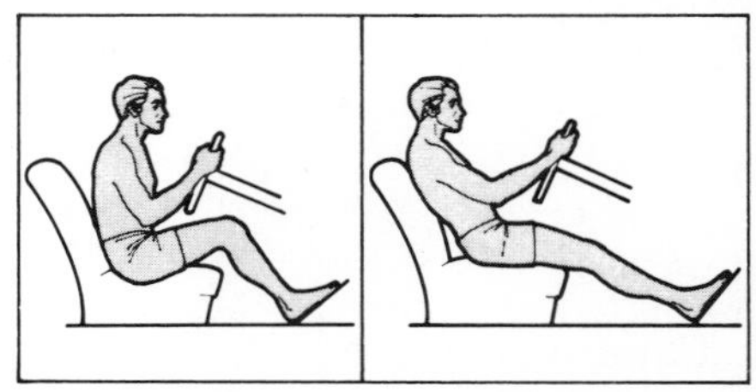

Correct Incorrect

Use a firm seat with a padded plywood or special seat support. Sit close to the wheel with knees bent. On long trips, stop every one to two hours and walk to relieve tension and relax muscles.

Proper positions for the basic activities of daily living to help prevent back strain and injury. (Reprinted with permission: Riker Laboratories, Northridge, CA.)

is felt results from the disc pressing on the nerves that come and go from the spinal cord.

The disc acts as a pad, separating the bones and cushioning the spine from pressure exerted when we stand upright. Shaped like a donut, it is composed of a tough outer covering and a soft inner portion. *Herniation* occurs when the outer covering weakens, allowing deformities in the normal circular shape of the disc. It may thought of as a bubble forming on an automobile tire when the inner tube bulges out of a tear in the outer tire. A slipped disc is thus usually not the product of the disc having moved, but of a deformity in the normal disc shape.

The bulges that occur in the disc then may press on the nerves that exit from the spinal cord. The result is pain, along with changes in normal neurological functioning, including loss of sensation in the lower limbs or groin, weakness in the legs or feet, a change in bowel or bladder function, or a change in normal sexual function.

It is not entirely clear why some people develop disc disease while others do not. Often the X rays of the bones of the spine will look abnormal, yet the discs will be normal. In other cases the X ray will look rather normal, and yet there will be serious disc disease. Most cases of disc rupture occur in the thirties and forties, although it is possible for it to occur in later years.

The initial treatment of debilitating back pain, with or without evidence of disc disease and nerve involvement, is usually bed rest. It is important to lie flat on the back, on a hard mattress, with a board between the box spring and mattress. If possible, it is best to stay flat continuously, which means using a bedpan to urinate and defecate. This is extremely constipating, so that measures like stool softeners, high-fiber diet, and increased fluid intake will be needed. Do not take mineral oil and Colace together.

Muscle spasm in the back may be relieved by antispasmodic medication. Local heat and vibration may also be helpful. Bed rest is psychologically difficult for almost everyone. It is normal to feel helpless and depressed. Yet it is worthwhile to be aware that it is better than traction or surgery, which are often necessary if bed rest fails. One to two weeks of uninterrupted bed rest usually serve as the initial form of treatment.

Sometimes severe spasm or pain must be treated with traction. This means lying flat with fifteen to thirty pounds of weight applied to the legs. After one or two weeks of bed rest (with or without traction), careful movement with a back brace support and/or crutches may be tried. If this is successful, a slow process of rest and exercise (like Williams exercises) should be initiated. A common problem is that people try to return to normal activity too rapidly and reinjure themselves. It is essential that the return to work, sports, and any form of lifting are done very gradually and with extreme care.

If rest does not work, myelography and surgery are the next steps. A *myelogram* is a form of X-ray test in which dye is injected into the spinal cord and films are taken of its passage from the lower back towards the head. Areas where the cord is being pressed upon because of disc disease or other problems may be seen on the myelogram. The myelogram is a useful and relatively safe tool that most surgeons require before contemplating an operation. It is questionable whether the test is worthwhile if no surgery is anticipated. Thus, before having this test, feelings about having surgery should be discussed.

It is estimated that less than 10 percent of people with ruptured lumbar discs must have surgery. With rest and patience, most people will respond to conservative measures. Surgery might be a preferable treatment under the following conditions:

- intractable pain that is emotionally debilitating
- loss of sensation or strength that impairs a normal life-style, including work and important recreational and interpersonal activities
- persistent alteration of normal bowel, bladder, or sexual function
- emotional or economic factors that make continued bed rest impractical

Fractures

A fracture, or broken bone, occurs when excessive force is applied to the bone. This can occur with falling, in traumatic accidents, in sports, or in response to certain diseases like tumors and nutritional deficiencies. Most people can recognize a broken bone. Pain, swelling, and often a visible deformity in the area of the break are the signs.

A fracture should be treated promptly by a trained medical person. Generally, this involves a cast to prevent further movement and injury, and rest. Some stress, even on an injured bone, will promote healing. For example, limited pressure on a leg fracture can be obtained by using a walking cast three to four weeks after the injury. A medical provider will be able to advise about the level of activity that is appropriate during the healing process. In general, fully healed bone is as strong as the bone prior to the injury.

A potential danger when a cast is fitted for a fracture is swelling that may impair blood flow to the affected area. Anyone treated in the emergency room and sent home with a cast should look for some important signs. First, be aware that swelling can be expected to occur for twenty-four to forty-eight hours after the injury. Increased pain, loss of sensation or warmth to the extremities (like fingers, hands, toes, or foot), redness, or red streaks on the skin are signs that the cast is too tight and cutting off circulation, that there is an impediment to the nerve supply, or that an infection has developed. Report them immediately.

There are four important rules for care after a fracture:

1. Elevate the extremity. If it is the arm, raise it on a pillow above the level of the heart. If it is the leg, keep it comfortably raised on a stool, and be sure to place a pillow under the knee to prevent muscle strain. These measures will reduce swelling.
2. Ice the injury for twenty-four to forty-eight hours. Avoid wetting the plaster cast by placing ice in a plastic bag and then loosely wrapping it around the cast in the area of the fracture. This helps reduce both pain and swelling.
3. Take adequate amounts of pain medication so that pain symptoms are fully controlled. Do not drive a car or operate machinery while taking these medications, as they produce drowsiness.
4. Report any numbness, pins and needles, severe pain, or change in color or temperature of the extremity *immediately*. Do not take extra pain medication in the hope that these symptoms disappear. These are signs that the cast is too tight, and unless refitted, permanent injury to the tissues may result.

Spine

With age, and often in conjunction with weight gain, comes an increased likelihood of fractures of the vertebrae that make up the spinal column. These fractures are not breaks in the bone in the same sense that we think of breaks in the arms, legs, or hips. Usually they are small injuries that do not cause the spinal column to move out of proper alignment. Treatment usually involves only a few days of bed rest.

After the injury it is common to have narcotic-containing pain medications prescribed by a physician. All of these medicines are constipating, as is bed rest. To minimize this effect, increased fluid intake, a high-fiber diet, and stool softeners prescribed by a care giver are helpful.

Fractures that occur in the neck are more serious than those lower on the spine, and they require more careful medical care. Without complete stabilization of these injuries, paralysis and death may result. A longer period of bed rest and a support to protect the neck are usually necessary.

Hip

Hip fractures are the most common serious orthopedic injury in people over fifty-five. This is especially true

Using a Crutch, Cane, or Walker

Many people feel unsteady when they walk. This may be because of an injury, stroke, or Parkinson's disease, or after an operation. There are aids available to provide steadiness and help one walk farther and with greater ease, but unfortunately, many people feel they will be negatively stigmatized if they use one. Too frequently a person in need of, but reluctant to use, a crutch, cane, or walker falls and suffers unnecessary and debilitating injury. It is far better to use one of these aids and be safe and mobile than to risk injury or stay at home, unable to get around the house or go outdoors.

Proper fit

Regardless of the type of appliance, the rubber tips at the bottom should be in good condition and wide enough to provide stability. Recommended size is 1 to 1½ inches (2.5 to 4 cm) in diameter at the bottom. Replacement parts can be obtained at a pharmacy.

The appliance should be the correct height. To adjust them:

Cane: Stand with the cane about five inches (12.5 cm) from your side. Your wrist should be straight and the height of the cane should allow a twenty- to thirty-degree bend in your elbow.

Crutches: Crutches should be fitted with your hands on the grips, wrists straight, and arms bent at a twenty- to thirty-degree angle. The top pad should rest two inches (5 cm) *below* the armpit. *Do not rest your armpit* on the crutch. Your weight should be supported on your hands, not your shoulders, to prevent possible damage to the nerves and blood vessels that run under the arms.

Proper use

Walker: The standard aluminum walker is light and extremely simple to use. Stand with your body in the walker, close to, but not touching, the appliance. Pick it up, place it in front of you, and take a *normal* step into it. Always place the four legs of the walker down at the same time; use your arms to help support your weight and steady your balance. You should always *lean forward* into the walker, never backwards. The back portion of the appliance has no stability.

Cane: A cane should be held next to your body, about five inches (12.5 cm) to the outside of your small toe. Your elbow should have a twenty- to thirty-degree bend, and your wrist should be straight.

A cane is meant to *share* your body weight. If one leg is weaker than the other, the cane should be held by the arm on the *stronger* side. Thus, if your left leg is weak or unsteady, carry the cane on your right side. Your body weight can then be distributed between the cane and the weaker leg. If both legs are equally weak or unsteady, it does not matter which hand holds the cane.

Crutches: The crutches should be adjusted to the proper height. Relax your shoulders: the weight should be on your hands, not armpits. To walk, place the crutches in front of you and walk into them. To prevent the crutches from slipping, take small steps and hold them with force exerted towards your body. The more you spread the crutches to your sides (away from you), the more *un*stable they will be.

—Patty Marcus, RPT

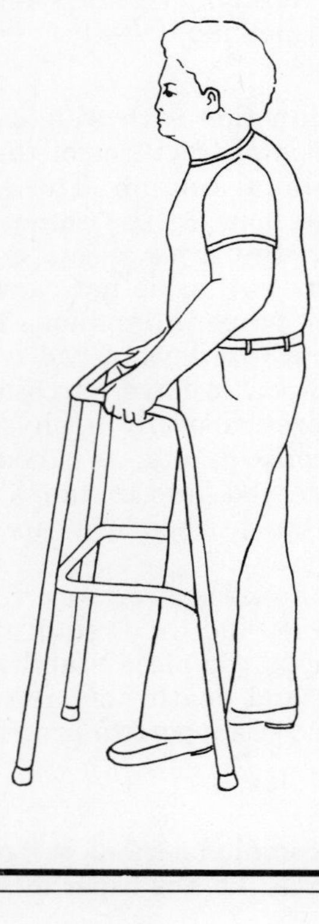

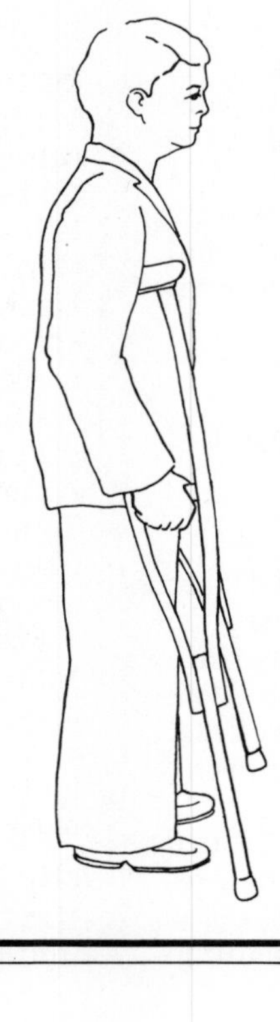

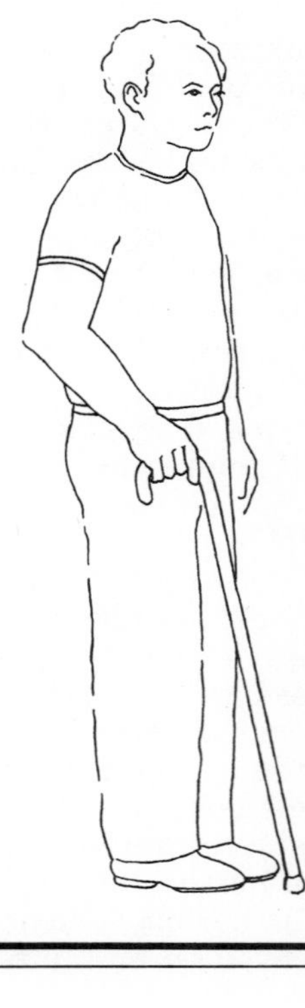

for women, possibly because of the weakening of the bones that occurs after menopause (osteoporosis).

These fractures often occur in conjunction with falls, although it is often unclear whether the fracture causes the fall or vice versa. Sometimes, however, these fractures occur without a fall or other traumatic accident.

The signs of a hip fracture may be dramatic or subtle, depending on the extent of the break. Usually there is pain in the area, swelling, shortening of the leg, and a tendency to hold it rotated outward. Some patients, however, are unaware of the fracture until it is discovered through an X ray. Pain in the hip area should be examined by a medical provider.

The treatment of hip fractures depends on the location and severity of the injury and to some extent on the preference of the orthopedist. Limited fractures may be treated by eliminating all weight-bearing for at least two to four weeks until there is no pain. During that period of time, the leg should not be raised in the straight position nor used as a lever to help change body position. Once X rays show that healing is under way, limited weight-bearing with a walker will help promote further healing. Usually these fractures heal well. Sometimes, however, they require surgical placement of a prosthesis to support the bones.

After surgery it is essential to watch for and report to the surgeon any pain, increased temperature in the area of the fracture, fever, limitation of movement, or discoloration. These are potential signs of infection, slippage of the prosthesis, or poor alignment of the bones. —D.A.

Metabolic Bone Disease

Our bones are in a dynamic state in which minerals and other basic constituents are continuously moving from bone to blood and back again. Our bones are constantly being formed, shaped, and reformed in response to stress and nutritional changes in the entire body. This dynamic structure tends to weaken as we age. This is especially true for women after menopause (see Chapter 3), but may also be true for men, and it is common in people who are bedfast because of other illness. It is felt that this process results primarily from changes in estrogen level for women after menopause, but other factors such as nutrition and exercise may be involved as well.

Two types of illnesses produce weakening of the bones: *osteoporosis* and *osteomalacia*. In osteoporosis there is a relative lack of *protein* in the bone, and sufficient calcium cannot be added to make protein-calcium substances that create the strong and resilient structure of bone. In osteomalacia the *minerals* are in short supply, and there are insufficient amounts of calcium and phosphorous to make strong bone. Osteoporosis is more common than osteomalacia in people over fifty-five.

The many potential causes for osteoporosis include thyroid disease, multiple myeloma (a form of cancer that originates in blood-forming cells of the bone marrow), and acromegaly (a disease that produces enlargement of the bones). By far the most common form, however, occurs after menopause or if a woman's ovaries have been surgically removed. The skeleton slowly begins to weaken, producing changes in posture and increasing the chance of fracture. These fractures commonly occur in the back, hip, and wrist.

Osteomalacia results from the loss of calcium or phosphorous through the kidneys or from a deficit in the dietary intake of these minerals. Another cause is a lack of sunshine, since sunshine is needed to convert a chemical in the skin to the active form of vitamin D, also necessary for normal bone formation. Osteomalacia is generally more readily treated than osteoporosis, because it is relatively simple to take in added calcium and phosphorous through improved diet or with nutritional supplements.

Osteoporosis that occurs after menopause is not quite so simple to correct. As Dr. Rothchild has pointed out in Chapter 3, there are many factors to consider in the decision to prescribe estrogens. I want to add that osteoporosis is a process that usually develops over many years, perhaps twenty to thirty. Starting to take estrogen replacement at age sixty-five or seventy does not necessarily reverse this process. In some cases it does help, but the side effects must be weighed against the risks. Women who are on estrogen replacement should continue to have regular examinations by a physician so that these potential side effects can be caught early. —J.C.

Contractures

Contractures of the arms and legs occur with disuse and atrophy of the muscles responsible for their movement. Most often this occurs after a stroke, but impairment of blood flow or nerve supply to a limb after an injury will also produce contractures.

Each joint has at least two opposing sets of muscles that move it. One set will pull in one direction, and the other set will pull the joint back in the opposite direction. This pairing is necessary because a muscle can only move in one direction, to contract. Contractures occur when a stronger, more dominant set of muscles remains unopposed by its counterpart muscles. For instance, the lower leg is moved by two sets of muscles. The calf muscle contracts to pull the leg backward; the thigh muscle has an opposing effect to move the lower leg forward. With disuse, or after injury, the calf muscles tend to pull the foot downward and the toes forward. This common type of contracture can be prevented (or at least minimized) with exercise. A physician or physical therapist can demonstrate how to do these exercises, and they can be performed on someone who has had a stroke or injury. They should be begun as soon as possible, because the longer the wait, the more difficult and painful the problem will become.

Three simple sets of exercises can be employed after a stroke or injury that affects the lower extremity. Before beginning, get medical clearance from a physician and instruction from either a physical therapist or medical provider. These exercises require two people: the injured person and a helper.

Ankle: Start with the injured person lying on his or her back. Place your left hand under the shin and gently lift the leg off the bed. Place your right hand on the ball of the foot and *gently* push the foot back toward the head. Hold it flexed for approximately ten seconds, but release tension before if this is painful. Repeat this exercise with the other foot. Do each foot

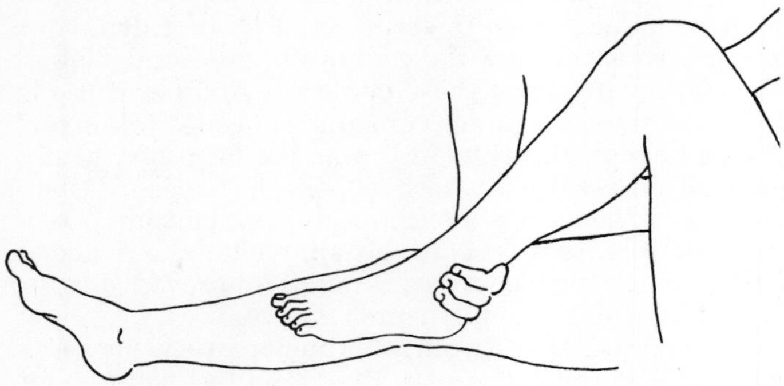

Ankle exercises to prevent contractures.

five times and repeat the entire excercise routine three to four times each day.

Knee: Start with the injured person lying on his or her back. Hold the ankle in one hand, and place your other hand on the underside of the thigh, near the knee. Lift the leg off the bed and bring the back of the heel toward the buttock. Then slowly straighten out the leg. Repeat ten times with each leg. Do this routine three to four times daily. Do not push the leg exercise past the point of pain.

Hips: To exercise the right hip, place the injured person on his or her left side. When exercising the left hip, the person should be on the right side.

Begin by exercising the right hip. Place your left hand on the lower portion of the right buttock, and place the knee in the crook of your right arm (at the bend of your elbow). Gently push your left hand toward their buttock and simultaneously slowly stretch the right leg backward (towards you) by moving your right arm toward your body. Repeat this ten times and perform three to four times daily.

Knee exercises to prevent contractures.

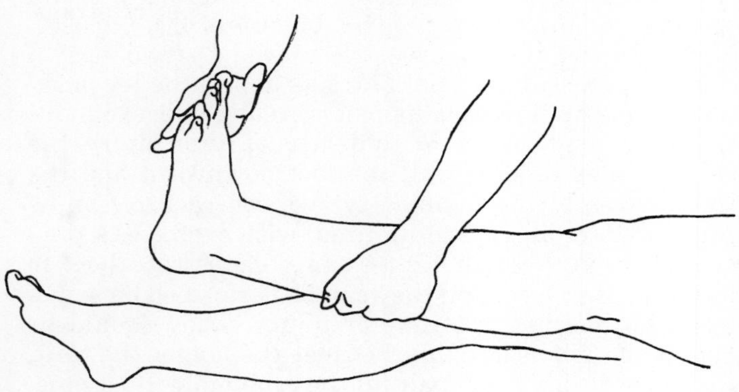

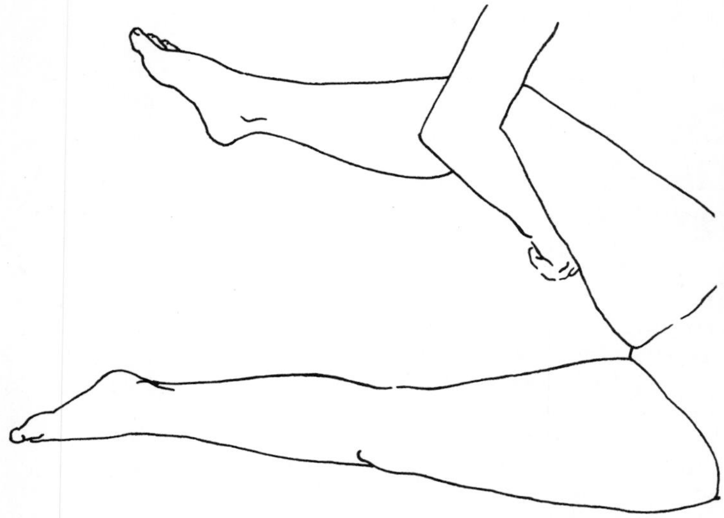

Hip exercises to prevent contractures.

Repeat the exercise for the left hip by having the person turn over and reversing the position of your arms.

❋

Orthopedics literally translated means *straight child,* but the surgical replacement of joints, the effective treatment of fractures, and the care of minor injuries like sprains and strains has made enormous improvement in the quality of life for people over fifty-five as well. With more people engaging in vigorous activity in later years, the need for the skills of the orthopedist is increased. Sports medicine clinics are valuable resources for young and older athletes. The orthopedist can provide information on the type of equipment to use, how to train, and how to avoid injuries. Although injuries can occur at any age, with some basic precaution, vigorous physical activity can be a part of everyone's life. The advances of orthopedic surgery can help people with arthritis regain the movement in painful joints as well. As Dr. Coblyn has pointed out, there is simply no need for most people to be limited by the common problems that affect the bones and joints.

—D.A.

Chapter 19
The Nervous System

Hank Pizer, PA-C

It is a popular, but untrue, myth that getting older means losing one's mental faculties. People use the word *senility* rather loosely to refer to the small episodes of forgetfulness or slight confusion that happen to people at any age but seem more frequent as we grow older. But true senility (*senile dementia* is the clinical term) is a neurological disease; it is *not* the result of getting older. It is a complex disease process with many possible causes, and one that can sometimes be successfully treated with proper medical therapy.

Mental decline is not a normal part of aging. We know that IQ remains fairly constant throughout our lives and that people can be productive at work and at hobbies at any age, particularly if they stay socially and physically active.

In the last twenty years, remarkable advances have been made in our understanding of the nervous system and in our ability to diagnose neurological diseases. We have been helped by the relatively new X-ray technique, the CAT scan (Computerized Axial Tomography Scanner is the complete name), which links the technologies of X ray and the computer. Great strides have also been made in neurochemistry, helping us understand the chemical basis of brain functioning.

Many of the medical problems that affect the brain in people over fifty-five appear to be a result of hypertension and atherosclerosis. Both subjects have been treated elsewhere, in Chapter 13, *The Heart,* and Chapter 8, *Nutrition.* I would like to reemphasize that good control of blood pressure and reducing the level of cholesterol and fat in the body can have a positive effect in reducing the chance of stroke and other problems of the nervous system. Controlling diet, exercising regularly, and receiving medical care for hypertension, if needed, are measures that we all can take to help prevent illness and to improve overall health.

Stroke (Cerebrovascular Accident)

Strokes are the third most common cause of death in the United States for people between the age of fifty and eighty. After eighty it becomes the number two killer. Men and women seem to be equally affected, and the risk increases in those who have diabetes, hypertension, or hyperlipidemia (elevated blood levels of cholesterol and fats). Recent years have seen some decline in the incidence of stroke, presumably because of better control of high blood pressure.

A stroke (sometimes called a "shock" by lay people) occurs when the normal blood supply to an area of the brain is interrupted. The brain is an extremely active part of the body (from a metabolic point of view), and it cannot tolerate more than a few minutes of impaired blood flow. Thus, any area deprived of its normal blood supply will quickly become injured and the tissues will die. Since these cells cannot grow back, an area of permanent injury results.

Most strokes are caused by formation of a clot (called a *thrombus*) in the brain. These clots appear typically in areas where the blood vessels are already narrowed and irregular as a result of atherosclerosis. Sometimes these clots form in the blood vessels of the neck and travel upward into the brain.

The nature and degree of loss of functioning that occur with a stroke depend on what part of the brain is affected. In general, injury to the left side of the brain affects movement and sensation on the right side of the body, and for most people, speech function as well. Conversely, if the right side of the brain is involved in the stroke, sensation and movement on the left side is likely to be impaired. This is because the nerve fibers that supply the body cross as they enter the brain.

High blood pressure, heart disease, previous transient ischemic attacks, diabetes mellitus, and atherosclerosis are all factors that increase the likelihood of stroke. Getting older does not necessarily mean one is more likely to have a stroke. In all likelihood, rather, it is the increased risk of acquiring one of the factors listed that predisposes people over fifty-five to cerebrovascular accidents. That is why the risk of stroke can be reduced by preventing these problems or controlling them once they have developed.

When a Stroke Occurs

A *stroke in evolution* is the medical term for the period of time when a stroke is occurring, during which the normal blood supply to the brain tissues is interrupted. It is an extremely frightening time that usually lasts from minutes to hours (rarely days). The symptoms vary in severity and type, depending on the area of the brain that is affected. They may include: loss of speech, disorientation, loss of sensation or muscle function, or alteration of normal bowel and bladder control.

Currently no medical treatments have been shown to be effective during a stroke in evolution. It is nonetheless important to be in the hospital so that heart, respiration, kidney function, and blood pressure can be assisted with supportive measures if necessary.

Once the stroke is finished, it is called a *completed stroke,* and the process of rehabilitation begins. For some people lost function—whether it is in movement, speech, or sensation—returns within a period that varies from a few days to as long as several months. In general, however, impairments of movement and speech that do not improve at all in one or two weeks are not likely to do so at all. Paralysis that remains after five or six months is likely to be permanent. Nonetheless, the goal for every person who has had a stroke is rehabilitation by a team of physicians; nurses; physical, occupational, and speech therapists; and counselors, the last of which help with the emotional aspects of recovery. This team approach has succeeded in helping many people recover function of lost abilities and develop strategies for learning new ways to compensate for losses.

Family Support

A stroke can be as devastating emotionally as it is physically. The person who suffers the stroke usually feels depressed, frustrated, and helpless. Loved ones have similar feelings: uncertainty about the future, guilt, remorse, and anger. Yet it is essential that in the time immediately after the stroke, family members approach the future with optimism and provide support for each other and the stroke victim. Their presence, along with the efforts of the rehab team, can impart a sense of hope that encourages the person to participate fully in the rehabilitation process.

Understandably, this is not easy. Initially the impairment of mental faculties may make the stroke sufferer seem different: removed, confused, and emotionally unpredictable. Being confined to a hospital bed, away from the familiar environment of home, exaggerates this, as does uncertainty about future recovery of physical and mental functioning. Will the stroke victim be dependent? Will major financial changes burden the family? Through all of this, it is worthwhile to remember that partial, or even complete, function can return in the weeks ahead. Only time will tell, and optimism helps in the rehabilitation effort.

Most hospitals are committed to involving the family in the care of the patient who has suffered a stroke. This should include counseling from the social service staff, which may include a social worker, psychologist, or psychiatrist. The attending physician is also a valuable resource. Families and the stroke victim should not have to deal with this crisis alone.

❝ There were very few tears shed at my father's funeral. Our tears had been shed during the four endless years of his illness. We all felt a tremendous sense of relief and gratitude that at long last he was free of his body and pain.

The day was warm and sunny. My mother sat at the graveside, loath to leave after the service was over and only immediate family remained. She told us that they had chosen the grave site because a tiny new tree had been planted there, and she liked to think that it would shade their graves someday. Now, forty years later, the tree, tall and majestic, shed a soft, green light over the new, raw grave. "Now I am ready to graduate," my mother said, and she rose and came away.

My father was always an independent man, a free spirit who adventured—gold mines, oil wells, wild schemes. Along with this he was a devoted and faithful husband and father. On all his adventures, he took my mother, my brother and me, and my great-grandparents, who lived with us. Wherever we traveled, home and security were where my father was.

A strong, vigorous man into his nineties, he woke at dawn, went marketing very early in the morning for the best and freshest food. He had, in very old age, taught himself to cook and produced delicious meals for himself and his wife. At the stockbrokers' office where he spent his mornings, he was the fountain of wisdom for the other board watchers. His wise advice on stocks and bonds was much in demand, and he did very well for himself. He was the patriarch of the family—my brother's family in Florida and mine in New York—very much loved and enjoyed by his children, grandchildren, and great grandchildren.

Suddenly, at ninety-four, he was struck down by a massive stroke. It left his mind clear, his memory on the whole unimpaired, but his entire left side was completely paralyzed. His every need and want had to be attended to. He was confined to a hospital bed and wheelchair. He valiantly tried, with great pain, to regain some of his body through physical therapy, but it was completely frustrating and to no avail.

My mother, aged ninety-three, watched over him in the hospital with the love and tenderness and courage that she had demonstrated through seventy-three years of marriage. During the four long years of his paralysis, even after the physical therapists had given up, she kept on, making him try to move an arm, a finger. She read to him and asked him questions, keeping his mind alert and alive in his almost dead body. He had never been a demonstrative man, but he said to her, "You are my life," and she was. She is a deeply religious woman with a strong faith. Near the end, even she, who never really accepted the fact that he could never improve and who could not in good conscience hope for his death, said, "Let God take care of him." When my father could no longer speak, or hear her, she sat beside him, hour on hour, holding his hand firmly, waiting for the moment when he summoned the strength to press hers.

As his daughter, I had a special relationship with him. He had expected my brother to follow in his footsteps, to be as strong and motivated as he was. Somehow his feeling for me was very different. His love was undemanding. Whatever I did pleased him. I always knew that whatever I became, whatever befell me in life, he would be uncritical, always there for me, a safe haven. When I telephoned my father over the many years of our living a continent apart, he always answered, "Hello darling." No one ever said "darling" in a way that moved me so deeply. Even as a seventy-two-year-old grandmother, I still felt like a beloved child.

During the years of his illness and physical decline, I knew what his brave front covered: the deep humiliation of being so helpless, of not being able to control bodily functions, of depending on nurses and attendants for everything. Once, from the depth of his agony, he cried out to us, his family, "Please don't abandon me!" As though we could or would. He was never out of our thoughts.

I found myself brooding on the unfairness of it. I felt a terrible responsibility to help him out of his tortured life. As he became more and more ill, cancer was found, and it became a question of what would come first, terrible intractable pain or death. My mind was filled with imagining finding a pill that would let him forget and drift off to an endless sleep.

My last visit to him and my mother in Florida was six weeks before his death. I sat all day at his bedside, taking my mother's place, holding his hand and willing him to sleep, to sleep forever. He would open his eyes and look to see that I was still there before he drifted off into unconsciousness, only to wake again. I sat, willing him to die, the father I loved so much, but his tough old heart beat on, still fighting for life.

I had to go home to my husband and family, but I was living unconsciously on a very superficial level. My real life was there in that hospital room with my parents. I felt a terrible, overwhelming responsibility and a feeling of guilt and helplessness. Somehow I should save him from this tortured time.

One night I couldn't sleep. I paced the house from dark room to dark room until morning came. I felt that I should be with my father, that I should be holding him in my arms, as he held me when I was his child. Now he was my child, and I was far away. Even if he was unconscious, on some level he would know I was there, helping him cross that threshold, keeping fear from him as he had kept it from me so many times. Early that morning the phone rang. My brother said, "This is the call." I wasn't surprised. I had been there all night.

My husband and I, our children and grandchildren flew to Florida the next morning. We stood at the graveside with my mother, my brother, and his family, not weeping, our hearts filled with thankfulness that at last he was free. My brother said that he felt our father, wherever he was, was now ready for new and exciting adventures.

After the funeral all of us—children, grandchildren, and great-grandchildren—met at a grandson's home where a feast had been prepared. My mother sat in a large armchair, like the queenly matriarch she is. One by one during the day each of us sat with her and told her how much we love her, how we respect her fidelity and character. What an example she has been to all of us—seventy-three years of faithful marriage, through thick and often thin, in sickness and health, literally until death parted them. She sat giving wise advice to grandchildren and great-grandchildren who live far away and see her seldom. They all had questions and problems that they felt she could solve for them. We all know that she is a special spirit who has an open line to "up there." There was such an outpouring of love and gratitude. She had kept us all from feeling too guilty about living far away and not sharing her burden by making us feel that it had not been a burden to her, but a labor of love that she needed to do herself.

It was a beautiful day of renewing family ties. It was an opportunity to show my brother and his wonderful, generous wife and children who lived near my parents how much we appreciate the unfailing responsibility and care they gave over the difficult years. Young cousins who rarely saw each other felt the warmth of belonging to each other. We older ones in our seventies watched our children and grandchildren experiencing the wisdom and warmth of our mother, who was a legend in our own families.

All day we talked and talked and retold stories of Grandpa's adventures from the time he came to America from the old country, at the age of five, and earned his first dollar selling newspapers. Stories of his adventures in Oklahoma and Mexico drilling for oil, the gold mine he bought in Arizona, his ups and downs. How magically he ended up and could insure independence for himself and his wife in their old age. How they indulged their love of giving presents, giving to charity, and helping those in need.

When the evening came, my husband and children and grandchildren flew back to New York. It had been a long day, a day none of us would ever forget. My mother said it was a good day, my father would have loved it, and so did she.

I stayed on with her for several weeks. I knew she needed to mourn and we would cry tomorrow. I had written a letter every day to my parents for years, assuaging my own guilt at being so far away when they were so old, so she knew of all our family doings from day to day and felt very much a part of my family back in New York. I would help her through the next period when the shock and numbness wore off and she would face the reality of being without her husband.

As for me, I shall never think of my father as dead. As long as I am alive, he will be alive, as vivid in my memory and feelings as he has always been. Now I shall be able to feel the joy of him, unspoiled by the sadness of his suffering. I feel a tremendous sense of peace and relief. I remember countless happy moments with him and the strong independence and security that his love built into me. I know that a loving parent is forever and can never really die. ❞

—Anita Ravage, 73

Among the many decisions that may have to be made are: Should the stroke victim be transferred to a specialized rehab facility for continued care? Is a nursing home needed? Can home health aids, visiting nurse, or volunteers come into the home to help with care? Will transportation be needed to and from the hospital for additional physical, speech, or occupational therapy? Whenever possible, these decisions should be made by the patient and family with guidance from an experienced social service and medical staff. Family members should not have to bear this responsibility alone, nor should the stroke victim.

Family can help with the exercises and rehab work. In most situations the rehab staff can provide only a few hours of attention a day, but family members can learn how to help with the basic exercises to improve mobility and coordination even while the patient is still in the hospital. They can also work with the occupational therapist in helping the person learn to bathe, go to the toilet, eat, dress, and perform basic grooming.

When the stroke victim is home, the family has an even greater role in the rehabilitation process. At that point the person is likely to receive only a few hours of attention a week from professional staff, so the major effort rests with loved ones. This can be both a burden and a positive aspect of the rehabilitation process. Working on specific goals helps structure the time spent at home. It helps the person who has had a stroke feel that others care and that there is hope.

None of this is easy, and the results are not always positive. I suggest that a continuing relationship with the social service staff be maintained. There may be many moments of anger, frustration, and despair, and strategies for both adaptation and interpersonal communication will have to be developed. Too often one person in the family attempts to shoulder all the burdens, when instead they could be shared amongst the entire family, close friends, and support services. A skilled social service person experienced in the dynamics of family interaction may be helpful.

Transient Ischemic Attacks

Transient ischemic attacks are important warning signs that a stroke may occur in the future. It is estimated that these attacks precede strokes about 80 percent of the time, so they deserve attention from a physician.

A transient ischemic attack is an episode lasting from a few minutes to, rarely, a few hours in which there is some loss of function. Symptoms may be a loss of vision, confusion, a disturbance in normal speech, numbness in the arms or legs, tingling, or other change in normal sensation. The exact symptoms of the attack vary from person to person and depend on the particular area of the brain to which the blood supply is slightly impaired.

Treatment of transient ischemic attacks depends on the site of obstruction. If in an artery in the neck, it may be possible to repair the defect with surgery. If within the brain, medical therapy is generally used. Although the best form of therapy has yet to be decided on, aspirin taken at least three times a day has been shown to be effective for certain people. This is because aspirin prevents clotting of blood and reduces the likelihood of a major interruption of blood flow through an already narrowed vessel. It is also important to control blood sugar, blood pressure, weight, and level of cholesterol and fats in the blood. Anyone who experiences confusion or has lost vision, sensation, or motor abilities, should report this to a physician.

Rehabilitation after a Stroke

Rhona Selkowitz, RPT

A comprehensive rehabilitation program should begin promptly after a stroke. Unfortunately, this is not always done, and the stroke victim loses time and mobility and may develop feelings of despair and dependency that make the rehab effort more difficult. The message of this discussion is to alert loved ones to the early need for a rehabilitation program and to avoid the depression and diminished self-worth that lying in bed brings.

Stroke rehabilitation should be performed as a team effort with participation of physician, physical therapist, nurse, occupational and speech therapist, counselor, and patient. The family of the stroke patient should also be involved. The premise is that each individual can achieve his or her maximum potential with a cooperative effort. It is to be hoped that a lifestyle can be reconstructed that does not differ appreciably from the way the patient lived prior to the stroke.

The Rehab Team

A number of professionals contribute their skills to the rehabilitation effort.

Physiatrist: A physician who specializes in rehabilitation.

Nurse: A licensed professional who cares for the medical needs of the patient.

Physical therapist: A university-trained, licensed professional whose approach is similar to the physiatrist, that is, to prevent loss of function, develop strategies for compensating for loss, and work on exercises and other programs for improving function.

Occupational therapist: Also university-trained and licensed, focusing on the recovery of abilities in the activities of daily living, such as washing, dressing, eating, and the like.

Speech pathologist: University-trained and licensed to work with communication losses.

Social workers: Licensed, postgraduate-trained professionals who help with emotional adjustments, family arrangements, placement into skilled nursing facilities, and coordination of supportive services for the home.

The Rehab Process

Rehabilitation should begin as soon as possible. Initially it will involve passive exercises, called passive range of motion, in which the therapist moves the paralyzed limb. This prevents tightening of the affected joints and improves circulation (see also Chapter 18, *The Skeleton*). Local heat can be employed to reduce pain and further improve circulation. It must be applied cautiously to prevent burns, since people who have had strokes cannot always sense hot and cold.

If voluntary movement is to return after paralysis, there will be a period of spasticity This means that the muscles appear to resist the passive movements initiated by the therapist. During the period of spasticity, the therapist may apply cold packs to aid in stretching the spastic muscles.

If voluntary movement returns, the next step is to work on achieving finer, more coordinated movements. The ultimate stage of rehabilitation improves strength with more exercise. Not all people progress past spasticity, however. Most patients and families want to know whether more function will return, but this question is extremely hard to answer. The longer the period without improvement, even with a good rehabilitative effort, the less likely the chance of more function returning.

Many devices, such as slings, suspension apparatus, splints, and braces, can help with rehabilitation. For instance, a sling elevates the arm to reduce swelling that develops in the hand or wrist. It can also prevent dislocation of the shoulder that may come with disuse. Instruction in the use of these devices should be provided for family members before the patient returns home.

It is common for stroke victims to lose an area of vision, the ability to maintain balance, or the sense of cold or touch. Part of the rehabilitation process, therefore, involves teaching the patient to be aware of these perceptual losses. Friends and relatives can help by positioning themselves in the patient's field of vision and by reminding them of the position of their body.

Loss of sensations brings with it the risk of developing sores in areas of sitting and lying. The patient must be taught to be aware of this danger. Family can help by turning and moving the person off pressure spots.

Strokes also affect mental function. It may be difficult to remember, judge, interpret language, read, write, and communicate with others. This is an important part of the work of the speech therapist, who can also teach the family skills for working on these losses when the person is home.

The degree of independence a person achieves varies

Self-Help Aids

Many aids can be purchased at a hospital, medical supply store, or pharmacy that can help people with disabilities lead independent lives. A medical provider or physical or occupational therapist, as well as the proprietor of the establishment that sells the product, can instruct on their use. The approximate cost listed may vary in different parts of the country, and it is worthwhile to do some comparison shopping before purchasing the product. Some products may be covered under insurance or Medicare. Check before you purchase.

Hygiene Aids

Bathtub transfer seat	$20
Bathtub safety rails	$15–20
Toilet safety rails	$18–25
Raised toilet seat	$20
Grab bars	$10

Dressing Aids

Wire tool with extended handle to aid one-handed buttoning and unbuttoning	$2–5
Velcro tape for clothing, to eliminate buttons, snaps, and zippers. 1 × 36 in. (2.5 × 92 cm)	$2.95
Elastic shoelaces—do not require tying (per pair)	$2
Stocking aid	$7–15

Kitchen and Household Aids

Paring board for mounting food; has nail extensions to hold food for one-handed cutting and peeling	$8–12
One-handed rolling pin	$5
One handed can opener	$50
Suction cups to hold kitchen equipment firmly in place	$5
Reaching aid: metal extension tool for securing objects that are hard to reach	$15

Eating Aids

Built-up utensils for poor finger control or grip (set of 4)	$12
Side cutter fork: side of fork has cutting edge	$4
Nonslip pad to prevent sliding of plates, glasses, bowls, 16 × 72 in. (41 × 184 cm)	$32.95

with the amount of damage that the stroke inflicts and the effort at rehabilitation. Attitude—mental and emotional—determines a lot of what ultimately happens. The more positive the feelings of the family and staff, the more likely the patient will keep a positive attitude and make rehabilitative progress.

Self-Help Aids

Medical supply stores stock many devices that can help a person maintain independence. Some aids help with personal hygiene, others with dressing, eating, and household functions. The physical or occupational therapist and the physiatrist can provide information about helpful aids. They should also be able to instruct the family and stroke patient in their use.

Much equipment, like wheelchairs, may be rented or obtained on loan from organizations like the Veterans of Foreign Wars. The accompanying chart lists some of the more common aids and their approximate price. This price may vary in different areas. Do some comparison shopping before purchasing any item.

Parkinson's Disease

Parkinson's disease or Parkinson's syndrome is the most common disease of the central nervous system in older people. Probably about 1 percent of those over fifty are affected, between 200,000 and 1,000,000 persons. It is named for James Parkinson, a London physician who first described it in 1817.

Parkinson's disease is really a group of symptoms that includes rigidity of the muscles, tremor, weakness, slowing of movement, immobility, and emotional depression. The degree to which one person is affected with these symptoms differs, and for the most part we do not know why a given individual becomes affected. The tremor is the most easily recognized part of the syndrome. It is a rhythmic motion, most often of the hands, which looks as if the person were "rolling pills" between the fingers. Since there are no laboratory tests to confirm Parkinson's, the clinical symptoms of the disease provide the diagnosis.

Because there is as yet no known cure for Parkinson's disease, medical treatment is directed at relieving the symptoms. A number of drugs can be used to do this. One type of drug, the anticholinergics such as Artane and Cogentin, reduces the tremor and muscle rigidity and, to a lesser extent, the weakness that occurs. These may, however, also cause blurred vision, dry mouth, occasional dizziness, increased heart rate, vomiting, confusion, hallucinations, and other adverse effects. They should not be used by those who have glaucoma.

Benadryl and other antihistamine drugs, often prescribed for people with allergies, may be used in conjunction with the anticholinergic medications to help reduce the tremors and muscle rigidity. They may produce drowsiness, which means one should not drive or operate machinery when taking these drugs.

Sinemet, a combination of levodopa and carbidopa, has also been used to treat Parkinson's disease. It supplies dopamine, a protein important to the brain, that is deficient in Parkinson's sufferers. Unfortunately, high doses of Sinemet may produce a number of adverse effects, including dizziness when standing, nausea, vomiting, difficulty eating, depression, memory impairment, and unusual and involuntary movements. In addition, some common drugs, such as aspirin, tranquilizers, barbiturates, and some diuretics, should not be taken along with Sinemet. Any questions about particular medications should be discussed with a medical provider.

Foods and Drugs to Avoid with Levodopa

Foods high in pyridoxine (vitamin B_6) and certain medicines interfere with the action of levodopa. If you are uncertain about a drug or have a question about your diet, discuss this with your medical provider.

Foods

avocado
bacon
beans (legumes)
beef liver
bread enriched with vitamin B_6
breakfast cereal enriched with vitamin B_6
bran enriched with vitamin B_6
kidneys
milk, whole, dry, and skim
milk, malted
nuts
peas
pork
salmon, fresh
tuna
wheat germ
yams
yeast

Drugs

aspirin
barbiturates (Seconal, Nembutal, phenobarbital)
methyldopa (Aldomet)
phenothiazines (Thorazine)
monoamine oxidase inhibitors (Eutonil, Nardil, Parnate)
reserpine (Serpasil)
anticholinergics (Artane, Cogentin)

Levodopa, when taken as a single agent (Larodopa, Dopar), acts and produces side effects similar to Sinemet. Moreover, vitamin B_6 (pyridoxine) and foods rich in B_6 interfere with levodopa for reasons that are not understood. The above chart lists foods that are rich in vitamin B_6.

A fifth medication used to treat Parkinson's is called amantadine (Symmetrel). It was first used to treat Type A influenza and by chance was found to reduce the tremor, rigidity, and weakness of Parkinson's syndrome. As with other medications, however, it has significant adverse effects, including slurred speech, insomnia, depression, confusion, and upset stomach. These side effects do tend to be less severe than with the other anti-Parkinson drugs, however.

Because all of these drugs are potentially harmful, all side effects and symptoms should be reported to a medical provider. In general, sufferers of Parkinson's disease should expect to start with low doses of these medications and to increase them gradually. For instance, Sinemet may be initially taken as a 10:100 combination, two times a day. It can then be increased by one tablet every three or four days, to a dose of three to six tablets of 25:250 strength. In other words, both the number of tablets and the strength of the preparation will be increased. Also the total dose may be divided up into four or more daily administrations, which may also help minimize unpleasant side effects. This is something that should be done only in consultation with a physician.

Parkinson's sufferers should be encouraged to follow four rules to help maintain function:

Stay active. This will help prevent unnecessary weakness, immobility, or contracture of the limbs. Some basic exercises to prevent or control contractures are presented in Chapter 18, *The Skeleton.*

Adapt activities to aid, rather than aggravate, the disability. Use a walker or other appliance. Be careful to avoid falls. High straight-backed chairs and couches aid in sitting and getting up to a standing position. Get used to clothing that has simple snaps, rather than buttons and other closures that are difficult to work with.

Take advantage of massages, warm packs to tight muscles, and physical therapy. All will aid in diminishing muscle pain. They also help loosen tight muscles and make daily activities easier.

Continue to be active in work, hobbies, and social interactions. Parkinson's does not diminish mental faculties until the disease is very far advanced. Thus, although one may have difficulty in movement, one still has an active, alert, and sensitive mind. All customary and enjoyable intellectual activities should be continued.

Senility

Senility is something that most of us fear, yet consider an inevitable part of aging. The negative social images laid upon the elderly have caused us all to expect mental decline with advancing years. In fact, senility is not a normal part of aging; it is a disease process that is being more accurately understood all the time.

Two types of senility are most commonly seen. The first is produced by many small strokes, and is called *multi-infarct dementia.* (An infarct is an area where tissue has died because of impairment of blood supply to the cells.) *Alzheimer's disease* is the other common form of senility. It results from changes in the cells that make up the outer layer of the brain (the cerebral cortex). The majority of senile individuals have Alzheimer's disease.

Senility develops gradually, which means the first signs are often quite subtle. Only close family and friends are likely to notice. Such personality changes and alterations of habits as a lack of initiative, depression and moodiness, irritability, inability to perform routine tasks, and subtle memory loss. With more advanced disease comes difficulty with thinking, inability to maintain attention in conversations and work, defective memory, speech impediments, and impaired judgment. Often the usual social graces are lost; failing to button one's clothes, and soiling the bed and/or undergarments are signs of this. Sometimes people lose their wallets, pocketbooks, and other valuables; leave the stove on in the house; or have repeated accidents. When the problem is very far advanced, there will be a loss of bowel and bladder control, a loss of virtually all intellectual functions, difficulty speaking, and an inability to care for oneself.

There are many known causes of senility. Some have to do with injuries, infections, drugs, and poor nutrition. More causes are being studied. If you suspect that a friend's personality, habits, or life-style is changing

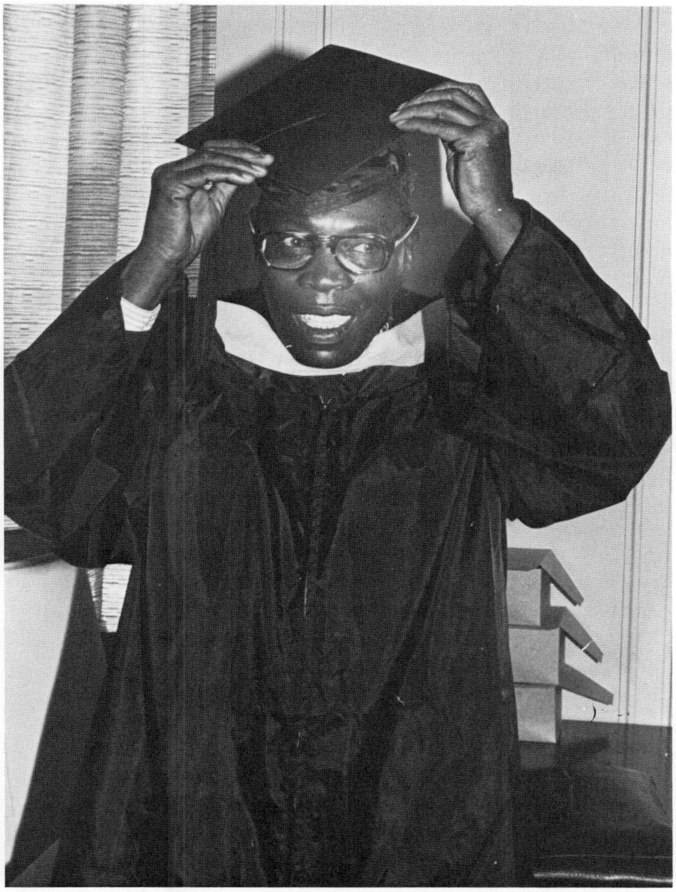

in one of the ways mentioned above, you should encourage him or her to see a physician or other medical provider. Senility can be reversed in some situations with the right kind of medical treatment. Also, the agitation, fear, and depression can be relieved with medication and a plan for involving the person in regular social and physical activities.

People who find their mental faculties changing often withdraw socially. They lose track of time and become confused. Others can help by reminding them of the time, day, and place, and by encouraging them or helping them to dim lights at night (helps reduce confusion), keep the home and environment filled with familiar objects, change gas appliances to electric, and lock medicines up. They may need help with money matters and with seeing that the home is free of potential dangers. The goal should be to keep friends and loved ones out of institutions and in familiar environments for as long as possible, since institutionalization often aggravates the confusion and depression.

If you have additional questions concerning how families can help with this problem, you may want to write to: Alzheimer's Disease and Related Disorders Association, 32 Broadway, New York, NY 10004.

Headaches

Chronic headaches are an extremely common problem for all adults. But headaches that begin in later years may be signs of serious underlying illness and should not be overlooked. Although over 90 percent of headaches are related to muscle tension, 10 percent result from a number of more serious causes, including inflammation of the blood vessels in the head, disturbances of metabolism, and sometimes tumors. Contrary to popular belief, high blood pressure and difficulty in vision are not particularly common causes of headache.

The current theory is that headaches are caused by electrical stimulation or traction on one of the sensitive areas of the skull. This may be one of the cranial nerves that traverse the brain, the membrane that covers the brain, or the blood vessels within the brain itself. Tension in the muscles of the neck can also produce headache. Certain foods have been known to cause allergylike reactions and produce headaches. Caffeine in coffee, tea, and soft drinks and MSG (Accent) in Oriental and other packaged foods are particularly common headache-producers, and avoiding them may stop the headaches.

Any new, persistent, or "throbbing" headache deserves medical attention. For most people the medical examination will rule out one of the more serious causes.

There is more to do for tension headaches than taking large amounts of aspirin. Such techniques as biofeedback, massage, yoga, and meditation have been shown to be effective in controlling tension. Good counseling that provides strategies for dealing with tension may also be helpful.

In any case, it is worthwhile to explore these possibilities before resorting to chronic use of aspirin or aspirin substitutes.

Brain Tumors

Tumors that arise within the brain itself are not common in people over fifty-five. Tumors of the lung and other areas of the body do spread to the brain, however. Cancer that develops in one organ and spreads to another is called *metastatic* cancer. This is not a neurological disease per se, although cancer can affect the nervous system in its spread throughout the body.

Usually brain tumors begin subtly and produce symptoms only as they enlarge and place pressure on the brain. Often a first sign is headache upon waking in the morning or one that interrupts sleep at night. There may also be a sudden onset of seizures, changes in vision, or persistent nausea and vomiting. All of these signs should be investigated by a medical provider.

The medical treatment for these tumors is not promising at this point. If the tumor is small, cure may be obtained by surgery to remove the mass. Radiation and chemotherapy are employed to extend life and relieve symptoms. Headaches, seizures, and other symptoms can be controlled with medication. As with other serious cancers, good counseling and hospice intervention are helpful to the individual and the family and should be sought out (see Chapter 5, *Hospice*).

Peripheral Nerve Disease

Sometimes people notice a change in the normal sensation in the hands or feet. The symptoms may be numbness and tingling, pins and needles, alteration of the normal sensation of temperature and pain, or weakness. All of these signs point to a problem with nerves that supply the extremities.

There are many potential reasons why this occurs, but *none* is a normal part of aging. Diabetes, alcohol abuse, specific vitamin deficiencies, kidney failure, drugs, and cancer are all potential causes. Sometimes a narrowing of the channel through which the nerve that supplies the hand runs (called *carpal tunnel syndrome*) can produce weakness or altered sensation in the palm and some of the fingers. Many of these problems can be successfully treated, either with diet, medications, stopping medications, or in the case of nerve entrapment in the hand, surgery.

It is also worthwhile to develop strategies to prevent injury to the hands and feet, including wearing warm socks and gloves in cold weather to prevent frostbite, using a thermometer to check wash and bath water before immersing hands and feet (the water should not exceed 100° to 110°F—38° to 43°C), and wearing properly fitting shoes and checking feet for blisters or areas where there is rubbing.

There is no evidence that the nerves become more sensitive with advancing years. Alterations in normal sensation are a signal of possible neurological disease and require a full medical examination.

Many people erroneously still believe that the decline of mental functioning is an inevitable part of aging. It is not, and study after study demonstrates that older people are mentally alert and productive in work and play throughout their lifetime. Therefore, we should never consider memory loss, changes in daily behavior, or impaired functioning as anything but a sign to see a medical provider. It is hoped that the myth that losing one's mental faculties is inevitable will die off like many of the other unfortunate images that we have of aging.

Chapter 20
The Blood

Blair Ardman, MD

Blood is the substance that fills our arteries and veins and is responsible for delivering oxygen and nutrition to all the organs and tissues in our bodies. It is also the main carrier of waste products that are ultimately removed through other specialized organs. Along with these basic functions, blood has multiple other jobs to do. It is an integral part of our immune system, a carrier of hormones that provide signals for many metabolic activities, and a part of a complex system for body temperature regulation.

Blood is not just a liquid. It is composed of blood cells and a fluid called *plasma* in which these cells live. The cells in the blood are of three main types; *red* blood cells, *white* blood cells, and *platelets.* Red blood cells carry oxygen, white blood cells function as a major part of our immune system, and platelets are essential for normal clotting of blood. They comprise about 40 percent of the total blood volume; plasma makes up the other 60 percent. All the blood cells in adults are normally made in the bone marrow, which might be thought of as the blood factory. The bone marrow is located inside of certain bones in our bodies. Plasma is composed mainly of water but also contains salt, proteins, minerals, and other substances. With this basic background in mind, along with some more facts to be presented throughout this chapter, you will be able to understand why problems occur in the body when there are abnormalities in the blood and why these abnormalities cause illnesses with particular symptoms.

Anemia

Anemia may be defined simply as less than a normal amount of red blood cells. The normal amount varies, depending on one's gender. For practical purposes, a normal amount is 40 percent of total blood volume. This is determined by taking a specimen of blood in a glass tube and putting it in a centrifuge, a device that rapidly spins the blood so that the heavier red blood cells settle out to the bottom of the tube while the lighter plasma remains above.

At this point, you might be wondering what happened to the other cellular components of your blood, namely the white blood cells and the platelets. They are still there but normally represent only a small portion of the cells in the blood and have nothing to do with anemia per se. There are roughly one thousand red blood cells for each white blood cell and twenty-five red blood cells for each platelet in normal blood. When a tube of blood is spun down, the platelets and white blood cells settle out in a thin layer between the red blood cells and the plasma.

Anemia is not itself a disease; rather, it is a sign of an underlying disorder or disease in the body. Many disorders and diseases can cause anemia, and they all do so through one or a combination of three general mechanisms: by causing decreased production of red blood cells in the bone marrow; increased loss of red blood cells from the body; or increased destruction of the red blood cells within the body. In other words, if you do not make enough red blood cells or if you lose more than you can make, you will become anemic. The accompanying chart should give you an idea of some of the disorders and diseases that can cause anemia and by which of the above three general mechanisms that they do so.

The symptoms of anemia may be caused by the anemia itself or may be overshadowed by the symptoms of the underlying disease causing the anemia. To confuse matters more, anemia may give absolutely

Anemia

The following table lists most of the causes of anemia according to the means by which it is produced.

Decreased Production
Vitamin B_{12} deficiency
Folic acid deficiency
Iron deficiency

Increased Destruction
Sickle cell anemia
Lupus erythematosus
Drugs
Inherited genetic diseases
Chronic diseases
  rheumatoid arthritis
  diabetes
Thyroid disease
Drugs
Malnutrition
Leukemia
Myeloma
Tumors
Inherited genetic diseases
Kidney disease
Chronic infections of bones, lungs, and other organs

Blood Loss
Ulcers
Tumors in the stomach or intestines
Menstrual cycles
Disorders of blood clotting (hemophilia)

no symptoms at all. Some people walk around with less than half the normal amount of red blood cells and show no symptoms from their anemia; other people are quite symptomatic if they lose only 10 to 15 percent of their red blood cells.

The actual symptoms of anemia are quite general. They include fatigue and weakness and, in more severe cases, dizziness and fainting spells. It must be emphasized that these symptoms are not specific for anemia, but they will cause a physician to suspect anemia among other possible disorders. A thorough history and physical exam, along with appropriate blood tests, should tell the doctor if a patient is anemic, as well as indicate the probable cause.

The treatment of anemia is directed toward correcting the underlying disorder that causes it. The most common cause of anemia in people over fifty-five in Western society today is an underlying chronic disease. This kind of anemia results from a poorly functioning bone marrow, a sick red blood cell factory if you will, made ill by the chronic condition. Anemia caused by chronic disease is relieved by treating the underlying illness.

Another important cause of anemia is iron deficiency. Contrary to popular belief, iron deficiency is not caused by an inadequate intake of iron in the diets, at least not in Western society. The vast majority of cases of iron-deficient anemia result from blood loss. This can be either an obvious blood loss, such as in women who are menstruating, or it can be hidden or silent blood loss, such as bleeding in the gastrointestinal tract (esophagus, stomach, intestines, rectum). Most people with this problem are not aware that they have been bleeding, usually because the amount of blood loss is small and occurs over a long period of time. The problem could be anything from an ulcer in the stomach to a tumor in the large intestine or rectum. Therefore, in an adult, iron-deficiency anemia is a sign that there might be trouble inside, and it requires a complete medical evaluation to find the cause of the blood loss. The presence of iron-deficiency anemia in an adult indicates internal bleeding until proven otherwise.

Iron pills or liquid is the treatment for anemia per se, but neither will treat the underlying cause of anemia. Identifying the cause of the anemia is the physician's important job. Occasionally, even after a rigorous evaluation including barium X rays of the stomach and intestines and direct examination of the rectum and sigmoid colon, the cause still cannot be found. But many times a bleeding site can be located, and proper treatment can then be administered.

Deficiency of folic acid or vitamin B_{12} or a combination of both can cause anemia. Folic acid can be found mainly in green leafy vegetables, and vitamin B_{12} is found in foods of animal origin (meat, eggs, and milk). Anemia caused by folic acid deficiency is usually seen in poorly nourished individuals, in particular those who consume more alcohol than food. It can be also seen in people who overcook their vegetables, especially in large amounts of water, which destroys or removes most of the folic acid from these vegetables. Vitamin B_{12} deficiency can occur in people with digestive disorders and in people who have had part or all of the stomach or part of the small intestine removed. These two organs are important for the absorption of the vitamin. Late middle-aged and elderly people who have never had surgery can also develop B_{12} deficiency and its corresponding anemia. In this case the culprit may be a disorder in which certain cells in the stomach fail to secrete a protein essential for vitamin B_{12} absorption in the intestines. Anemia caused by vitamin B_{12} deficiency is usually insidious in onset and may take up to five to six years to become clinically apparent. This is because the human liver normally has vast stores of this vitamin that can be utilized by the body and the bone marrow.

The treatment of anemia caused by folic acid deficiency is folic acid, usually in pill form. The treatment of anemia caused by vitamin B_{12} deficiency is vitamin B_{12}, by injection. Supplemental folic acid and vitamin B_{12} are of no benefit for treating anemia that is not caused by a deficiency of either one of these particular substances. A monthly vitamin B_{12} injection is for people who have documented vitamin B_{12} deficiency. If a person is not deficient in vitamin B_{12}, the money spent getting these injections could, to put it mildly, be better spent. The same holds true for iron supplements for iron-deficiency anemia and, for that matter, for any vitamin or replacement medicine for any deficiency state.

Leukemia

Leukemia is a term from the Greek meaning, literally, white blood. It is a malignant disorder of the blood-forming elements in the bone marrow, in which too many white blood cells are made but ironically fail to develop into fully mature white blood cells. There are several different types of leukemia because there are several different types of white blood cells, any or all of which can become malignant cells. Not all of these types of leukemia affect adults. Because it is an illness that has captured the public's eye, however, and because it can be rapidly fatal, leukemia will be discussed in general terms in this chapter. Be aware that some types of leukemia can now be cured, and many types can be controlled to a reasonable extent. In fact, almost no other area in medical research has progressed so far in so little time as has the study of how to cure leukemia.

The damaging effects of leukemia can be understood if you remember that the major function of white blood cells is to help fight infection. If these cells do not function properly, either because they are immature or because there are just too many of them (or both), they fail in that task. One of the symptoms of leukemia is the inability to fight what might, in a healthy person, be considered a minor infection. Even more important, when someone who has leukemia contracts a serious infection, it might well cause death. Medical science today has developed powerful antibiotics and an incredible technology that can help people with leukemia heal from these infections, but sometimes these artificial aids cannot do enough.

Another major problem caused by having too many abnormal white blood cells is a tendency to bruise easily, and even to bleed. There are a few reasons for this, but the most important one has to do with the third type of blood cell, the platelet. Platelets are also made in the bone marrow; they are responsible for clotting blood and maintaining the integrity of some of the blood vessels in our circulatory system. Leukemia can and frequently does cause a significant decrease in the number of platelets that circulate in the blood and thus interferes with their function. This seems to happen because they are simply crowded out by the malignant white blood cells. In other words, the leukemic cells take over the bone marrow and push out the other cells that are responsible for making platelets (and red blood cells, for that matter). The result is a low platelet count, anemia, and an increased tendency to bleed.

Malignant white blood cells have the capacity to settle in many different organs and fluids of the body, such as the skin, liver, spleen, lymph glands, lungs, spinal fluid, and brain. These cells, once settled, continue to divide and grow into actual tumors and create symptoms specific to the organ system they invade. This can happen at any time during the course of the illness.

Rampant infections with very high fevers, uncontrollable bleeding, and rapid deterioration of a previously healthy person can all be part of leukemia. No wonder it has been such a dreaded illness in the past and still is regarded an extremely serious disease by the medical profession. But it is important to recognize that some leukemias can now be *cured* with proper therapy and not all leukemias need to be treated, since certain kinds may progress so slowly that they never seriously endanger the life of the person who has the disease. Chronic lymphocytic leukemia is such a type. Even if the type of leukemia is aggressive, a person may still be able to enjoy a year or two of good-quality life.

Treatment of these diseases should be confined to specialized centers that have expertise in these conditions. There are many different forms of therapy, and new applications are being tried continuously in the hope of improving survival and eventually finding a cure. For almost 70 percent of people with acute granulocytic leukemia, a type of leukemia that used to be rapidly fatal, some period of remission is now possible. This, however, involves many techniques and drugs, and it is hoped that in the future better treatments will be discovered. Slowly the survival rate is improving in these diseases.

It is becoming more apparent as every year goes by that there are probably multiple causes of leukemia. As of this writing, there has been no proven cause of any single type of leukemia in humans. Viruses, heredity, exposure to chemicals, drugs, and exposure to radiation have all been implicated, but none has been proven as the single cause for leukemia. It may well be that a specific cause for this illness in humans will never be found, and as with many diseases in medicine, the cure for it will precede the complete understanding of the illness itself.

Myeloma

Myeloma is a malignant disease of the plasma cell, the blood component responsible for making antibodies. It is more commonly found in middle age and after. In a way similar to leukemia, myeloma (also known as multiple myeloma) causes major problems with the ability to fight infection. As the abnormal plasma cells grow in the bone marrow, they replace normal bone marrow cells and the antibodies these malignant cells produce function either poorly or not at all. Therefore, an early sign of myeloma can be a pneumonia that just will not get better, typifying a breakdown in the body's immune system.

Another common symptom of myeloma is low back pain. Since myeloma is a disease of middle-aged and elderly people and low back pain is a common problem in these age groups as well, this symptom alone is not enough to suggest the presence of myeloma. If low back pain exists and anemia is also found in the course of a routine blood test, however, a physician will suspect myeloma and investigate further. Why is anemia an important associated factor? As you may have guessed, myeloma cells, along with crowding out the normal plasma cells in the bone marrow, also crowd out the cells responsible for making red blood cells.

As with leukemia, myeloma may be a mild chronic disease, or it may run a rampant course. Also similar to leukemia, myeloma can be treated, and the treatment can provide significant relief from the symptoms and even improvement of the actual illness. Strictly speaking, there are no known cures for this disease, but here as well the research is active, and answers will be forthcoming in the very near future.

The Role of the Hematologist

There are many less common medical problems that affect the blood-forming cells of the bone marrow and the entire blood system. These problems usually require a trained hematologist, a physician who specializes in disorders of the blood. Hematology is a medical specialty that requires postgraduate medical training. Most large hospitals and teaching facilities have hematologists who are available to treat these specific medical problems. They are usually employed in consultation with a family medical practitioner or through the hematology clinic in a major hospital in your area.

Chapter 21
The Hormones

Blair Ardman, MD

Hormones are complex biological substances (proteins and steroids) produced in a variety of organs and tissues throughout the body. They are essential for the regulation of body functions, and they affect virtually all tissues of the body active in metabolism. For example, growth hormone is produced by the pituitary gland located in the brain. It is vital to the growth of bones and other tissues, as well as to the development of many organs during the first two decades of life. Cortisol, a hormone produced in the adrenal glands, significantly affects the body's metabolism of fats, sugars, proteins, and water throughout life. It also influences the immune system. The roles of at least twenty-five hormones in the human body have been well defined. The presence of many more hormones is inferred, but these have not been fully isolated and studied.

For people over fifty-five, two extremely important hormones affect health: insulin, which is produced in the pancreas and is involved with diabetes; and thyroid hormone, produced in the thyroid gland in the neck. Although other hormones are important for normal functioning, they are not commonly linked with illness and need not be discussed here.

Diabetes Mellitus

Diabetes mellitus is best known for its characteristic elevations of blood sugar (glucose). It is often called sugar diabetes and is extremely common in Western society. In the United States, it is the seventh leading cause of death, and the number one cause of blindness (see Chapter 10, *The Eyes*). Increasing age brings a greater chance of becoming disabled with diabetes. It is a serious problem that should never be ignored. People with diabetes generally fare better if they understand the nature of their problem and develop daily routines for optimal adjustment.

Above all, diabetes is a very complicated disease that affects virtually all the parts of the body. Its immediate effect is through damage to the blood vessels, which impairs blood flow and therefore produces problems as varied as stroke, heart disease, blindness, skin diseases, kidney disease, infections, and loss of sensation in the hands and feet. The exact process by which this damage occurs is unknown, as are the reasons why some people get one or more of these complications while others do not. There is a tendency to accept some of the potential signs of diabetes as a normal part of the aging process. They are not and should be thoroughly investigated by a medical provider.

It is worthwhile to divide diabetes into two groups of diseases: juvenile onset (JODM) and adult onset (AODM) diabetes. As its name suggests, the juvenile form begins in childhood. It is characterized by a deficiency in the production of insulin in the pancreas. The adult onset form is different because the pancreas can produce insulin (often increased amounts), but the hormone does not effectively perform its usual task of facilitating the entrance of blood sugar (glucose) into cells. In other words, in these diabetics there seems to be a resistance to the normal operation of the insulin. We do not know exactly why this resistance to normal insulin function occurs, but whatever the reason, the result is elevation of the amount of sugar in the bloodstream.

Symptoms

The symptoms of diabetes include increased thirst, increased frequency of urination, and sometimes weight loss in the face of normal eating. Other symptoms include a tendency towards infections, especially in the urinary tract and vagina in women, as well as in the skin. Injuries often do not heal readily, there is an increased likelihood of early cataract formation (see Chapter 10, *The Eyes*) and a decrease in the normal ability to sense heat and cold.

Diagnosis

The test for diabetes begins with an analysis of a blood and urine sample. In diabetics sugar is "spilled" into the urine, and this can be detected with a test in the physician's office or even at home. If the first blood test shows an abnormally high level of sugar, it may have to be followed up by a *glucose tolerance test,* in which the test subject drinks a quantity of sugar mixed with water and the tester obtains blood samples over a few hours, then analyzes them for blood levels of glucose and insulin.

Treatment

The initial treatment for adult onset diabetes is to lose weight, because the majority of diabetics are overweight and this seems to contribute to their insulin resistance. In fact, for many people this alone may correct their diabetes (see Chapter 8, *Nutrition,* for a discussion of the dietary treatment of diabetes). Adding a regular exercise program to the effort to lose weight has a positive effect as well. No one should attempt to diet, however, without the counsel of a medical provider or nutritionist experienced in working with people who have diabetes. They can help plan food intake and schedule meals to avoid the problem of low blood sugar (*hypoglycemia*), which is a dangerous possibility.

In addition to dietary management, some people will require medical treatment with insulin, taken by injection. Insulin is by no means always required in treatment of adult onset diabetes, but it may sometimes be needed. Insulin cannot be taken by mouth because it is a protein and would be broken down by enzymes in the digestive system. It is made commercially from the pancreas of cattle and pigs; most preparations contain some combination of both animal forms. Pure insulin from either cattle or pigs is available, but only for people who are allergic to the standard mixed type. It is also more expensive. In the near future, pure human insulin may be available by mass production from bacteria through recombinant DNA technology. This will probably reduce the cost as well as eliminate allergic reactions.

Most people with diabetes can achieve reasonable control of blood sugar using one or a combination of two types of insulin. NPH or Lente insulin provides coverage for a twenty-four-hour period. For people who "spill" sugar with NPH, regular insulin, which is faster acting, may be added. Choosing the appropriate dose of insulin depends on activity level, the presence of other illness, and incidence of unusual stress. Exercise may *decrease* the insulin requirement; illness, like an infection, may increase the need.

A relatively new innovation is the insulin pump. It may be worn externally or implanted under the skin. It senses levels of blood sugar, delivers the correct amount of insulin, and works to prevent symptoms of fluctuating blood sugar levels like alterations in vision and tingling and cramps in the legs. It is not yet known whether this innovation will help prevent the long-term complications of diabetes, especially the effects on the blood vessels.

There is considerable controversy now about the appropriate role of oral hypoglycemic medications in treating diabetes. These drugs, taken in pill form, are intended to lower blood sugar. Although commonly used in the past, mounting evidence suggests that they increase the risk of heart attack and have other adverse side effects. In most medical centers, the tendency now is to use insulin if medical treatment is necessary. Four commonly prescribed oral medications are: tolbutamide (Orinase), chlorpropamide (Diabinese), acetohexamide (Dymelor), and tolazamide (Tolinase), all of which have similar effectiveness. Those concerned about the possible long-term effects of these medications should discuss this with their medical provider.

Hypo- and Hyperglycemia

An injection of insulin removes sugar (glucose) from the bloodstream. If too much insulin is taken or if one does not eat enough, the blood sugar level may be lowered too far (*hypoglycemia*). Alternately, if not enough insulin is taken, the blood sugar level may become abnormally high (*hyperglycemia*). People with diabetes often have problems in regulating and maintaining the right level of glucose in the bloodstream. The human body is extremely sensitive to changes in blood sugar levels, especially those that are too low.

Hypoglycemia is extremely common when people with diabetes undergo stress or unusual physical activity or when they skip meals and still take their insulin. Symptoms include profuse sweating, fainting, and cold, clammy skin. An attack of hypoglycemia can be corrected by ingestion of sugar in almost any form, including juice, sugar water, soft drinks, or candy.

Hyperglycemia occurs when the insulin dose is insufficient to remove excess glucose from the bloodstream. There is an increase in the level not only of blood sugar, but also of its toxic breakdown products. The effect of prolonged high blood sugar may be coma and death. The signs of hyperglycemia are dry skin and tongue, a "sweet" acetone smell on the breath, spilling large amounts of sugar in the urine, and an alteration of normal mental functioning.

If someone has these symptoms but you are not sure whether their blood sugar is low or high, you can try to give them some sugar water or juice. If they do not revive mentally, it means blood sugar is high. They will not be harmed by this small amount of extra sugar, but they should be seen immediately by a trained medical person. Hyperglycemia is dangerous and requires prompt treatment, often in the hospital.

To avoid these complications, especially low blood sugar, it is important for diabetics to eat three regular meals a day, plus a snack if they start to feel any weakness, fainting, increased heart rate, or become cold and sweaty. Even when the diabetic is sick, the normal amount of calories, as well as insulin, must be provided.

Foods like table sugar, soft drinks, candy, and many desserts provide large quantities of free sugar that are rapidly absorbed into the bloodstream. This produces large swings in blood sugar, which may be dangerous for diabetics. These sweet foods should be avoided. A diet that is rich in both protein and complex carbohydrates including whole grains and foods high in fiber will supply a constant supply of energy and reduce the chance of hypoglycemia. (See also Chapter 8, *Nutrition*.)

Other Considerations

Diabetes produces effects on the eye. Diabetics should therefore see an ophthalmologist regularly, at least once a year, if not more often. Untreated diabetes can produce blindness. With appropriate treatment, however, damage to the eye can often be prevented. It is essential that treatment be initiated early in the disease process (see also Chapter 10, *The Eyes*).

Since loss of perception of heat, cold, position, and pain commonly occurs in the feet of people with diabetes, it is particularly important for them to protect the feet from injury. This means wearing properly fitting shoes and socks, and appropriate foot care. A podiatrist can help with this. To prevent burns while bathing, diabetics should keep a thermometer beside the tub or washbasin and measure the water temperature before immersing hands or feet. Temperatures greater than 100°–110°F (38°–43°C) should be avoided. Since healing of injuries is impaired in diabetes, it is necessary to *prevent* injuries.

For more information concerning diabetes, contact the American Diabetes Association, 18 East 48th Street, New York, NY 10017.

“ I am seventy-two now, born and raised in the United States. I have been working since I was twenty, married at twenty-five, and work has been a central theme in my life. I think that is because so much of my youth was changed by the Depression. In my family there were six boys and three girls—I was the eighth—and I had to contribute to my family. I have only one sister left, who is now eighty.

Three and a half years after I was married, we had our first child. I was panicky about being a father, and I remember that I felt we couldn't afford a family. I was working for eighteen dollars a week, and my rent was fifty dollars a month. So we had to give up the apartment after the baby was born. I went to live with my mother, my wife and the baby went to live with her mother. After awhile my wife came to live with my mother, but it was very difficult. After two full years, in 1939, we were finally able to get our own apartment.

In 1942 our second child was born. Times were different then because I was making money. Also this baby was planned. By 1944 we bought our own home, and we stayed there for the next five years. By that time I had my own business, things were going well, I felt very close to that second child, and she was very easy to raise. I stayed in my own business until 1969, all told twenty-five years.

Then I sold it, and I thought that I might retire. One of my salesmen bought my business, and he offered me a job as a salesman. In three months he was out of business. I think that it was a question of fast women and slow horses. At any rate, I wanted to continue to work, so I called several people and got a job in the same field, as an outside salesman. When I first sold the business I thought that I would retire and live a whole different kind of life. But when I was home for two weeks, I thought I was going out of my mind. I had nothing to do. I would watch TV, read a little, and get tired. Even now I have little patience for being home. I take one week off in December and one week off in July. After three or four days, I get very restless. I don't particularly care to travel or do the other kinds of things that men who retire seem to want to do.

In 1967 I had my annual physical checkup, and I was told that I had diabetes. I had no symptoms at that time, but my blood tests showed high sugar. At first I was put on a sugar-free and low-starch diet, but this did not help. Later I was on insulin, although I was still unaware of having any symptoms. But I trusted the doctor then and I still do.

In 1975, in the early summer, I had an uneasy feeling after dinner one night. I had been fine during the day, but I felt like something was sitting on my chest. I called the doctor, was sent to the hospital, and placed in intensive care for a heart attack. I was in the hospital about three weeks and was due to come home when the toes on my foot became numb. It was diagnosed as a blood clot, and I had two surgical procedures performed.

After I got home from the hospital my toes became gray and then turned black. I was sent to a surgeon, who said I would need an amputation. Shortly afterwards my leg was removed below the knee. After the operation I had phantom pains, and I was very frightened about having an "iron" leg. After a while I was fitted with a plastic prosthesis and began to adjust. I didn't mind walking on it, but when I looked at it I still sometimes became frightened. I had to learn to walk and to get up stairs with a cane or by holding on to the handrail.

But I still could not stand being around the house and not working. By Christmas I went back to work. Even when I was in the hospital I called my customers. My motto is If the Car Goes, I Go.

About three months ago, while driving, I got double vision. I actually saw two cars coming. I stopped the car and realized that if I closed one eye, I could see normally. I made it home and called an optometrist. He said, "Your eyes are fine, see an ophthalmologist." The ophthalmologist said, "Your eyes are fine, see a neurologist." The neurologist said, "You have a nerve condition, caused by your diabetes and age." I still was determined to continue working and doing all of the other things that I had to do.

In spite of all of this, I sleep well, I manage all of my own bodily functions, and I take care of myself. I hate to buy clothes or go to the barber, but that is no different from before. I love my wife, children, and grandchildren, and I am happy when they come home. Of all of the things that have happened, the death of my grandson in a car accident has been the hardest for me. I can't get over that. I do have a granddaughter, whom I adore.

When my wife goes out alone, if she doesn't get home until late, I get anxious. She's only playing bridge with her friends, but I think, "What if something happened to her?" I don't know what I would do. What would I do if I were alone? Who would have me? I guess that I would probably sell the house, but where would I go? I have made my will, but I haven't discussed it with anyone. These things are very hard for me.

Overall I feel accepting about my medical problems and committed to keep on working. I don't need the money, but I need to keep on going. I'm going to be seventy-three years old and I want to keep on for as long as I can. I feel that it's my world because I'm in it. ”

—Alex Kellerman, 72

Thyroid Disease

The *thyroid gland* is located in the neck, just below the Adam's apple, or larynx. It secretes thyroid hormone, which is integral to the regulation of the body's metabolism. Sometimes this gland underproduces hormone *hypothyroidism* or overproduces it *hyperthyroidism*. Either irregularity can cause many symptoms that need medical attention.

In the newborn, for instance, deficiency of thyroid hormone causes *cretinism* (retardation of growth and mental functioning). Later on in life, the symptoms of thyroid disease may appear insidiously and affect one's general well-being. Because thyroid hormone regulates so much of body metabolism, abnormalities can mimic senility or other mental disorders. Proper recognition and treatment can often reverse these symptoms.

Thyroid Deficiency (Hypothyroidism)

Lowered levels of thyroid hormone produce symptoms of lethargy, cold intolerance, constipation, and in more advanced situations, weight gain, coarseness of the hair and skin, and nonspecific muscle aches. If left untreated, heart disease, anemia, and problems with the nervous system, including emotional problems, may arise.

There are many potential causes for failing thyroid function in adults, but often the cause is not determined. In some people an enlarged gland, called a *goiter*, is an initial sign. But this may also be a sign of excess thyroid production. Because iodine-enriched salt is now widely used, iodine deficiency is no longer the major cause of goiter it once was in Western countries. In any case any lump or change in size of the gland should be brought to the attention of a medical provider.

The diagnosis of thyroid malfunction is based on symptoms, physical examination, and a simple blood test that is safe, painless, and relatively inexpensive.

The treatment of hypothyroidism is replacement of the deficient hormone. There are many preparations on the market, but most agree that the pure, synthetic drug is best. Its strength is uniform, and it has very few inactive contaminants that may produce an allergic reaction.

Treatment will produce a slow reversal of symptoms and must be continued for the rest of one's life. Surgery can be employed to reduce the size of the goiter, but it is usually advised only if the enlarged gland presses on the airway or makes swallowing difficult.

Thyroid Excess (Hyperthyroidism)

Sometimes the thyroid gland overproduces hormone. The symptoms of this problem include an enlarged thyroid gland, tremulousness (shaking, tremor, quiver), nervousness, palpitations of the heart, heat intolerance, weakness, fatigue, and weight loss. There may also be thinning of the hair, brittle nails, bulging of the eyes, insomnia, nightmares, and often dreams about death.

The most common type of thyroid overproduction is Graves' disease, named after the Irish physician who first wrote about it. Other illnesses may produce hyperthyroidism, however, and this problem requires a full medical evaluation by a trained medical person.

This investigation begins with a blood test for the different forms of the hormone that can be found in the bloodstream. If an abnormality is found, a thyroid scan is usually performed next. This involves injecting a radioactive dye into the blood and following its course through the gland.

There are essentially three forms of therapy for hyperthyroidism: drugs that block the production of thyroid hormone; radioactive iodide that destroys the hyperfunctioning thyroid tissue; or surgical removal of most or all of the thyroid gland.

Most older people usually start with radioactive iodide, whereas surgery is often tried in younger people. Because there are so many potential underlying causes, it is hard to generalize about treatment. The type of therapy that is best should be discussed with a physician. For those who have a tremor, a drug called Inderal may also be employed (see Chapter 25, *Common Medications,* for information on Inderal).

Therapy should establish normal thyroid function and abolish the symptoms. Unfortunately, the development of bulging eyes (*exophthalmos*) and changes in vision may not be helped with medical therapy. Surgery, radiation, and certain other medications are available to treat the eye problem.

✽

The problems of diabetes and thyroid disease in people over fifty-five can be easily detected and are generally amenable to medical treatment. This takes a mutual effort on the part of the patient and the medical provider. In the long run, a full, active, and productive life can usually be enjoyed.

Chapter 22
The Skin, Hair, and Nails

Barbara Maloney Turner, RN, NP

The skin is more than just a covering. It is a dynamic organ that protects the body from injury, retains water, regulates body temperature, contains an important reserve storehouse of energy, and is a visible sign of emotional and physical health.

Few of us think about taking care of our skin until we begin to notice illness or the effects of aging. Later on in life, many people tend to become fixated on wrinkles and sags and to become resentful of gray hairs and aging nails. We have become overly conscious of these signs of aging, perhaps because of advertising, which promotes beauty aids through the faces and images of the young.

In addition, it is unfortunate that the cosmetic industry continues to place emphasis on the care of the skin, hair, and nails with expensive, sometimes ineffective or harmful products. The care of the skin, hair, and nails is something that we can all do for ourselves with a minimum of time, effort, and expense. Most measures are extremely simple and depend mostly on regular care at home. Possibly more than with any other organ system of the body, we can control the aging process of the skin, hair, and nails.

The Skin

The skin consists of three layers: the *epidermis,* the *corium* (or *dermal* layer), and the *subcutaneous tissue.* The outermost layer, or epidermis, protects us from injury, chemical irritation, bacterial infection, and the general effects of sun, wind, and weather. Lubricating glands, hair follicles, and the nails are outgrowths of this layer. The dermis, which lies below the epidermis, gives strength and elasticity to the skin. And in the deepest layer, or subcutaneous tissue, a layer of fat insulates, cushions, and provides a reserve of energy.

During aging the epidermis thins as the result of years of exposure to the environment and the gradual slowing of the body's ability to replace damaged skin cells. This produces slower healing but is not a danger to our health. The dermis ages as well, becoming more coarse and calcified and losing some fibrous connective tissue and lubricating glands. The deepest layer also diminishes in fat and water content.

These changes produce a loss of elasticity, the diminished ability of the skin to return to its normal shape after a pinch or pull. We also perspire less, and this may make temperature regulation in extremely hot climates more difficult. Dry skin is often a problem because of the loss of lubricating glands that reside in the skin. Sometimes this produces itching and cracking, which usually can be prevented with regular application of a bland lubricating cream.

Care of the Skin

Care of the skin should be a lifelong process that begins when we take measures to prevent diaper rash in our children and continues through adult life. This care should take into consideration what we put on our skin each day.

As a general rule, try to use as *little* soap as possible, since all soaps denude the skin of its natural lubricating oils. Soap that is used daily should be of a nondrying variety. Dove, Basis, Alpha Keri, and Neutrogena are examples of the many nondrying soap products available. Ask your pharmacist which nondrying soap is the best buy in your area.

The water used for daily bathing should be warm, never hot. Adding oil to the bath water will also help restore lubrication. Mineral oil and baby oil are inexpensive and just as effective as more expensive oils. Be *careful* when getting in and out of the tub if you use oil, because the tub surface and your hands and feet will be slippery.

It is a good idea to rub bland lubricating cream on your skin after you bathe; it is especially important if you have used a harsh soap and hot water to remove grease or other contaminants. Emollient creams that soothe, soften, and impart moisture should also be used on skin exposed to sun, wind, and harsh weather. Regularly cream the neck, face, hands, and during the summer or in warm weather climates, the arms and legs. Petrolatum, Nivea, Eucerin, Lubriderm, and Keri are examples of the many brands of emollient creams on the market. If these creams make you feel greasy and uncomfortable during the day, use them at night before going to sleep. They will be completely absorbed when you awaken the next day.

Women who use makeup are advised to use a hypoallergenic brand. Clinique and Almay are two common types, but there are many to choose from. If you are uncertain, ask your pharmacist if a particular makeup is hypoallergenic. Also, try using an emollient cream under your makeup. It moistens the skin, is inexpensive, and will make it easier to remove the makeup. You should remove all makeup *every day* so that your skin can breathe, lubricate, and clean itself.

You can help to slow down the effects of aging by protecting your skin from extremes of weather, sunlight, and chemicals in the environment. The ultraviolet rays of the sun cause sunburn and seem to hasten the signs of aging. In the presence of some drugs, in particular certain antibiotics, diuretics, and antihypertensives, sun exposure can produce a hypersensitivity reaction in the skin. If you are concerned about a medicine you are taking, ask your medical provider before getting sustained sun exposure. The photosensitivity reaction looks like a moderate to severe sunburn, with blistering and swelling.

Chronic sun exposure not only produces wrinkling, sagging, and other aging effects, but also increases the likelihood of skin cancer. It is difficult to say what chronic exposure consists of, since different people have varying levels of skin pigment that protect them from getting skin cancer. The amount of sun you get depends on the intensity of the sunlight (ultraviolet rays), which depends on the season, climate conditions, and geographical location. We are all exposed to the sun almost every day. It comes into our houses and buildings through windows, and outside it shines on us and is reflected back onto us from sidewalks, snow, water, glass, and sand. All of this, in addition to moderate sunbathing at the beach a few days a week in the summer, could be considered chronic exposure over a lifetime. People with fair skin and light hair will experience sun-related changes sooner than individuals with darker skin, who can tolerate more exposure before burning.

It is neither possible nor healthful to avoid all contact with the sun. It is advisable to avoid severe sunburns. When going out in the sun to work, relax, or swim, using sunscreen creams and covering your body with clothing and hats are extremely important. The most effective sunscreen creams contain PABA (para-aminobenzoic acid). Pabanol and PreSun are two of the many brands that contain PABA. They come with a number beside their name, which indicates the amount of protection that the cream provides. For example, if the cream has a number 15 after the name, it will take fifteen times the amount of exposure to create a burn as if you stayed in the sun without any protection. The higher the number, the more the protection. Choose the strength of the sunscreen you need according to the way your skin usually reacts to sunlight, and use a stronger cream until you build up a tan. Sunscreens should be applied before going out into the sun and after sweating or swimming. Be aware that they may cause some discoloration of light-colored fabrics.

Cosmetic Surgery

Many people are curious about facelifts and other cosmetic surgery to look younger. The choice rarely involves medical considerations and is therefore a personal matter based on individual feelings. A facelift will not make you look ten or twenty years younger, although it may give you a more refreshed and vigorous appearance.

Surgery for a facelift usually takes about four hours and requires hospitalization for about three days. Complete recovery takes about two weeks, during which the bruises heal and all the sutures are removed. The risks are infection and, uncommonly, injury to the nerves supplying the area operated on. The face may not be entirely symmetrical after the procedure.

The results depend on the condition of the skin prior to the operation. A plastic surgeon can give a good indication, but no guarantee, of what the face will eventually look like. The effect should last five to ten years, but this again depends upon the condition of the skin before surgery and the care taken of it afterwards.

The cost of a facelift varies with geographical location, the length of hospitalization, the fee of the surgeon, and the occurrence of complications. It ranges from five to eight thousand dollars and is almost never covered by standard medical insurance. It is, however, tax deductible.

Steroid Skin Creams

The treatment for many skin problems, especially inflammation caused by allergy or other sensitivity reaction, is often steroid creams. When people hear the word *steroid*, they often think of the dangers associated with taking these potent drugs by mouth or by injection. These adverse reactions and side effects include: bleeding ulcers, weakened bones, infection, cataracts, glaucoma, weight gain, and alterations in normal body chemistry. The use of steroid creams is, however, only rarely associated with these problems.

The advantages of these medications, called *topical steroids*, are that a very small amount is effective, they require no special storage, and they are used locally (where the problem is). Often prescribed steroids are fluorinated, which makes them more potent (Lidex, Synalar, Valisone). The amount of fluorinated cortisone in most available preparations is from 0.025% to 0.2%. The lower-percentage medication is usually chosen for beginning treatment. Absorption of the medication and potency are increased when the area under treatment is covered with a plastic wrap. Sometimes this form of treatment produces side effects like those associated with oral administration of steroids: fluid retention, hypertension, gastritis, thinning of the skin and easy bruising, increased likelihood of bone fractures, the masking of signs of infection, difficulty fighting infections, and changes in skin pigmentation. These side effects rarely occur unless steroid treatment is continued for long periods of time. When the drug is discontinued, function usually returns to normal. Long-term use of steroid creams should therefore be employed only in serious illness and under the careful supervision of a trained medical professional.

Several over-the-counter steroid preparations like Lanacort and Cortaid contain nonfluorinated hydrocortisone. The amount of cortisone in these creams is 0.5% or 0.5 milligrams per gram of cream. The nonfluorinated creams provide less antiinflammatory action than the fluorinated brands.

Premalignant, Nonmetastasizing, and Metastasizing Lesions

The various categories of disordered skin growth are often poorly understood by the average person. Unfortunately, this often produces anxiety when individuals are told that they have an abnormal skin lesion. Three terms are usually employed: precancerous or premalignant, nonmetastasizing, and metastasizing.

Precancerous lesions are not yet truly cancerous but are abnormal and have the potential to develop into cancer. The term indicates that the skin has been damaged and that the cell looks abnormal when examined by the pathologist. An example is *actinic keratosis*, which in up to 25 percent of cases may develop into a malignancy called *squamous cell carcinoma*. Clues to recognizing precancerous lesions are areas of skin, often sun and weather exposed, that develop a change in color, texture, size, or appearance.

Nonmetastasizing skin lesions are those cancerous growths that do only local destruction. They spread laterally on the skin but do not invade underlying structures. An example of this type of lesion is the *basal cell carcinoma.*

Metastasizing lesions are those that have the potential to spread throughout the body. They do this by penetrating the skin and spreading to lymph nodes and the internal organs. *Squamous cell carcinoma* and *melanoma* are examples of metastasizing lesions.

The type and degree of malignancy depends on many factors: size and age of the lesion, its origin on the skin, and pathology of the tumor. It is not possible to fully explain these factors here. What is essential is that any change in the normal color or texture of the skin be reported promptly to a medical provider. Skin that has been termed "sun damaged" or precancerous should be protected from further sun exposure. The next sections provide a description of the three most common forms of skin cancer: basal cell carcinoma, squamous cell carcinoma, and melanoma.

Basal Cell Carcinoma

The most common of all skin cancers is the basal cell epithelioma. These lesions are seen most frequently in fair-skinned, light-haired, middle-aged individuals, but they may be seen at any age. They, like many of the premalignant lesions are also more common on the sun-exposed areas of the body. Basal cell tumors are slow-growing tumors that destroy the soft tissue in which they grow. They rarely spread, however, to any area other than that which immediately surrounds the tumor.

The lesions usually are raised, firm lumps (called *nodules*) with a pearly looking border. There may be a large number of blood vessels within the lesion, and the center may be depressed, providing the appearance of a tiny crater. Ulceration generally occurs if the lesion is allowed to grow.

The treatment for basal cell cancer is complete removal. A small surgical incision is employed, which must take a margin of normal tissue. This ensures that all of the cancer has been removed. Unless the lesion is in an area of skin fold or wrinkle, some scarring will result. The lesion should be analyzed by a pathologist, who will type the tumor and tell if a satisfactory margin of normal tissue was removed. Sometimes X-ray therapy and electrodesiccation and curettage are employed to remove the growth.

The site of the lesion should be checked every six months by a medical provider for possible recurrence of the tumor.

Squamous Cell Carcinoma

Squamous cell carcinomas, unlike the slow-growing basal cell lesions, may progress rapidly to destroy normal tissue. They occur most often in middle-aged and elderly people and are often preceded by leukoplakia (see Chapter 11, *The Ears, Nose, and Throat*), actinic keratoses, and other precancerous lesions. Occasionally they may even spread to the lymph nodes and internal organs. Because of this, early treatment is essential.

The lesion often begins as a dry growth on a hard, round base. Eventually this turns into a little ulcer with a rolled-looking border. When the lesion appears on the mucous membranes of the mouth or tongue, it looks like a bleeding ulcer.

The treatment of choice is surgical removal, as described for the basal cell lesion. X-ray, radium, and electrodesiccation are sometimes employed for small lesions. If the tumor has spread, it may be necessary to treat lymph nodes and other organs. After treatment the skin should be checked regularly for reappearance of tumor and be protected from exposure to the sun.

Melanoma

The most malignant and dangerous cancer of the skin is the melanoma. It rapidly spreads to the internal organs of the body, including the brain and nervous system, producing death. Melanomas are found on the skin and mucous membranes. They are more common in fair-skinned individuals, women, and people from age thirty to sixty. It is possible, however, for most anyone to develop a melanoma.

The lesions vary in size and shape, but they tend to be pigmented (melanin is the pigment that colors skin) in a mottled black, blue, or brown fashion. They usually are highly irregular in shape and often will bleed, ulcerate, and rapidly change their size and shape.

The treatment of a melanoma is early and complete removal. The lesion should be analyzed by a pathologist, and in most cases a series of tests will be ordered to look for potential spread to other areas of the body. The type of treatment used after excision of the lesion depends on the grade of the tumor and the evidence of spread. The care of this problem should be undertaken in consultation with an oncologist (a cancer specialist).

Melanomas often develop from moles or lesions that appear to the lay person to be a mole. For that reason any mole should be examined once by a medical provider and then reexamined periodically. If the mole changes in size or shape, bleeds (especially through a small trauma like the rubbing of a belt, bra, jewelry), or changes in color, it should then be immediately reexamined. The most effective form of therapy is catching melanomas before they can spread to the internal organs. Also, try to avoid traumatizing moles by pulling the hairs out of them or shaving over them. If they are a problem, they should be surgically removed by a medical provider.

Glossary of Common Skin Problems

There are many problems of the skin that occur in people over fifty-five. Some are purely cosmetic, whereas some like skin cancer, are potentially serious. This is a listing of some of the common ailments, including a description of their appearance, treatment, and potential risks. Use this as a reference guide along with the care of a medical professional. The specialist who cares for skin problems is the *dermatologist.* Many common problems, however, can be adequately cared for by your family medical provider or an internist.

Chilblains

Chilblain is caused by exposure to the cold and is most common in people who have poor circulation. This occurs most frequently in the hands, feet, and head. The areas exposed to the cold, including ears, face, hands, and feet, first become red and swollen, then develop a reddish-bluish color along with burning and itching. The color disappears when pressure is applied to the area, and the skin will feel cool and somewhat damp.

Treatment includes bathing affected areas with lukewarm water and massaging gently with warm oil each day. Electric heating pads on low settings can be used to gently and slowly warm the skin.

Prevent chilblains by protecting the skin against cold, injury, and dampness. Wear warm socks, gloves, hats that cover the ears, and a face mask or scarf. Wear socks in bed. Avoid extremely cold weather, and stop smoking, which impedes circulation.

Cutaneous Horn

Cutaneous horns are premalignant lesions usually seen in individuals with a long history of sun exposure. They are hard, dry projections which, as their name implies, look like a horn sitting on a round base. They may develop from actinic keratoses, seborrheic keratoses, or squamous cell growths.

The horn should be removed and sent for biopsy.

Dry Skin (Xerosis)

With aging comes a loss of the number and activity of the lubricating glands that produce oil to cover the skin. The dryness of homes heated in cold weather climates, excessive bathing with hot water and harsh soaps, the sun, wind, and weather all contribute to dry skin problems.

Dry skin causes itching, a signal to replace lost oil. The itching is usually most severe on the arms and legs and may be aggravated by bathing, washing dishes, chemicals, or hot water. If it is not treated, the skin will become reddened and cracked, and eventually eczema may develop.

There are some simple measures to prevent this problem:

1. In the winter bathe somewhat less frequently than in the summer, use cooler water, and bathe for shorter periods of time.
2. Use a mild, nondrying soap.
3. Add oil to your bathwater, and after your bath add lubricating oil to your skin. Remember, oil will make the tub slippery.
4. Try lowering the temperature of your house to a level that is comfortable when you are wearing a sweater.
5. Increase the humidity in your house with an inexpensive room vaporizer, or place pans of water on your radiators, stove, or heat vents. Houseplants also humidify the air.
6. Use an emollient cream over itchy areas and on the entire body a few times a day.
7. If itching progresses to red, cracked skin, it is time to consult a medical provider. You may have eczema.

Eczema

Eczema usually follows untreated dry skin. It may also be a reaction to skin irritants like wool and detergents. It is more common in people who have allergies like hay fever or who are prone to allergic skin reactions like poison ivy. All types of eczema are made worse by stress.

Eczema is characterized by round, red or pink, scaly lesions. They sometimes become wet and are accompanied by intense itching. Common areas for these lesions are the hands, forearms, lower legs, buttocks, and neck.

Preventive measures are those described for dry skin. In addition, care should be taken to allow good ventilation of affected areas and to avoid prolonged exposure to dampness. Often when the lesions first develop, the use of an inexpensive emollient cream several times a day will clear them.

If these measures fail, a topical steroid is recommended. It should be used three to four times a day until the lesions disappear, usually in one to two weeks.

Areas that become infected may require antibiotic therapy. Antihistamines can be used to decrease the sensation of itching. Chlor-Trimeton, in two- or four-milligram tablets, can be purchased over the counter. Be aware that all antihistamines make you drowsy and may impair your driving or use of machinery. They may be taken at night to help promote sleep if you find that the itching keeps you awake.

Herpes Simplex

There is considerable confusion about herpes simplex infections, in part because of the rise in popular media coverage of this problem. There are two types of herpes simplex virus, Type I and Type II. Type I has been termed the nongenital kind, and Type II is often called genital herpes. Because the disease is spread through personal contact, however, these distinctions are becoming increasingly blurred, since, for example, Type II can appear in the mouth after oral-genital contact. The symptoms of both types of herpes simplex are essentially the same. The distinction between the two is based on laboratory analysis of the virus that causes the illness.

The virus is found in human secretions and spread through personal contact. After spreading, it may produce infection or lie dormant in the nervous system. The infection is then triggered by some factor, not well understood as yet, but usually associated with stress. Sun exposure, anxiety, physical stress, illness, and injury all may activate an infection. It is felt that 90 percent of people who have recurrent infections had a previous primary attack but were not aware it was caused by herpes.

The primary infection lasts from one to three weeks, during which time the skin reddens and forms clear blisters. The lesions are usually painful and can be transmitted to others through contact. Recurrent herpes attacks last from seven to ten days and may also be painful. When people have attacks, especially a primary attack, they may have fever, malaise, and other general symptoms of a viral illness. In addition, in anyone who is taking steroid medications (like cortisone), is being treated with chemotherapeutic drugs, or is in some other way immune-suppressed, the outbreak is likely to be more widespread, painful, and last longer.

Unfortunately, there is no curative treatment for

herpes simplex as yet. All measures are aimed at relieving pain with aspirin, antiviral, antiinflammatory medications, and narcotic pain relievers when necessary. Topical antibiotic creams may be necessary if the herpes lesions form a crust, indicating an infection with a bacteria. Some people try over-the-counter mouthwashes or gargling with plain salt water (one or two teaspoons in a glass of lukewarm water) two or three times a day. Some suggest taking lysine, an amino acid, to shorten the attacks. Lysine, taken as 500 milligrams four times a day, can be purchased over the counter. It is a normal constituent of protein and is not harmful. It has never been proven beneficial, however, in scientific testing. A new drug, acyclovir (Zovirax), has been developed to treat first-time herpes attacks. Application of this medication may promote more rapid healing of sores, but it will not prevent subsequent infections. (For additional information on herpes, see also the discussions in Chapter 11, *The Ears, Nose, and Throat,* and Chapter 17, *The Genitourinary System.*)

Keratocanthoma

This is a benign lesion associated with aging. It is significant in that it may resemble squamous cell carcinoma. Keratocanthoma usually occurs in sun-exposed areas of the body; however, it may also appear in the mouth. It is a small lesion, often appearing as small lumps with dry, depressed centers. It usually reaches full size in a few weeks and then spontaneously disappears in about six months.

Because it may resemble squamous cell carcinoma, it is advised that keratocanthoma be surgically removed. This surgery can be performed as an office or outpatient procedure, with local anesthetic. The lesion should be examined by a skin pathologist to confirm the diagnosis.

Liver Spots (Senile Lentigines)

Senile lentigines are commonly called liver spots, although they have nothing to do with liver. They are found most frequently on sun-exposed areas and are more common in fair-skinned individuals.

The spots vary in size and color and are benign in nature. Treatment involves removing or diminishing the size of the lesions for cosmetic purposes. One simple technique is to freeze them off with liquid nitrogen. A blister will form, which will flatten and fall off in two to four weeks. After treatment the area may be slightly lighter in color than the surrounding skin. Some formulas available by prescription will help to bleach the pigment and must be applied two to three times a day for several weeks to be effective.

Several advertised over-the-counter creams (Porcelana, Esotérica) are also available to lighten the spots. They do not, however, completely remove the lesions.

Monilia (Skin Yeast Infection)

Yeast is a normal inhabitant of the skin, mouth, and vagina. During hot weather and in areas of skin folds (under the breasts, in the groin and underarms), these organisms can produce local skin infections, called *monilia.* (When this occurs in the vagina, it produces a very common form of vaginitis; see Chapter 17, *The Genitourinary System.*) The symptoms are itching and redness. Infection may occur as a complication of antibiotic or systemic steroid therapy.

Infections can frequently be prevented by keeping the skin clean and dry. Wearing all-cotton underwear and applying powder to damp-prone areas is also helpful. Cornstarch is not recommended as it may encourage bacterial and fungal growth.

A prescription antimonilial cream, applied two to three times daily, is effective treatment of monilia. Since monilia may also be a sign of diabetes, blood sugar should be checked if the problem recurs.

Plantar Warts

The same virus causes all warts, but plantar warts, which occur on the feet, look different. They are usually flat or only slightly elevated and are different from calluses in that they interrupt the normal skin lines. They also tend to grow more deeply into the skin than warts in other parts of the body. Because of this, they commonly produce some discomfort in the foot.

Treatment of these warts should be performed by a medical professional. Usually this involves paring the warts down to normal tissue bimonthly and applying acid or podophyllin to the wart. It may take several treatments to dissolve the warts, and they may recur. Desiccation and sharp excision of the warts is usually not recommended because a resultant scar may produce additional discomfort in the foot.

People can help in their own treatment by periodically rubbing the wart with a pumice stone. Proper-fitting shoes and a padded ring (Dr. Scholl's) around the wart will relieve some of the pain produced by pressure from the wart.

Psoriasis

Most medical texts say that psoriasis is uncommon in the elderly. In my practice, however, where 90 percent of the clients are over fifty, it is a frequent occurrence. Psoriasis is a genetically inherited, chronic disease. Although a lot of research has been done on the problem, its cause is still unknown. It is known, however, to be aggravated by stress, trauma, and dry skin.

The lesions of psoriasis are raised, red patches that are covered with silvery scales. When scratched, these scales tear off, often leaving small bleeding points. The patches are most commonly found on the elbows, knees, scalp, and lower back, although all areas of the body may be affected. They may be confined to a few areas or may cover most or all of the body.

Local treatment is with topical steroids and tar preparations. After application a medical provider may suggest covering with a dressing.

Many over-the-counter items are available to aid in the treatment of psoriasis. Tar shampoos (Polytar, T-Gel, Tegrin, Subutone) aid in the treatment of scalp lesions and may be used daily if needed. Bath oils that contain tar (Balnetar, Polytar, Zetar) help in treatment of the lesions and in lubricating normal skin areas. Employ all of the methods listed for dry skin to treat skin lesions and prevent recurrence. Sun exposure is effective in the treatment of psoriasis for many people. Some people find that their lesions disappear completely during the summer months.

Systemic steroids may be needed if topical creams do not clear the lesions. The use of oral psoralens and daily irradiation with ultraviolet light (PUVA treatments) have been approved recently by the FDA for the treatment of the symptoms of psoriasis. These methods do not cure the disease but can relieve its symptoms. In some cases methotrexate is used. All of these measures have potential side effects and should be discussed with a medical provider before initiating therapy.

Seborrheic Keratoses

Probably the most common condition that we develop with aging is the seborrheic keratosis. These superficial lesions are very common in older people, although they may occur as early as age thirty. They are round, raised, of varied size, and have a greasy, scaly, crustlike consistency. They are usually yellow or tan when they first appear and become brown and black with age. The lesions are commonly seen on the head, shoulders, back and chest but may occur anywhere on the body.

Although these lesions are benign, treatment is usually undertaken for cosmetic reasons or because the lesion is in an area that is constantly irritated. Long-standing irritations, especially ones that bleed, should be shown to a medical provider. Treatment can be performed in a medical office or clinic, using a ringlike knife, called a dermal curette, or by desiccation. Both forms of removal can often be performed without anesthesia. Healing takes one to two weeks after removal and should leave a clean, smooth skin surface.

Shingles (Herpes Zoster)

Shingles, or herpes zoster, is common in people over fifty-five. It is caused by the same virus that causes chicken pox. Chicken pox develops in people who have no immunity to the virus, whereas shingles develops in people who are partially immune. In this situation the zoster virus probably lies dormant within the nervous system and is activated by an unknown stimulus. Interestingly, susceptible children who are exposed to herpes zoster often develop chicken pox; and less frequently, older people exposed to chicken pox may develop zoster. Unlike chicken pox, which almost always occur only once, shingles can recur again and again in the same individual.

Herpes zoster is caused by a different virus than herpes simplex. Zoster is usually not found on the genitals or in the oral cavity, where herpes simplex is often seen. And zoster is not known to be sexually transmitted.

The lesions of zoster are firm, tense blisters on a red base, which occur in a line. They are usually on one side of the body and are most commonly seen on the chest, although they may also occur on the face, neck, arms, lower back, and legs. Widespread eruption of these lesions, particularly on both sides of the body, may be a sign of an underlying malignancy or other serious illness. Any lesion on the forehead, near the eye, should be examined by an ophthalmologist. Pain in the eye and blisters on the nose are other signs of potential eye involvement. Eye involvement can lead to loss of vision.

Skin eruption usually lasts from one to two weeks. There may be pain before the lesions actually appear, and there is usually pain after the eruption. Treatment is aimed at relief of pain with analgesics, narcotics, and more recently, antiinflammatory drugs. Systemic steroids, taken early after the eruption, may be helpful in decreasing the post-herpetic pain. Local injections under the lesions may also be helpful in producing pain relief.

When the lesions first appear as blisters, cool wet compresses (tap water is sufficient) should be applied several times a day. Later, when the lesions become crusted, a topical antibiotic may be needed. Usually a medical provider should be consulted to help treat the pain and potential complications.

Skin Tags (Papillomas)

These benign flesh-colored or brown attachments to the skin resemble small, loose bags and are commonly seen hanging from the neck, eyelids, and under the arms. They are most commonly seen with increasing age and with obesity. People usually seek attention for cosmetic reasons or because the tags catch on jewelry and clothing and begin to bleed.

Treatment involves cutting them off at their narrow base with a pair of sharp scissors. If the base is large, a local anesthetic may be used. Bleeding is usually minimal and can be controlled with light use of an electric current (desiccation) or local pressure. Never attempt to remove them yourself, as this may produce infection and inflammation.

Stasis Dermatitis

Stasis dermatitis is a brown pigmentation of the skin of the lower legs and ankles caused by venous congestion. It is common in older people. Early signs include slight swelling of the lower leg, near the ankles, and a darkened discoloration of the skin. Eventually, as the condition worsens, the area may develop into a red, wet patch of eczematous dermatitis, which may ulcerate. These ulcers are usually seen just above the ankles and on the front of the legs.

Preventing the progression of this condition involves elevating the legs at frequent intervals during the day, keeping the skin lubricated, and wearing elastic stockings to encourage return of blood to the upper portion of the body. A medical provider should help in selection of the stockings, making sure they fit properly and instructing on a schedule for their use.

Treatment of eczematous dermatitis that follows stasis dermatitis involves staying in bed with the legs slightly elevated, wet compresses (tap water is sufficient) three or four times daily for twenty to thirty minutes, and application of a topical antibiotic-steroid mixture. A diuretic may be prescribed if the swelling is severe. Oral antibiotics may be needed to control infection.

Treatment of ulcers, if they occur, may be more difficult. Again wet compresses (using Burow's, Domeboro, or saline) and the application of various ointments and creams during the day may be necessary. Bed rest with the legs elevated is also usually needed. Any weight-bearing will increase swelling and slow the healing process. Any irritation to the feet or legs, such as poor-fitting shoes, will promote the recurrence of skin ulceration.

Varicose Veins

Most cases of stasis dermatitis are associated with varicose veins, an inherited condition in which the veins of the lower legs become congested and hardened.

The condition is aggravated by standing for long periods of time and by obesity.

The skin changes in color as described for stasis dermatitis, and there may be pain and swelling as well. The treatment is also similar in that rest, elevation of the legs, support hose, and a diuretic may all be helpful. If the condition cannot be controlled by conservative measures, however, an operation called *vein-stripping* can be tried.

In the vein-stripping procedure, an incision is made in the upper thigh and around the ankle. The vein to be removed is tied closed at both ends and then loosened from the surrounding tissue with a special instrument. Finally the vein is cut at both ends and removed from the leg. Blood flows to the tissues through new vessels (called collateral circulation) that form rapidly during the healing process.

Warts

Warts are benign lesions that seem to plague us regardless of age. They are viral in origin and can spread through the skin surface by touching and scratching. They are also contagious, spread by close contact with others. Some warts disappear spontaneously, whereas others must be removed medically. Even those that are removed may come back.

Warts project outward from the skin and are rough and cauliflowerlike in appearance. Some are brown or black and fingerlike; others are flesh colored or gray.

Warts may be removed in several ways. They can be removed with electric desiccation (touching with an electric current), curettage (scraping with a ringlike knife), liquid nitrogen, or various acids and chemicals. The procedure may have to be repeated any number of times, no matter what method is used.

People seek professional services for wart removal when they are large, unsightly, or uncomfortable. The decision to remove the wart is based on individual preferences. But if you have one wart removed, you should probably have all the warts removed since warts that remain contain virus that may spread to other areas of the skin. Two-thirds of all warts will fall off on their own.

The Hair

Hair is present on all parts of the skin except the palms, soles, nails, glans penis, and lips. The growth of underarm, pubic, facial, and body hair is influenced by sex hormones, inheritance, and aging.

Hairs grow from hair follicles in the epidermis, all of which are formed before birth. Hair grows in cycles, which include a resting and a growing phase. The average period of growth ranges from two to six years. Scalp hair grows at a rate of 1/100 inch (0.35 mm) per day and the average density ranges from 1,200 to 2,200 hairs per square inch (6.5 cm^2).

Care of the Hair

Good hair care is similar to care of the skin. Frequent washing and hair dryers tend to dry out the natural lubrication of the scalp and make the hair dry, brittle, and easily split. Hair dyes also cause dryness, splitting, and generally "worn out"-looking hair; they may, in sensitive people, produce allergic reactions. Brushes with synthetic bristles and tight hair curlers can also damage hair.

To keep your hair looking and feeling healthy, use a mild, nondrying shampoo. Soapless shampoos (Dara) and tar shampoos can also be effective. Surprisingly, baby shampoos are quite strong and should be diluted before being applied to the scalp. I suggest diluting baby shampoo with an equal amount of water. Dandruff shampoos are potentially drying to the hair. Try a soapless tar shampoo as a substitute.

Hair conditioners should be used a few times a week to combat the drying effects of shampoo, harsh weather, dry-heated homes, and hair dyes. Hair conditioner need be applied only to the ends of the hair, not directly on the scalp. Most hair dyes irritate the scalp to some degree. Sometimes these reactions are severe and prolonged. This is because the dye cannot be completely removed from the hair by washing (it has to grow out), and its presence produces a continual allergic reaction.

Hair Loss

Male pattern baldness, common with aging, occurs because of hormonal changes and genetic influences. Usually this is seen as thinning on the sides of the head (temporal area) and thinning or complete loss of hair on the top of the head. This process usually begins during the late twenties and accelerates with age. It can occur in women, although it is far less common. When it does, it may also be accompanied by coarse hair appearing on the chin and upper lip. This is felt to result from a decrease in female hormone production (estrogen) and a relative increase in the concentration of male sex hormone (androgen) that occurs after menopause.

Hair may thin and be lost in other parts of the body as well, most commonly the abdomen, the pubic region, and the underarms. Related to hormonal changes, it occurs most often in women but may also occur in men. Loss of hair in a small or localized area of the body may, however, be caused by illness. Hair from the lower legs is frequently lost in sufferers of peripheral vascular disease because the loss of blood flow to the area interferes with the growth of the hair from the epidermis, where it receives nutrition.

Loss of hair on the head may also be caused by acute illness, anxiety, or drug reaction. The baldness produced by these causes may be complete but more often is seen as patchy hair loss. It is often temporary. When hair is lost from chemotherapeutic drug treatments (like Adriamycin) or from radiation therapy to the head, regrowth may not take place.

Hair is sometimes lost along the front and back edges of the scalp because of pressure from curlers and tight-fitting hats. Repeated pulling of the hair, either through rough handling, brushing, or nervous habit may also produce hair loss. Persistent pressure, usually seen when people are bedridden following surgery or illness, may also produce hair loss. Since there are so many potential causes for hair loss, it should be investigated by a dermatologist.

Hair Transplants

Thinning and loss of hair is a common aspect of aging. As with the use of hair dyes, the decision to try hair transplanting is largely cosmetic, with some medical ramifications. They are, however, usually not applicable to hair loss from chemotherapy, poor nutrition, and other diseases.

The *pinch graft* involves taking small plugs of healthy hair follicles from a part of the scalp where hair is growing and transplanting them to an area of little or no hair growth. The procedure takes about two to three hours and is performed under local anesthesia. It must be repeated three to four times, until the desired area is filled in.

Another method is the *whole thickness graft,* which takes a one-inch (2.54-cm) strip of hair from the back of the head to an area of no growth. The skin is loosened during the procedure, and the entire strip of hair is removed and carefully placed into the area of no growth. The donor area is closed with stitches so that no seam or area denuded of hair can be seen. A third option is to have a hairpiece sewn into place. This procedure should usually be performed by a plastic surgeon or dermatologist.

All of these procedures are generally safe, but the results vary with the amount of area to be covered and the extent of the hair remaining. Since these procedures are cosmetic, they are rarely covered by insurance. Anyone considering a hair transplant should understand the cost involved before beginning the course of therapy.

Graying

Probably more than any other aspect of aging, graying of scalp hair produces tension and anxiety. Graying is the generalized loss of pigment in the hair. It is determined by our genes, and it is something that we cannot prevent. Moreover, it is not an overnight occurrence that signals getting old. For most people it is a gradual process that begins in the late twenties and thirties and becomes increasingly apparent as more hairs turn to gray.

The only cure for graying is dyeing. This is a cosmetic decision. Be aware that dyes dry the hair and may produce allergic reactions. It is hoped that we will begin to look more favorably upon graying as we change our attitudes towards aging.

The Nails

The nails, an appendage of the skin, are composed of three parts: the *body* (the part we see and feel), the *free edge* (which extends away from the body), and the *root* (which lies under the skin surface). The nail body lies in a soft, modified portion of the dermal layer of the skin, called the *nail bed.* The portion of the bed that lies near the root is called the *matrix.* The nail grows through multiplication of cells in the root and is held on at the sides and root by skin folds. The whitish crescent near the base of the nail, which is usually seen on the thumb and covered by the nail fold in the other fingers, is called the *lanule.*

Nails grow about 2/100 inch (0.5 mm) per week. Usually growth is somewhat faster in the summer and slower in the winter. Fingernails grow about four times faster than toenails. The white spots seen on the nails develop from minute air bubbles that form during the growing phase.

Care of the Nails

Caring for your nails is easy and takes only a few minutes two or three times a month. If you have poor circulation in your hands and feet or are diabetic, nail care is even more important, and you may want to employ the services of a podiatrist for the care of your toenails.

As with the care of your skin and hair, the most important part of nail care is to avoid harsh and drying soaps and chemicals. Cleaning of the nails can be done regularly by soaking fingertips and feet in a nondrying soap for a few minutes. This softens the cuticle, as well as loosens dirt.

Only four tools are really necessary for nail care, although a variety of products are available. Use an orange stick for pushing back cuticles, an emery board or file for smoothing, a sharp scissors or nail clipper for trimming nails, and a cuticle scissors for trimming the cuticle. The cuticle should be trimmed only if it is torn.

After you have soaked your nails, gently push back the cuticle toward the base of the nail. Trim the nail edges that are jagged and smooth them by using an emery board or file. File in one direction only. Between manicures, try soaking your nails in mineral oil or baby oil for five to ten minutes once every two weeks. This will replace lubrication of the nails and cuticles removed from soap and water.

Drinking gelatin or soaking your nails in gelatin has never been proven helpful for making nails stronger or healthier looking. In addition, while some manicurists say that nail polish provides support and protection, there is little evidence to support this.

In general, strong, healthy nails come with good nutrition. The strength of nails, however, varies among people, often on the basis of heredity. If your nails occasionally break, this is not necessarily a sign of illness. Keeping them trimmed will help prevent breaking.

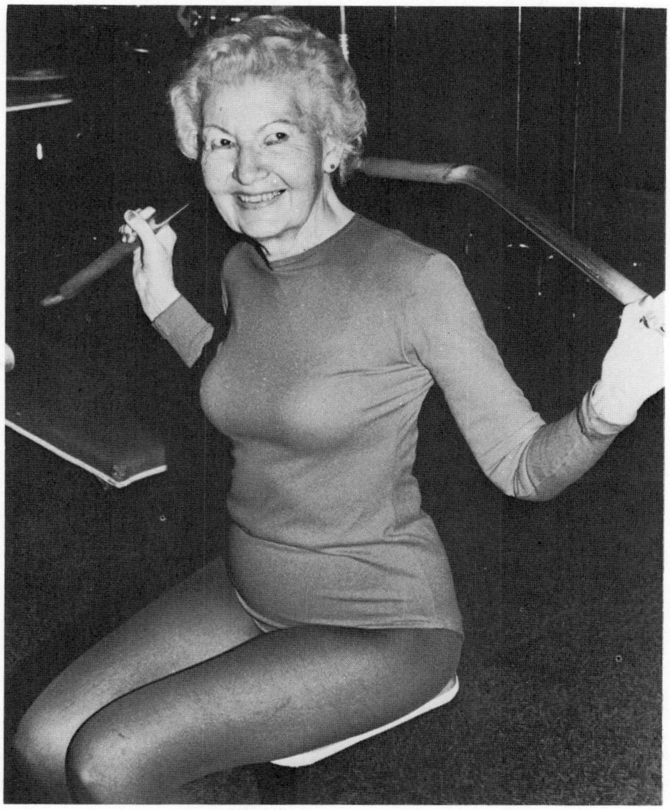

Care of toenails that are permanently thickened (often a result of limb paralysis or diminished circulation) should be performed by a podiatrist. They may be difficult to cut, and an inexperienced person may injure the sensitive skin of the feet.

Disorders of the Nails

A number of changes in color and texture of the nails pose either a medical or cosmetic problem. Most of the time they are caused by exposure to detergents, chemicals, and weather.

Soft or fragile nails and nails that split at the ends can be caused by excessive use of nail polish, nail polish removers, or exposure to detergents and chemicals. This is an external problem, which means that it is not a sign of underlying disease. The best treatment is to protect your hands while washing dishes, working around the house, and on the job. If you use nail polish, it should be on an intermittent basis. Like the skin, nails need to "breathe." Similarly, the continued use of nail polish remover along with the polish dries and damages the nail.

Sometimes, however, soft and brittle nails are caused by a problem with the matrix. This may be genetic, or caused by a disorder yet to be discovered. In this situation there is usually little that can be done other than protecting the hands and nails during work, washing, and activities around the house. Although it offers no proven benefits, some suggest drinking gelatin to strengthen the nails. One package of unflavored gelatin (like Knox) mixed with water or fruit juice daily for three months is worth a try. This is harmless, and supplies a small amount of protein to the diet.

Pitting of the nails caused by eczema will usually go away with the same treatment recommended for the skin. It will, however, take about three months for the nails to grow out and the cracks and pits to be displaced by normal-looking nails. Psoriasis, like eczema, is treated by the medications used for the skin. It is often more difficult to clear this up in the nails; again it will take at least three months for normal-looking nails to grow in.

Thickening of the toenails may be caused by continued rubbing from poorly fitting shoes or the effects of diminished circulation caused by peripheral vascular disease or paralysis. The conditions are not treatable with any form of medication. If your circulation is normal, be certain that your shoes fit correctly. A podiatrist can help choose properly fitting shoes and also help trim the toenails.

In some uncommon situations, brittleness of the nails may be caused by illness. Hypothyroidism and vitamin A and B complex deficiency are examples. Symptoms of these disorders will appear in other areas of the body as well, however, and these other symptoms will normally bring the person to a medical provider. Treating the thyroid problem or taking vitamins will correct the nail disorder.

Green nails are caused by a type of fungus called *monilia* (or yeast) and are treated with oral antifungal agents (usually oral nystatin). *Pseudomonas,* a type of bacterium, may also produce green nails and is treated with one of a number of antibiotics. *Tinea,* another type of fungus, produces discoloration of the nails, thickening, and detachment. It is more common on the feet but may also occur on the hands. An antifungal agent called griseofulvin is the treatment of choice for this infection, which may be extremely difficult to eradicate. The medicine is taken daily for three months. If the nails are removed, the infection may only require one month of medication. The infection often returns after the medication is stopped.

White spots, as previously mentioned, are caused by air bubbles that appear during nail formation. There is no treatment for this, but they will grow out. *Beau's lines,* however, are white lines or furrows across the nail that indicate the possible presence of illness when the nail was forming. Tuberculosis, syphilis, heart disease, emotional problems, radiation therapy, malaria, and other illnesses have been implicated in the production of Beau's lines. Again, there is no treatment for the lines, but they will grow out in about three months.

Clubbing of the nails looks as if the nail has taken on the shape of a back of a spoon. This may be a sign of long-standing lung disease and is not treatable with measures aimed directly at the nails.

Most nail problems, however, are not caused by serious internal disease, but result from exposure to chemicals, soaps, detergents, and polish. These problems can be prevented or treated with simple measures designed to protect the nails from further insult and to allow the nails to regrow normally.

✽

Healthy skin, hair, and nails are important to us because they say so much about beauty and self-image. Yet, despite all of the advertising and publicity that surrounds the aging, beauty, and care of these parts of the body, it is often true that the most basic approach is the best. I have tried to give the message that simple measures—using bland creams, avoiding excessive dyes and other harsh chemicals, and bathing with mild soaps, things that we can all do for ourselves—are more important than expensive and elaborate beauty treatments. With these simple procedures, all of us can maintain healthy and attractive skin, hair, and nails throughout our lives.

Part IV

Emergency and First-Aid Guide

Providing help to someone who is injured or ill does not usually involve the heroic measures that we see on television and in the movies. Generally it means keeping a clear head, calling for professional help, and providing warmth, empathy, and reassurance to the distressed person. Anyone who has worked in emergency care will attest to the importance of these basic comforting measures.

You can also learn some important medical techniques to help others. They include stopping bleeding; initial treatment of burns, head injuries, heat exposure, sprains, and strains; and providing basic life support in the face of heart or respiratory emergencies. You do not need a medical background to learn these techniques, but you should take a course on first aid to master them rather than trying to pick them up through a book alone. In almost all communities throughout the United States, the Red Cross, American Heart Association, hospitals, and local service organizations teach these basic courses. The material in this section is designed to supplement a training course, not to substitute for it. These courses are extremely important, especially for people over fifty-five who are more likely to suffer a heart attack or other emergency. Learn these techniques: they may help you save a life.

As important as providing medical and emotional support is knowing what constitutes an emergency and how to use the emergency care facilities in your area. These questions are addressed in the beginning of this chapter. If you or a loved one have the symptoms described, seek emergency medical attention promptly. You should know about the availability of ambulance transportation, paramedic care, and the health care facility near you *before* you need their help. Further, know your rights as a patient and insist upon them when you receive care. Knowing about these things before you have an emergency will help you and your loved ones get the best care possible in the most timely fashion.

Chapter 23
Emergencies

Neil Robertson, PA-C, EMT

What is an emergency? This is not an easy question to answer. Recent publicity, especially on television, encourages us to think of the emergency room (ER) as a place where dramatic events take place, calling for high-speed rescue, high-technology diagnosis, and daring treatment. The medical care system, on the one hand, makes money off rather routine problems that come to the emergency room, which make up the largest number of patient visits. And yet they often criticize people who come to the ER with minor complaints. It is not surprising that this double message adds to the layperson's confusion as to what an emergency is and when to seek help.

I do not necessarily believe that the emergency room is only for the gravest of illness. It is not always easy to know when one is seriously ill. Being frightened, having pain, or being emotionally distressed are kinds of emergencies, even if one is not seriously ill. In fact, most people visit emergency rooms for that reason. For instance, I recently saw a man in the ER who had just discovered a lump in his testes. To him this was an emergency, although he did not need emergency care.

If you find that you have to go to the emergency room, you should expect considerate, thorough, and rapid treatment. I have worked in ERs and know the frustration of staff, who are often overwhelmed by minor complaints. But I have been more upset and saddened by the person who was seriously ill and failed to seek treatment because he or she did not want to bother anyone. The symptoms and problems of older people may be time-consuming for the professional staff, and all too often these professionals are young and not entirely understanding of the problems of older people. These are poor attitudes, and you should be firm about your desire for thorough, personal, and gracious care.

To you, your problem is an emergency. Often you will need to be firm and resolute in your approach to the professional staff. I know that it is easy to feel timid. One feels that complaining will compromise care by alienating the staff. Yet it is still necessary to be clear, direct, and assertive. Medicine is a service profession, and the staff is there to serve.

The answer to the question, then, is that an emergency is any time when a person is in pain or frightened and the simple measures that have been tried do not relieve the problem. You may want to call your family doctor first, to see if some help can be obtained over the phone. But, if you cannot reach that person (or do not have one), go to the emergency room of the nearest hospital.

Getting to the Emergency Room

Before an emergency occurs, you should know how you are going to get to the ER should you ever have to. Rehearse. Learn the route if you plan to drive, or work out a transportation network with friends or relatives in your community.

There are a number of possible emergency services in your community. Realize that none of them is likely to respond with a physician in the ambulance or emergency vehicle. You are likely to see someone who has first-aid experience and training only. In general, these practitioners are not trained in making a diagnosis (although they can make some assessment of the problem) or rendering treatment. Some states are trying to establish a procedure for the administration of treatment by radio order from an ER physician, but this is evolving slowly.

You are likely to encounter one of the following trained people.

- **First-aid graduates,** trained by the American Red Cross, have the lowest level of training.
- **Emergency medical technicians** (EMT) have at least eighty hours of training, often with more advanced training in splinting, oxygen therapy, and evaluation of the patient. They must pass a national examination.
- **Paramedics** are emergency medical technicians with advanced training. Their training places emphasis on cardiac and respiratory emergencies, and in some situations they administer treatments.

All of these professionals should be identified by a patch or name tag and should be willing to describe the level of their professional training.

What to Take to the ER

To maximize the quality and speed with which you obtain your care, be sure to bring these items to the emergency room.

- Your **Medic Alert bracelet** or other identifying items.
- Your **medications.** The bottles are best, but a list of medications with dose and frequency will be satisfactory.
- Evidence of your **medical insurance,** like a Blue Cross or Medicare card.
- Do *not* take unnecessary valuables like jewelry or a watch.

Arrival at the Emergency Room

When you get to the emergency room, you should expect a prompt analysis of your problem by a trained professional. This may not be a physician, but someone who is trained in *triage* (a French word for a battlefield process that divides the wounded into categories based on the seriousness of their condition).

You may become quite distressed if you feel others are being seen before you. This delay should be based on the triage process: someone who is more ill is being

When to Seek Immediate Emergency Care

It is not always easy to know when to seek emergency care. Below is a list of possible situations where such care is advised. Although you may have one of these symptoms and not actually have an emergency, seeking professional care is prudent and may in some cases prevent unnecessary serious illness or loss of life. Seek emergency care if any of these signs are present:

- chest pain that lasts longer than five minutes, especially (but not only) if it is behind your breastbone or radiates down either arm or into the neck; is crushing, tearing, or ripping in quality; is accompanied by nausea and vomiting, sweating, or shortness of breath
- profuse bleeding, including from the rectum, vagina, or urinary tract
- vomiting blood or "coffee-ground"-stained material
- coughing up blood
- a seizure or convulsion when you have never had one before
- a serious headache, especially if it is worse than any headache previously felt or is accompanied by alteration in normal vision
- an injury to the head that produces loss of consciousness
- loss of consciousness not caused by trauma or in someone who is known to have diabetes
- unexplained or sudden difficulty breathing
- any sudden paralysis of a limb, numbness or tingling; or sudden loss of vision
- a traumatic eye injury
- pain in the eye and/or alteration of vision

attended to. If you feel that you have been forgotten or your condition is more serious than was assessed, be persistent. There are two people who may help you. In larger hospitals a *patient care representative* or *ombudsman* is often on staff to deal with patient complaints. In smaller hospitals bring your complaint to the *head nurse* or *administrator* on duty. The emergency room administrator may be available to help with this as well. If you have a complaint that is not handled satisfactorily while you are receiving treatment, write a letter afterwards to the hospital stating your grievance. This is the way that consumers can make changes in hospital policy. Usually these letters are followed up. The chart on the next page lists your rights and standards of care that you are entitled to.

When you see the triage provider, advise that person of the following:

- your *current* medical problem, with a brief history of the immediate events just prior to your symptoms; for instance, "I have had a pain in my abdomen for three hours, and I vomited twice"

Getting to the Emergency Room

Know where your local emergency room is and how you are going to get there *before* you have an emergency. Make arrangements with an ambulance service, fire or police department, or family or friends who will be able to assist you if you need immediate medical care.

Some potential services in your area include:

Private ambulance service: Traditionally not well trained but are gradually improving in service and training. May also be expensive. Contact the ones in your area before an emergency to see if they will take a check, will bill you, accept Medicare or Medicaid, know how to reach your home. Ask also about the level of training of their personnel.

Fire department rescue vehicles: Personnel may or may not be well trained in emergency care (however, often are trained in Red Cross techniques) and may or may not be able to transport you to an emergency room. It may delay your treatment if they have to call an ambulance. They are generally less costly than private ambulance service.

Volunteer ambulances: This may be the only alternative in rural areas. The staff is usually very dedicated but may not be especially experienced. The cost varies but is usually less than a private ambulance.

Public professional ambulances: May be based in either a hospital or fire department. Generally, this is the most experienced group since they see more emergencies. Also, this service may employ paramedics with more advanced training. Depending on the city, however, may be overworked and understaffed. Fees vary but are often less than a private ambulance. Those who cannot pay may be eligible for consideration under the Hill-Burton Act, which provides funding for hospitals that treat patients who have difficulty paying for services.

Police vehicles: May vary widely in the training of personnel and equipment on the vehicle. A call may get you a fully equipped ambulance or a patrol car with little equipment. Many police departments are getting out of the business of providing emergency care. Investigate carefully. If you cannot reach another source of transportation, call them, but the wait may be the longest of all if they are busy with police duties.

Your Rights and Standards of Treatment

On the way to the ER (by ambulance)

When you use an emergency service, you become a patient, but you do not give up your rights as a person.

Before you are moved, emergency personnel should:

1. Question you about your medical problems.
2. Take your blood pressure, pulse, respiration, and, if necessary, your temperature.
3. Examine you briefly, but thoroughly (especially if you have been injured in an accident) based on the nature of your medical problem.
4. If you have been injured, you should not be moved unless you are first checked for tender or painful areas or possible fracture.
5. When you are moved, it should be done in a way that does not aggravate an injury, *especially* if you sustained injury to the back or neck. If you have had such an injury, you should be immobilized with special collars, straps, and boards to prevent further damage.
6. You have a *right* to privacy, dignity and to be informed of any procedures or medications *before* they are administered.
7. You have a right to safe transport. Excessive speed is not only unsafe, but can cause you anxiety and be a stress on your condition. Complain if you are frightened.

In the emergency room

Some of your rights in the emergency room are unique to that setting. Others apply if you are admitted to the hospital as well.

1. You have a right to expeditious care.
2. No one may jeopardize your condition by inquiring at length about your ability to pay.
3. Even if you cannot demonstrate an ability to pay, you *probably* cannot be denied emergency care. All public and private institutions that receive funds under the Hill-Burton Act (which provides funds to institutions that care for people who have difficulty with payment) must give a certain amount of free care. They are required to post this information.
4. If treatment is begun, it must continue until an emergency no longer exists. The hospital may or may not provide follow-up care. But you should:
   - ask if you need further treatment
   - be told what it will involve and where to get it
   - know what you must do to take care of it yourself
   - be informed of future problems that may arise and what you should do about them
5. You also have a right to know and should ask:
   - What your problem is, in terms you can understand
   - What test, treatment, or surgery the doctor wants to use, and why
   - What the alternatives are, and why the one that is being suggested is best for you
   - The names and training of the people involved in your care
   - If the procedure or medication is new or experimental
6. You have a right to know why you are being asked to wait and to receive a reasonable estimate of when you might be seen.
7. You have a right to privacy.

- all your previous illnesses, hospitalizations, and surgeries
- a list of your medicines, or give the bottles
- the name of your private physician; request that the staff contact that person

When you see a medical provider, be certain that he or she knows all of this information as well. Try to be *concise* as well as complete. The medical provider will direct their treatment to your chief symptom, so try to inform them of facts that pertain to this problem.

Preventing Emergencies

You cannot usually prevent the onset of an emergency medical problem, but you can help prevent accidents that might bring you to the emergency room. Accidents are one of the ten leading causes of death for people over fifty-five. Many can be prevented. Some strategies for preventing accidents are listed in the chart on the next page.

Emergency First Aid

The following guide includes information on the initial care of selected emergencies. This is not meant to be a comprehensive guide nor a substitute for formal first-aid training. I do not presume that you have prior training, and I urge you to enroll in a basic life-support course offered by either the American Heart Association or the American Red Cross. Further, I urge you to read this section and practice some of the techniques *before* an emergency occurs. If you are not prepared, it is extremely unlikely that you will be able to react with composure by reading a book.

Nervousness is normal when one is confronted with an emergency. I work in an emergency room and still have this feeling; I know my colleagues do as well. Nervousness need not prevent you from performing well—but panic will. Panic occurs when you have no training in what to expect or what to do. This is perhaps the most basic reason to enroll in a first-aid course.

In all emergency situations, the first step is to check the airway, breathing, and circulation as outlined in the section on rescue breathing presented later in this chapter. And I want to emphasize the importance of *reassurance* for anyone in distress. This can reduce pain and help stabilize the injured person. It is an essential aspect of providing good first-aid care.

Preventing Accidents

People over sixty-five comprise 12 percent of the population in the United States, yet suffer 23 percent of the accidental deaths. As people approach their seventies, accidents become increasingly common. In fact, they become one of the ten leading causes of death. Accidents can often be prevented with some simple precautions.

Falls

- Illuminate all stairways and put light switches at both the top and the bottom of the staircase
- Place night-lights or bedside remote-control switches in your bedroom; place night-lights in sockets in hallways
- Put sturdy handrails on both sides of stairways
- Tack down carpeting on stairs and use nonskid treads
- Remove throw rugs that tend to slide
- Arrange furniture so that it is not an obstacle
- Use grab bars on bathroom walls and nonskid mats or strips in the bathtub
- Maintain outdoor steps and walkways in good repair
- Have stairways and walkways shoveled to clear snow and ice; wear shoes and boots with soles that grip well

Burns

- Never smoke in bed or when drowsy
- Do not wear loose-fitting clothing when cooking
- Avoid very flammable synthetics in robes, nightgowns, and pajamas
- Set water heater thermostats so that water does not scald the skin
- Know your exits at home, office, and hotel in case of fire

Motor vehicle accidents

- On public transportation have your fare ready, so that you do not fumble for change
- On public transportation remain alert and brace yourself when a train or bus speeds up, slows down, or turns
- Do not carry too many packages so that you are off balance; have one hand free to grasp railings, safety straps, or handles
- Watch for icy or slippery pavement when leaving any vehicle; be alert for curbs and hazards like drains, hydrants, and street signs
- Allow extra time to cross streets, especially in bad weather
- At night wear light-colored or fluorescent clothing and carry a flashlight
- Wear a seat belt in automobiles
- Do not drive if you are tired, take medication that makes you drowsy, or are not feeling well

Adapted from "The Age Page," National Institute on Aging, U.S. Dept. of Health and Human Services

Bleeding

Most bleeding can be stopped with direct pressure applied to the wound. To arrest bleeding:

1. Apply direct pressure to the wound, using a compress-type bandage or clean cloth.
2. Elevate the extremity above the level of the heart if the bleeding is in an arm or leg.
3. If bleeding is profuse, you may have to search for the source. If you do not find it in short order, place the compress where you see the most bleeding and apply direct pressure.
4. Continue to apply steady pressure. Do not lift the bandage to check if bleeding has stopped. This may dislodge clots, producing additional bleeding.
5. If the wound bleeds through the compress, do not remove it. Instead, place another bandage over the first one and continue to apply pressure.
6. Monitor the person's breathing and pulse. Increased breathing and heart rates are signs of distress. Get medical help immediately. If there is no pulse or respiration, begin basic life support resuscitation (see *Rescue Breathing*).
7. Do not use a tourniquet unless the bleeding cannot be controlled with direct pressure. This may interrupt blood flow and cause the loss of the limb.

Pressure Points

If direct pressure fails to stop bleeding, apply pressure at a pressure point. These are places where a pulse can be felt as the artery passes close to a bone. A pressure point should be used only when direct pressure fails, since, like a tourniquet, you may interrupt blood flow and cause the loss of the limb.

Arm: Apply pressure on the inside of the arm between the biceps and triceps muscle. Use the flat side of your fingers to press the artery toward the bone. Keep the arm elevated.

Leg: Apply pressure on the front of the thigh just below the crease of the groin with the heel of your hand. Keep your arm straight and lean forward, using your body weight to maintain pressure. Elevate the bleeding leg.

Tourniquets

If both direct pressure and pressure points do not work, employ a tourniquet. This should be performed only if the person's life is threatened or if a limb has been amputated.

To apply a tourniquet:

1. It should be *at least* two inches (5.08 cm) wide.
2. It should be long enough to go around the limb twice, with some left over for tying.
3. It should be of strong material, for instance, a wide belt or sturdy cloth.
4. Place the tourniquet just above the wound, between the wound and the body.
5. Wrap twice around the wound, and tie a half-knot.
6. Place a sturdy stick or spoon across the knot, and complete a second half-knot over it.
7. Twist the stick until the bleeding stops but *no more.*

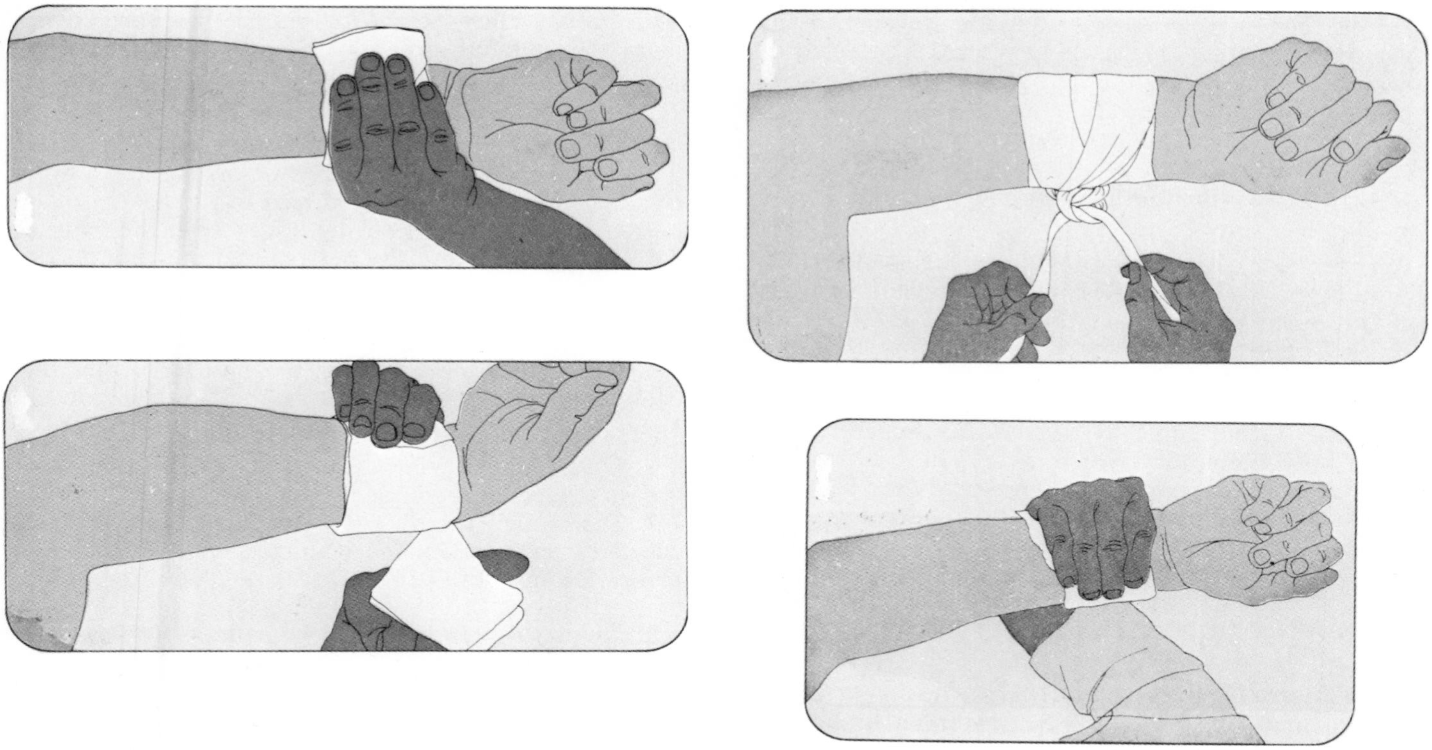

Techniques to stop bleeding.

8. Tie another knot, so the first knot will hold.
9. Once the tourniquet is in place, *never* remove it.
10. Attach a note, if possible, with the time of application.
11. Get medical attention immediately. Check for signs of shock.

Internal Bleeding

Suspect internal bleeding if someone has suffered a blow to chest or abdomen or if they are taking anticoagulant medication, such as Coumadin, which makes one more prone to bleed. Look for coughing of bright red blood, vomiting of bright red blood, passing dark or tarry stools, swelling of the abdomen, or signs of shock.

Immediately:

1. Check for breathing and pulse, and begin resuscitation if necessary.
2. Treat for shock.
3. Give nothing by mouth. There are *no* exceptions to this, no matter how thirsty the person is.
4. Get immediate medical attention.

Nosebleeds

Nosebleeds vary from minor to repeated, heavy bleeding that can be dangerous. There are only a few serious causes of nosebleeds, but repeated episodes should be evaluated by a medical practitioner. High blood pressure is a cause in rare cases.

To stop nasal bleeding:

1. Lean forward slightly and pinch the nostrils shut for fifteen minutes.
2. Release pressure slowly. If bleeding resumes, repeat the above.
3. If bleeding continues, pack the nose with cotton, lean forward slightly, and pinch the nostrils together.
4. If bleeding persists, place ice in a plastic bag, and hold against the nose. This will help constrict blood vessels and aid clotting.

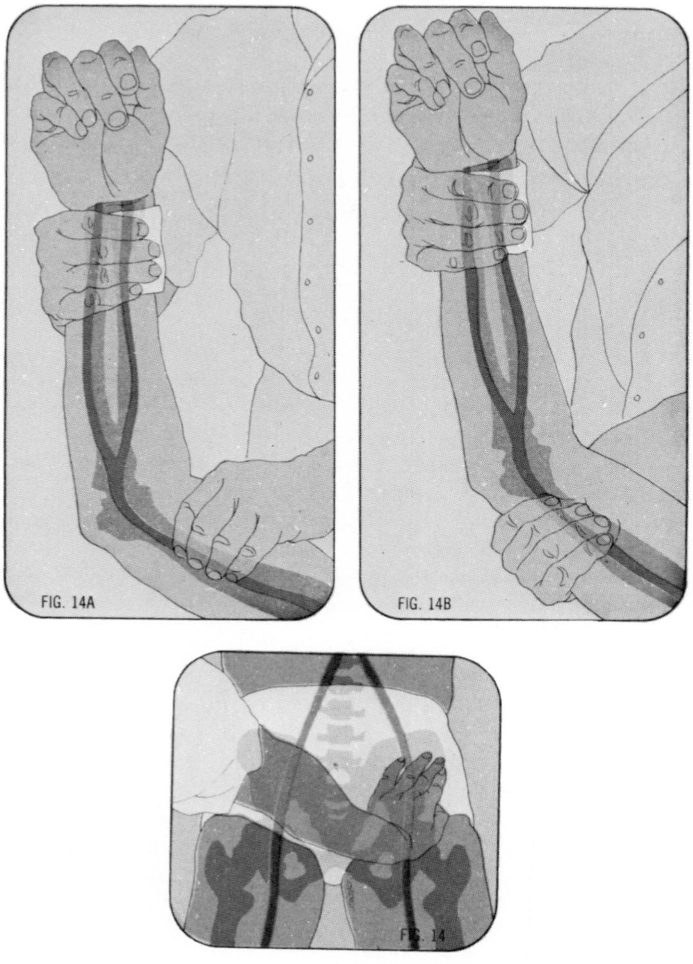

Using pressure points to stop bleeding.

5. Do not blow or pick your nose. If you feel that you have to sneeze, place a finger across the upper lip, beneath the nose, and apply light pressure. This will help to alleviate the feeling.

6. Avoid hot liquids and aspirin.

7. If bleeding persists or was sustained by a blow or injury, get a medical evaluation.

Burns

Burns may be caused by heat, corrosives, electricity, or sunlight. The goal of first aid is to prevent extension of the burn, relieve pain, and prevent infection and shock. Major burns are extremely dangerous. Fluid is lost, and the skin surface no longer provides protection against infection.

Burns are classified by degree. *First-degree* burns affect only the outer layer of skin. They are red and painful, may be slightly swollen, and do not blister or break the skin. *Second-degree* burns are red, often blotchy (red and white areas), and painful. They blister. *Third-degree* burns are potentially very dangerous. The skin will appear white, or charred and dry; there will be little or no pain. They require prompt medical attention.

Treatment of First-Degree Burns

1. Immediately place the burned area under cold running water. If running water is not available, apply a cold water compress or soak in a basin of cold water. Do not attempt to dry the skin. This prevents extension of the burn and reduces pain. Do *not* use ice or ice water. If no water is available, proceed to step 2.

2. Remove all jewelry.

3. Cover loosely with a clean bandage.

4. Never apply grease, butter or other ointments. This may retain heat and aggravate the burn.

Treatment of Second-Degree Burns

1. Cool the area by placing under running water, as in the treatment of first-degree burns.

2. Gently pat dry, but do not break, blisters.

3. Remove all jewelry in case of subsequent swelling.

4. Wrap lightly with clean bandage.

5. Do not apply grease, butter, or ointment.

6. Elevate the affected limb above the level of the heart.

7. Facial burns, if caused by flame or smoke, may cause damage to the lungs. Look for singed eyebrows and nostril hairs, burned lips, or soot in the mouth or nose. Seek *immediate* medical attention for facial burns.

8. Second-degree burns should usually be evaluated by a trained medical person.

Treatment of Third-Degree Burns

1. All third-degree burns should receive prompt medical attention. Take the person's pulse, and evaluate breathing. You may have to initiate basic mouth-to-mouth resuscitation and/or external heart massage.

2. Do not remove burned clothing that has adhered to the skin.

3. Immerse burned area under gently running, cold tap water, or apply cold cloth. Immerse in basin with cold water if necessary. Do not use ice or ice water.

4. Cover with clean bandage.

5. Elevate burned arm or leg above the level of the heart. If burn is on face, keep person upright.

6. Do not allow person to walk if the burn covers more than a small area.

7. Get emergency medical attention *immediately*.

If Someone's Clothes Are on Fire

1. Do not grab him.

2. Use a thick drape, throw rug, or blanket. Throw this over him, and command him to lie down.

3. If the person will not lie down, keep the blanket between yourself and the person, and pull him to the ground.

4. Roll him in the wrapped blanket.

5. Extinguish smoldering clothing with cool water.

6. If the face is burned or the nose or throat has been seared, keep the person in a sitting position.

In Case of Electric Shock or Burn

1. Do not touch the person if he is still in contact with the electrical source.

2. Disconnect person from electrical source with a wooden stick or other nonconducting object. *Never* use metal. Do not stand in a wet area. If necessary, disconnect fuse or circuit breaker.

3. Evaluate breathing and heartbeat. Begin resuscitation if necessary, without delay.

4. Get immediate medical attention. Electrical burns can run an invisible course along the route of the current.

In Case of Chemical Burns

Chemical burns in the home may be caused by drain openers, ammonia, or other corrosives.

1. Immediately flush area with large quantities of cool water. If outside, use a garden hose. Inside, use the shower. While flushing, remove clothing saturated with offending substance.

2. Persist in flushing for at least fifteen minutes to remove the chemical.

3. Check label of substance for specific instructions.

4. Do not use lard, butter, or ointments to cover the burn. Use only cool, clean compresses.

5. Get medical attention, especially for any burn to face or eyes.

Rescue Breathing

Anyone who has stopped breathing or has stopped having normal heartbeats needs immediate resuscitation, including rescue breathing (artificial ventilation or mouth-to-mouth breathing) and, if necessary, external cardiac massage. In the section that follows, instruction is given on how to open the airway and provide ventilation. This is useful when breathing has stopped but an effective heartbeat remains. Remember, however, no breathing means that the heart will stop beating within a minute or two.

We will not give instruction in external cardiac massage because the American Red Cross believes that the combination of rescue breathing and external cardiac massage is too difficult to learn from a book, and that the latter technique may be dangerous if performed improperly. Faulty technique may produce fractures of the ribs and puncture of the lungs. You should learn the complete skill; courses in cardiopulmonary resuscitation (CPR) are taught in most communities through the American Red Cross, American Heart Association, community groups, and hospitals. Learn this technique; it may help you save a life.

WHEN BREATHING STOPS

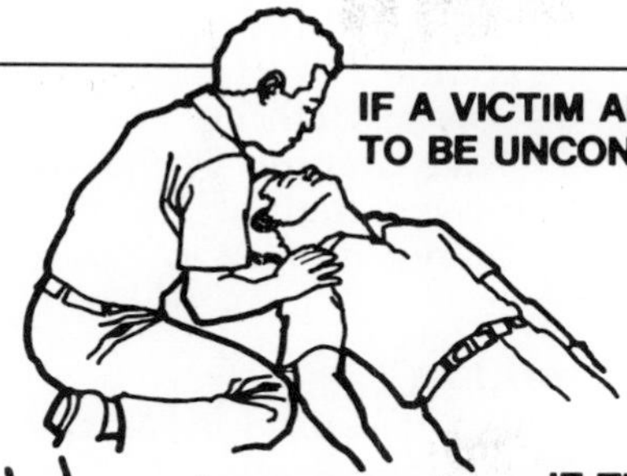

IF A VICTIM APPEARS TO BE UNCONSCIOUS TAP VICTIM ON THE SHOULDER AND SHOUT, "ARE YOU OKAY?"

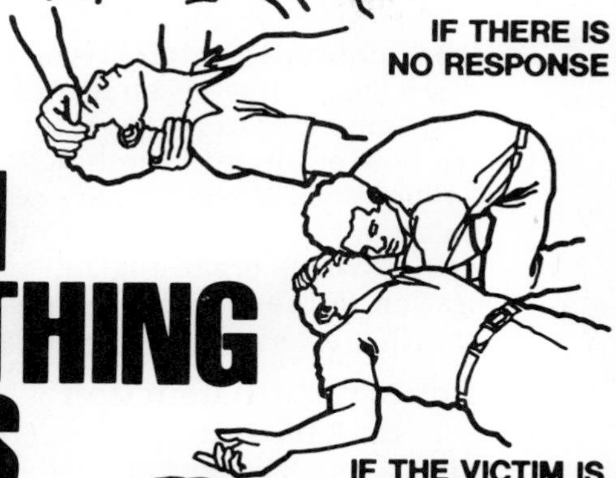

IF THERE IS NO RESPONSE TILT THE VICTIM'S HEAD, CHIN POINTING UP. Place one hand under the victim's neck and gently lift. At the same time, push with the other hand on the victim's forehead. This will move the tongue away from the back of the throat to open the airway.

IMMEDIATELY LOOK, LISTEN, AND FEEL FOR AIR.
While maintaining the backward head tilt position, place your cheek and ear close to the victim's mouth and nose. Look for the chest to rise and fall while you listen and feel for the return of air. Check for about 5 seconds.

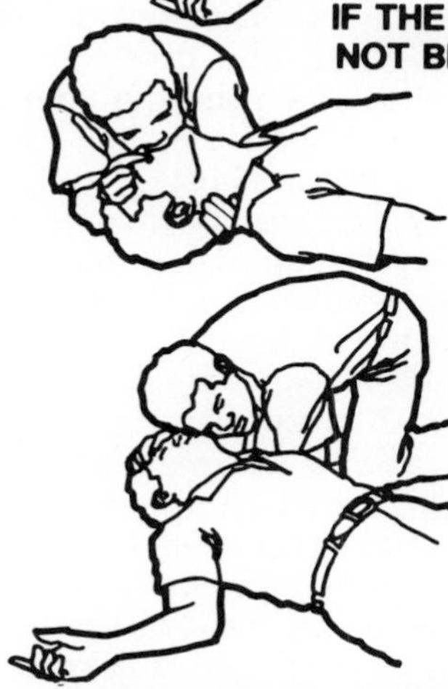

IF THE VICTIM IS NOT BREATHING GIVE FOUR QUICK BREATHS.
Maintain the backward head tilt, pinch the victim's nose with the hand that is on the victim's forehead to prevent leakage of air, open your mouth wide, take a deep breath, seal your mouth around the victim's mouth, and blow into the victim's mouth with four quick but full breaths just as fast as you can. When blowing, use only enough time between breaths to lift your head slightly for better inhalation. **For an infant,** give gentle puffs and blow through the mouth *and* nose and do not tilt the head back as far as for an adult.

If you do not get an air exchange when you blow, it may help to reposition the head and try again.

AGAIN, LOOK, LISTEN, AND FEEL FOR AIR EXCHANGE.

IF THERE IS STILL NO BREATHING CHANGE RATE TO ONE BREATH EVERY 5 SECONDS **FOR AN ADULT.**

FOR AN INFANT, GIVE ONE GENTLE PUFF EVERY 3 SECONDS.

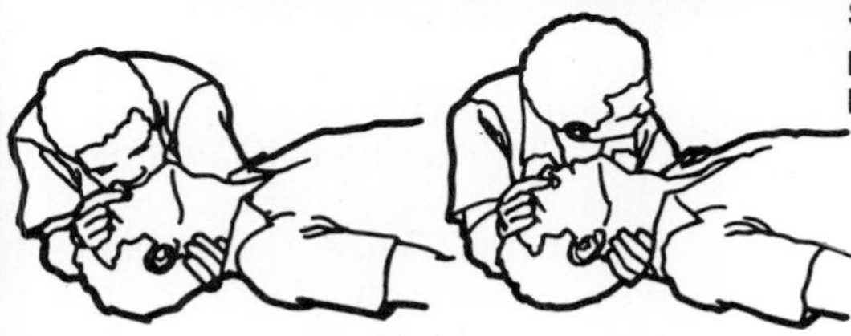

MOUTH-TO-NOSE METHOD

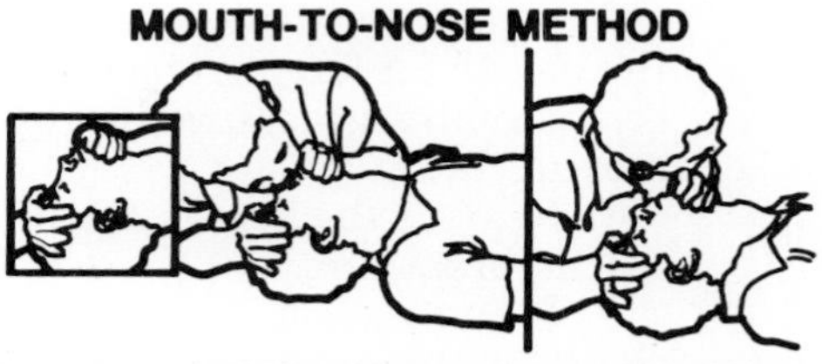

The mouth-to-nose method can be used with the sequence described above instead of the mouth-to-mouth method. Maintain the backward head-tilt position with the hand on the victim's forehead. Remove the hand from under the neck and close the victim's mouth. Blow into the victim's nose. Open the victim's mouth for the look, listen, and feel step.

For more information about these and other life-saving techniques, contact your Red Cross chapter for training.

American Red Cross

ARTIFICIAL RESPIRATION

Rescue breathing. (Reprinted with permision: American Red Cross.)

To perform rescue breathing:

1. Check to see if the person is conscious. If someone collapses, attempt to arouse him by gentle shaking, and ask, "Are you all right?" If there is a chance of head or neck injury, be very careful when you shake him.

2. Gently tip the head back until the chin is straight up. Place your hand under the neck to support the head. Check for breathing for at least five seconds. If there is breathing, you may see the chest rise and fall, hear air enter their mouth and nose, and feel air on your cheek.

3. If there is no breathing, give *four quick, large breaths,* as rapidly as you can, mouth-to-mouth. Do *not* let the chest fall between breaths. These are called "stair-step" ventilations because the chest rises in this pattern.

4. If air does not enter the lungs, there may be an obstruction to the airway. You will encounter partial or total resistance to your breathing efforts and the chest will not rise. The obstruction may be caused by the tongue or a foreign object and must be relieved. See *Choking,* below, for treating this problem.

5. Always continue to provide breaths. Try not to breathe too deeply or with excessive force. This can cause air to bypass the airway and pass down into the stomach, resulting in pressure buildup and eventual vomiting.

6. If vomiting occurs, turn the person onto his side and clear the vomitus from the mouth by sweeping two fingers in a cloth through the mouth. Reposition the head and neck and recommence breathing. Use less force and somewhat shallower breaths.

Chest Pain

Not all chest pain signals a heart attack. It is not always easy to know when to seek medical attention. If you are uncertain about what to do, it is usually wise to seek medical attention. Even if the symptom is not a sign of a serious problem, you will have reassured yourself and your loved ones.

If you or anyone you know has *any* of the following symptoms, get a prompt medical evaluation:

- pain behind the breastbone
- pain that is crushing or accompanied by a feeling of weight or pressure on the chest
- pain that radiates down the arm, into the neck, jaw, or abdomen
- pain accompanied by paleness, sweating, nausea, or vomiting
- pain that is sudden and severe, especially if accompanied by shortness of breath
- pain that is accompanied by indigestion and not relieved by two tablespoons of antacid
- pain that is accompanied by irregular, rapid (greater than one hundred beats per minute) heart rate or very slow (less than sixty beats per minute) heart rate
- pain that lasts for more than five minutes

If you, or someone you are with, has *any* of these signs, proceed to get emergency aid. If you think that this help will not be available quickly, go to your nearest emergency room.

En route or while waiting:

1. Monitor pulse and breathing.

2. Sit upright, or partially reclining, in a comfortable chair.

3. Loosen clothing.

4. Take nothing by mouth, except for nitroglycerin if you have angina.

5. Do not lie flat, as this may increase shortness of breath.

Choking

Choking is caused by partial or complete obstruction of the tubes leading to the lungs—the trachea and bronchial tubes. Often this is caused by food, especially when people have been drinking alcohol while eating. The immediate danger occurs if the object hampers the flow of air into the lungs.

Symptoms of choking are usually obvious. They are inability to speak, coughing, high-pitched crowing sounds when breathing in, and a red or blue discoloration to the face. If the person can speak, cough, or breathe, do not perform emergency measures.

Relieving Obstruction

1. Back blows: Stand behind the person and slightly to the side. Support the person with one hand under the chest, and give four sharp, rapid blows high up and between the shoulder blades with the heel of your hand. If possible, have the person's head below the level of the chest.

2. Abdominal thrusts: If back blows do not help, deliver four abdominal thrusts with the side of your fist. Deliver the thrust below the rib cage and above the navel. Do not strike the xiphoid (the lower portion of the breastbone), as this may cause internal injury.

3. If the person is unconscious, initiate rescue breathing as previously described.

4. If air will not enter the lungs, you will encounter partial or total resistance to your breathing efforts and the chest will not rise. This is a sign of obstruction to the airway, caused by the tongue or foreign object.

5. Reposition the head and neck and attempt to breathe again. If there is still an obstruction, turn the person on their side and deliver four solid blows to the midback, between the shoulder blades, with the flat of your hand.

6. Replace the person on their back and deliver four thrusts to the abdomen with the heel of the hand, as illustrated. Deliver these blows at a point located halfway between the navel and the edge of the lowest part of the sternum, the xiphoid process. Be careful not to thrust against the xiphoid itself.

7. Again, turn the person onto their side, and check the mouth for foreign objects, sweeping the mouth and/or manually grasping for the foreign object and removing it.

8. Replace the person on their back and again begin rescue breathing.

9. If ventilation is again unsuccessful, you have no choice but to repeat the sequence until you are successful.

Heat Stroke

Anyone who is exposed to heat or has impaired sweating or diminished body fluid stores (dehydration) may get heat stroke. Phenothiazine drugs and other tranquilizers, including Thorazine, Stelazine, and Mellaril, may also impair one's ability to handle heat exposure.

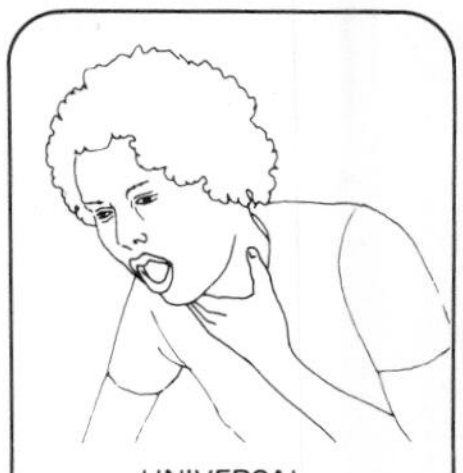
UNIVERSAL CHOKING SIGN

FIRST AID FOR CHOKING

If victim can cough, speak, breathe ➡ *Do not interfere*

If victim cannot cough speak breathe — *Have someone call for help. Telephone: ____________ (Number)*

TAKE ACTION: FOR CONSCIOUS VICTIM

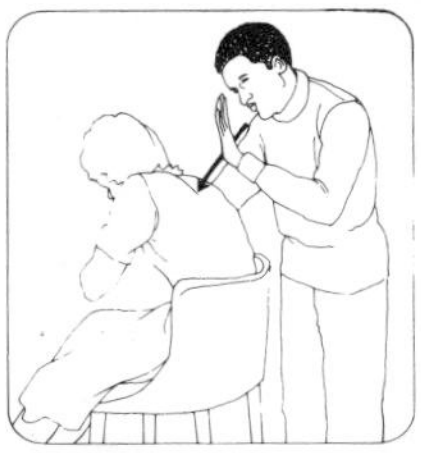
4 QUICK BACK BLOWS

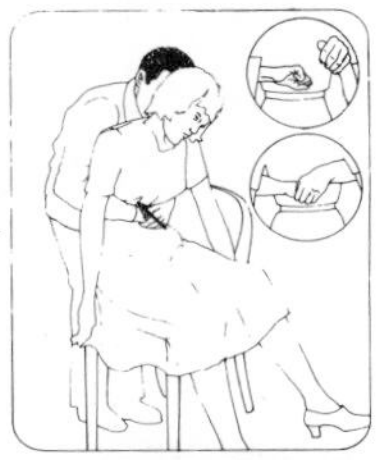
4 MANUAL THRUSTS

Repeat steps until effective or until victim becomes unconscious.

TAKE ACTION: FOR UNCONSCIOUS VICTIM

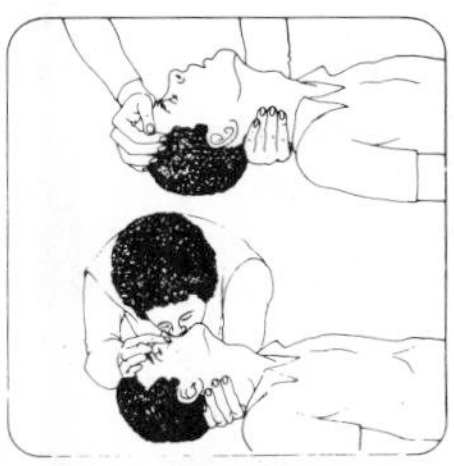
TRY TO VENTILATE

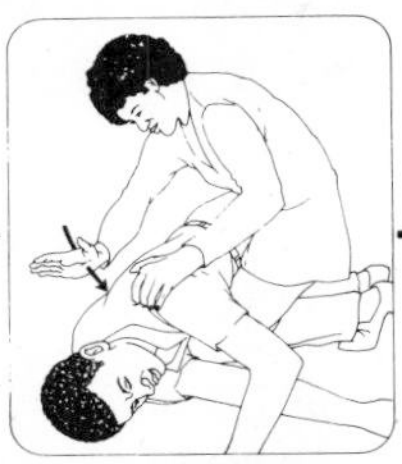
4 BACK BLOWS

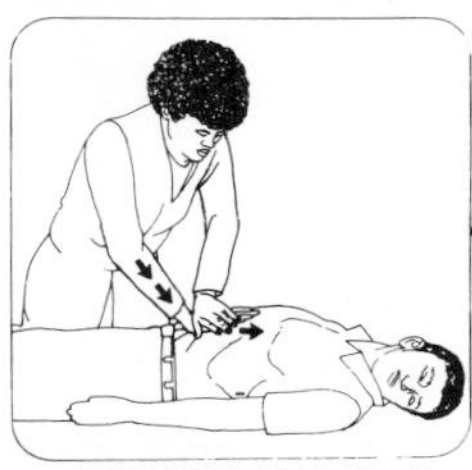
4 MANUAL THRUSTS

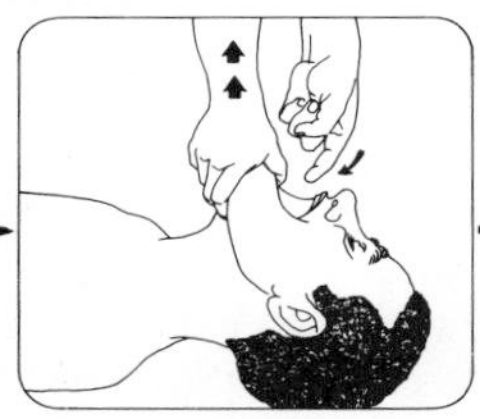
FINGER PROBE

Repeat steps until effective.

Continue artificial ventilation or CPR, as indicated.

Everyone should learn how to perform the above first aid steps for choking and how to give mouth-to-mouth and cardiopulmonary resuscitation. Call your local Red Cross chapter for information on these and other first aid techniques.

Caution: Abdominal thrusts may cause injury. Do not practice on people.

AMERICAN RED CROSS

Techniques to stop choking. (Reprinted with permission: American Red Cross.)

Warning signs of heat stroke are:

- elevated temperature, possibly in excess of 104°F (40°C)
- dry, warm, or hot skin
- dry tongue and mouth; absence of tears
- rapid, bounding pulse
- confusion

The object in treating heat stroke is to lower the body temperature. To accomplish this:

1. Undress the person.
2. Place victim in a tub of cold tap water. Do not use ice.
3. Check temperature every few minutes.
4. Avoid lowering temperature below 101°F (38.3°C).
5. If a tub is not available, sponge with cool water or alcohol or spray gently with a hose.
6. Give fluids, but avoid alcoholic beverages, tea, coffee, cola, and other caffeine-containing drinks.
7. You may use a fan to help in cooling.
8. Call for immediate emergency help. Take the person's pulse, and evaluate breathing. You may have to initiate basic mouth-to-mouth resuscitation and/or external heart massage.

Minor Injuries

Bruises

A bruise usually results from a blow that produces rupture of the small blood vessels under the skin. As the vessel breaks, it turns the skin red, then dark blue after clotting, and finally yellow-green as the blood is broken down and absorbed.

To treat a bruise:

1. Apply ice (in a plastic bag) immediately.
2. Elevate the limb to reduce swelling.
3. Leave ice on for fifteen minutes, then remove for fifteen minutes. Repeat.
4. After twenty-four hours, apply moist, warm compresses. This dissolves the clotted blood, increases circulation, and improves healing.
5. Take acetaminophen (Tylenol) for pain. Avoid aspirin for the first twenty-four hours, as it may inhibit blood clotting.
6. Any persistent bruising requires medical evaluation.

Foreign Bodies in the Eyes

It is quite common for a foreign object to be blown or rubbed into the eye. This is painful and potentially damaging if the object is allowed to scratch the surface of the eyeball. The following instructions apply to removal of an object from your own eye or someone else's.

First aid should be prompt. The eye should not be rubbed. Clean your hands before attempting removal. Never use a hard object like a match or toothpick to remove the object.

To look for the foreign substance, begin by pulling down the lower lid and moving the eye in all directions. This may dislodge the foreign body. If you see it, remove it with a clean handkerchief or other lint-free cloth. Do not use tissue paper or lint-shedding cloth that can leave additional debris in the eye.

If you cannot see the object, you will need to look under the upper lid. Follow these steps:

1. Grasp the lashes of the upper lid and pull gently away from the eyeball. This may dislodge the object and allow tears to wash it away.

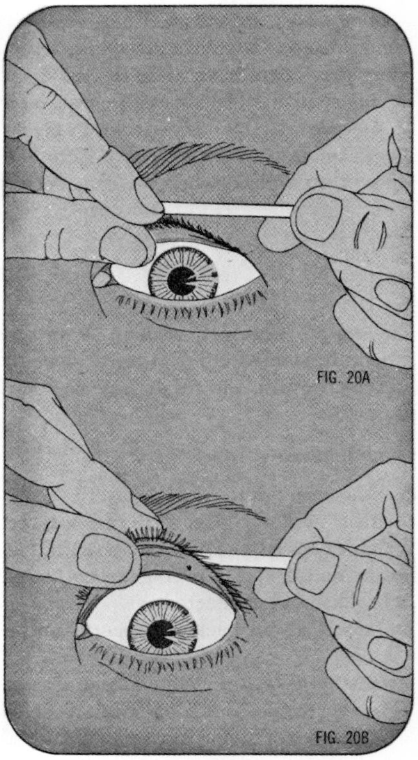

Removing a foreign body from the eye.

2. If this is unsuccessful, place a matchstick, firm swab, or other thin instrument along the *outside* of the upper lid, grasp the lashes, and gently turn the upper lid inside out. Look for the foreign body and remove with a clean cloth.
3. Flush with tap water using an eye cup, dropper, or a small bulb syringe.
4. If the sensation of a foreign body persists after ten or fifteen minutes, apply a clean dressing over the covered eye and obtain emergency medical attention.

If a more serious or penetrating injury to the eye occurs, such as a direct blow with a blunt object (fist, stick) or sharp object (BB bullet, glass), follow these steps:

1. Lie flat.
2. Cover *both* eyes with a clean dressing, attached by loosely wrapping with gauze or tape that completely encircles the head. Avoid putting any pressure on the eyeball.
3. Keep *both* eyes closed (so the unaffected eye does not move, causing the affected eye to move as well).
4. Get immediate medical attention and transport by stretcher, if possible.

Shock

Shock occurs when there is insufficient blood flow to the brain and other vital organs. It may occur in allergic reactions (bee stings), burns, severe heart attacks, injury, infection, in diabetes (see Chapter 21), or with heavy bleeding. The first aid measures often do not depend on the cause. The underlying cause will be established by trained medical personnel.

Some signs of shock are rapid, thready, or faint pulse; increased rate of breathing; change in mental functioning; cool, clammy, pale, or bluish skin; or a combination of these signs.

To treat shock:

1. Assess breathing and pulse. If necessary, initiate CPR.
2. Stop any obvious bleeding.
3. Keep person lying down.
4. Elevate legs eight to twelve inches (20 to 30 cm) off the ground. Do not elevate, however, if you suspect head or neck injury, spine injury, or if the person is unconscious.
5. Give nothing by mouth.
6. Get immediate medical attention.
7. Be reassuring.
8. Keep person warm.

Sprains

A sprain is a forceful stretching or tearing of ligaments, which support joints. Sprains produce swelling and pain and may appear black-and-blue. If there is discoloration, the ligaments may be ruptured, a sign to seek medical evaluation.

Applying an ace bandage.

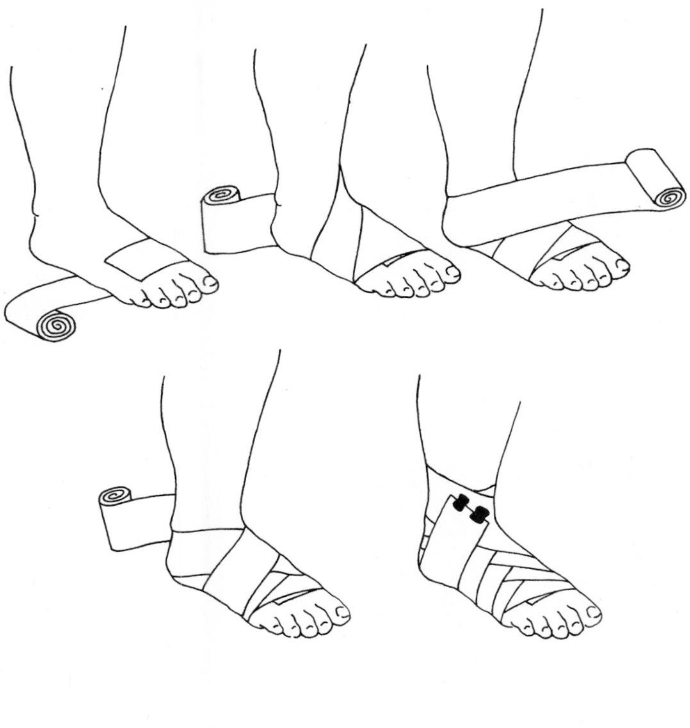

To treat a sprain:

1. Apply ice (ice pack or ice in a plastic bag), and cover with a towel for insulation. Alternate fifteen minutes on and fifteen minutes off.
2. Elevate limb above level of the heart.
3. Apply elastic bandage loosely around affected area. Fingers and toes should remain warm and have normal touch sensation.
4. If wrist, elbow, or shoulder is injured, support the arm with a sling.
5. If pain, swelling, or limitation of movement continues for more than a few days, obtain a medical evaluation.
6. If the affected area turns black-and-blue, seek immediate medical care.

First-Aid Supplies for Home or Car

The contents of a first-aid kit should be limited to a few simple items that you know how to use. The following items are useful for the emergencies discussed in this chapter.

- sterile gauze pads, four by four inches (10 by 10 cm), packaged individually, to stop bleeding (ten pads)
- heavy dressings, called ABD pads, for serious bleeding (six pads)
- two rolls of gauze bandage (Kerlix or Kling) to wrap injuries; these are self-adhering but do not stick to the skin
- adhesive tape in one- or two-inch (2.5- or 5-cm) width (one roll)
- cotton-tip swabs, to look under the eyelid for a foreign body (one package)
- scissors, for cutting bandages
- flashlight
- adhesive bandages of assorted sizes
- hydrogen peroxide for cleaning small wounds (one bottle)
- a three-inch (7.5-cm) elastic wrap for wrapping injured limbs; use carefully according to instructions given in text and by your medical provider
- eye cup, for rinsing eyes

Part V

Drugs and Medications

The importance of understanding *why, how,* and *when* to take medicines increases with advancing years. The older we are, the more likely we are to need one or more medicines on a regular basis. Although these drugs are often essential for maintaining a normal life, the risk of having an adverse reaction to medical therapy also increases with age.

It is therefore essential that people over fifty-five know about the use and action of drugs. We should be able to understand and recognize an adverse reaction to a medicine and be ready to report it *promptly* to our medical provider. This is an important part of being an astute consumer of medical services and may save your life or the life of someone you know.

This section is divided into two chapters. The first describes how drugs work and provides information for taking medicines. The second part is an alphabetical listing of common over-the-counter and prescribed medications used by people over fifty-five. Although it is not possible to list all the medicines that are available, we have tried to include those most commonly taken. Look up your medicines and become familiar with their use, dosage, and potential side effects.

Some general points:

- Keep a list of your medicines with you when you leave the house and spare prescriptions when you travel on vacation.
- Discuss all your medicines, their use, and possible side effects, whenever you see your medical care giver.
- Take your medications only as directed by your care giver. Do not skip days or add extra pills if you forget to take a dose or feel a new symptom.
- Do not trade or give medicines to friends.
- Keep your medicines out of the reach of children.

Chapter 24
Drug Guide

Rein Tideiksaar, PA, PhD

Taking drugs to gain relief from pain and discomfort and to cure illness is as old as humankind. Since World War II, however, the number and complexity of the drugs on the market have increased enormously. People over sixty-five receive 25 percent of all prescriptions for medications, even though they comprise only 11 percent of the population, and spend three times as much on drugs ($2.6 billion) as younger people.

The older you are, the more likely you are to be taking a number of medicines at the same time. Consequently, the medicines have a greater potential for interfering with each other or causing some kind of harmful or unpleasant reaction. This includes medications like aspirin and antacids that can be purchased without a prescription. Just because you do not need a prescription does not mean the drug is harmless.

For all these reasons, it is essential that older people understand more about their medications and how to be better drug consumers. Sometimes medical care givers are not as aware of the potential dangers as they should be. Of the more than seven thousand drugs on the market, only 25 percent of them were available when many physicians were in medical school. This places even more responsibility on the consumer. If you are taking a medicine, you should know the proper amount to take, what the potential side effects are, what its use is for you, and if there are special considerations in how you take it. For instance, should it be taken on an empty or full stomach? Does alcohol interfere with its action? Is it dangerous when taken with some other medicine that you need? The ultimate responsibility for drug use falls on you, since the drug is going into your body.

How Drugs Work

As we age, drugs affect us differently than when we were younger. In general, we are more susceptible to them and may need reduced dosages to maintain the proper effect and minimize side effects.

Most drugs are metabolized in the liver. As we age, the rate at which the liver accomplishes this process decreases. From a practical point of view, drugs such as Valium and Dalmane used frequently for anxiety or sleeping are eliminated more slowly from the body. This means less of the drug than used in the average person may be necessary to avoid feeling dizzy, confused, or unnecessarily drowsy.

Drugs are excreted by the kidney, which also shows some decline in function with age. Although this may not be important in normal circumstances, the diminished ability of the kidney to eliminate digoxin (used to treat heart disease) may increase its likelihood of having toxic side effects. If you take digitalis-type drugs, be conscious of any nausea, lack of appetite, or memory loss, and report it to your care giver.

Drug Reactions

Any unfavorable reactions to medication should be reported to a medical care giver *immediately*. Because the effect of drugs and adverse drug reactions may be cumulative, it is important not to delay in discussing symptoms with a family physician or other trained person. Unfortunately, both medical personnel and patients often attribute these symptoms to old age rather than to a drug. Thus, a symptom that would cause an immediate alert of a potential adverse drug reaction in a thirty-year-old person might be overlooked in older people. Be persistent with yourself, your loved ones, and your medical providers—do not take an unpleasant symptom for granted.

What are some clues that indicate an adverse reaction? The skin is a good indicator. If a *rash* develops after a medication is begun, it should be reported. Other frequent symptoms that warn of danger are *nausea, dizziness, unexplained irritability, confusion, visual difficulties,* and *stomach upsets*. Other side effects that pertain to specific medications are listed in the drug guide that follows (Chapter 25). Remember: the responsibility for being aware of and reporting these symptoms is your own.

Over-the-Counter Medications (OTC Drugs)

Vast amounts of nonprescription drugs have been introduced to the general public by the mass media. It is estimated that older people spend up to one-third of their drug dollar on OTC preparations. It is a myth that these medicines are completely safe. They are not: like prescription drugs they may cause unpleasant or dangerous reactions and may interfere with prescription drugs.

Moreover, people taking OTC medicines have usually diagnosed and are treating their own illnesses without medical assistance. Sometimes this hides symptoms of serious illnesses and delays prompt medical investigation and treatment. Never take OTC medications for prolonged periods of time when a symptom does not go away.

There are some important points to remember when taking OTC drugs. First, they may interfere with prescription drugs. Tetracycline, for instance, is an antibiotic used to treat infection. Iron supplements or antacids may decrease the amount of tetracycline that is absorbed from the stomach.

OTC drugs may be ill-advised for certain medical conditions. Antacids and laxatives often contain high concentrations of sodium, which may aggravate high blood pressure. Aspirin, found in over four hundred OTC medications, can contribute to excessive low blood sugar in diabetics who take insulin.

OTC medicines may cause unpleasant side effects. They are not harmless. Aspirin can inhibit blood-clotting and produce bleeding from the stomach. Cold preparations can cause drowsiness and dizziness. Know the potential side effects of any OTC medication before you take it by asking the pharmacist or a medical care giver.

Finally, OTC drugs may hide early symptoms of a serious problem. Do not medicate yourself to cover up a nagging symptom for any appreciable length of time. A simple rule of thumb is that you have a serious problem if you have to buy a second package of any particular product. Cough preparations used to cover up a chronic cough may delay the diagnosis and treatment of a respiratory illness like lung cancer or emphysema. Laxatives can cover up symptoms of a bowel cancer.

When you see your medical care giver, go to the hospital, or purchase a medication from a pharmacy, tell the professional who sees you about all your medications—including OTC medications; otherwise you may wind up with conflicting medications. Remember, OTC drugs, like all others, are potentially dangerous.

Generic Drugs

Whenever a drug company develops a new drug, it receives three names: the chemical name, which is usually not given on the label; the generic or official name, and the brand name. Aspirin, for instance, is the generic name, acetylsalicylic acid is the chemical name, and Bayer is the brand name for a popular painkiller. Unlike generic names, which usually are tongue twisters to ask for, brand names are short, easy to remember, and often suggest the pharmacological action of the drug.

It is the brand name that is used to advertise a drug to your medical providers. Tetracycline, for example, is a widely used prescription antibiotic. Your medical provider may write a prescription for this drug by its generic name (tetracycline), or may prescribe it under such brand names as Achromycin, Sumycin, or Tetracyn. Whether you receive this drug as a generic or brand name makes little difference in the drug's antibiotic effectiveness. All generic drugs must meet the official Federal Drug Administration standards for that drug for safety, strength, and effectiveness. So, by law, generic and brand name drugs must be equivalent both chemically and in the way they affect your body. The main difference between generic and brand name drugs is cost. Because brand name drugs are heavily advertised, they cost considerably more than generic drugs.

For example, Polycillin is a brand name drug that costs approximately twelve dollars for one hundred capsules. The generic form, ampicillin, costs four dollars for the same one hundred capsules. One way to hold down your drug costs is to encourage your medical provider to prescribe drugs by their generic names and to encourage your pharmacist to fill prescriptions with the lowest costing version of the prescribed drug.

At this point you may wonder why, since there is no difference between generic and brand name drugs, medical providers do not write far more generic prescriptions. Some medical providers may have more confidence in using products from large drug companies. Others may not be aware of the difference in price between a generic and brand name drug, or they may not be aware that a generic equivalent is available. Another factor is that the professional journals of medical providers advertise drugs by their brand names. Thus, medical providers tend to prescribe by brand names out of habit. As medical providers gain more understanding of generic drugs, generic prescribing will likely increase. The result will be a lower cost to you, the consumer.

Analgesics

Injury or discomfort to some part of the body is experienced as pain. With advancing years we encounter a number of physiological changes and diseases that render us susceptible to pain. Thus, with increasing age, there is a need for ways of alleviating pain. Analgesics, drugs that decrease pain, are therefore frequently taken for the relief of pain.

The two most frequently used over-the-counter analgesics are aspirin and acetaminophen (Tylenol). The successful management of pain depends upon your being aware of their uses as well as their abuses.

If used properly, both aspirin and Tylenol work equally as well in relieving the pain caused by minor injuries or tension headaches. Aspirin has an added advantage over Tylenol: it reduces inflammation (redness and swelling). So it works better than Tylenol against inflammation-causing conditions like arthritis.

Aspirin is probably one of the most useful drugs you can have around the house, but do not underestimate its dangers. Aspirin has a common side effect. It often irritates the stomach, causing bleeding. Tylenol does not have this side effect and often can be a substitute if stomach irritation or heartburn is a problem.

If aspirin is needed for its antiswelling effects, you can seek out an aspirin preparation that is enteric coated (a special covering that protects the stomach) to reduce stomach irritation. You can also try a buffered aspirin or aspirin mixed with antacids, although these products do not always prevent stomach discomfort.

Also available are innumerable prescription pain relievers (Motrin, Clinoril, Tolectin, Naprosyn). These drugs are chemically related to aspirin and are now being used as alternatives for people who cannot tolerate aspirin's side effects. Although the side effects of heartburn and bleeding from the stomach occur less frequently with these products than with aspirin, they are much more expensive and should be used as second choices to aspirin for the control of pain.

To ensure successful management of pain while taking aspirin, it is important to follow these instructions:

- Aspirin should be taken as directed by a medical provider.
- Never increase, decrease, or change the dose without specific instructions from a medical provider.
- Aspirin may cause stomach upset. If this is a problem, take aspirin with two tablespoonsful of an antacid or with meals. Report stomach upsets that continue or increase in frequency, to a medical provider.
- If you take aspirin on a routine basis, inform every medical provider you visit that you take aspirin on a regular basis.
- Remember that many over-the-counter and prescription drugs contain aspirin as one of the ingredients. If you cannot tolerate the side effects of aspirin,

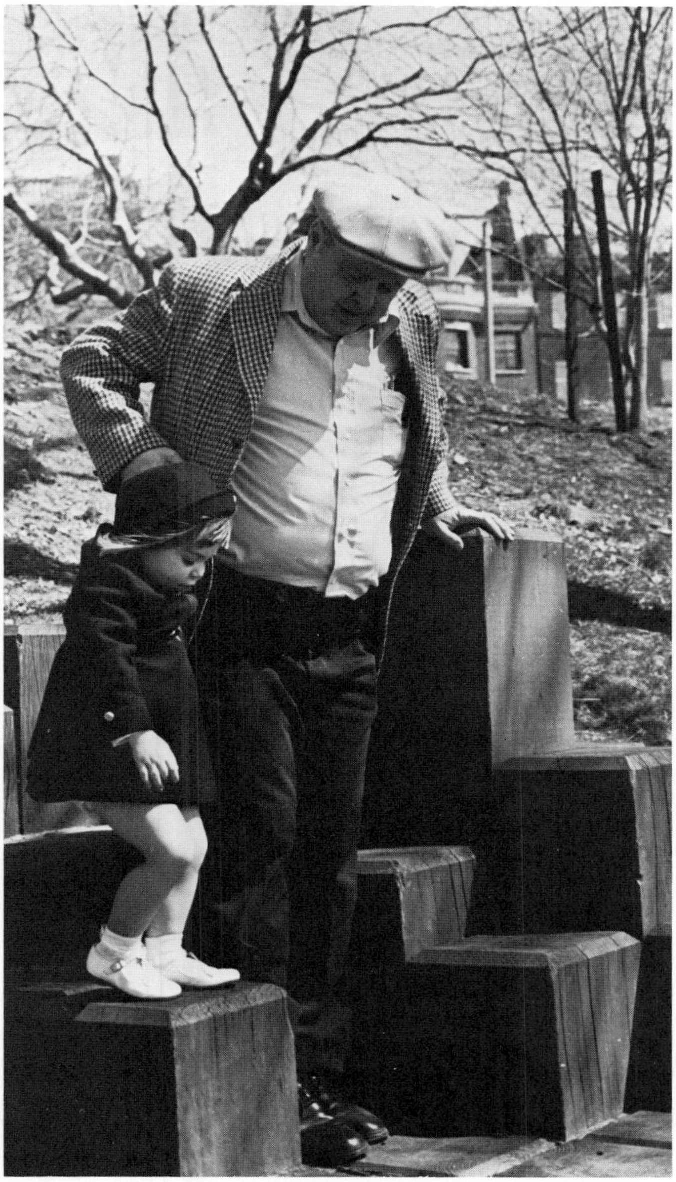

always ask your pharmacist if you are taking medications that contain aspirin.

- Report these signs to a medical provider if they occur:
  - blood-tinged or black bowel movements
  - blood-tinged vomit
  - ringing in the ears or difficulty in hearing
  - skin rash
  - heartburn or stomach pain

Alcohol and Drugs

Just how much a person is affected by the mixture of alcohol and drugs depends upon the amount of alcohol consumed and the types of medications taken. Not all drugs will interfere with that occasional evening cocktail. Of the most frequently prescribed drugs, however, a sizable majority of them contain ingredients that are known to adversely interact with alcohol. In addition, many over-the-counter drug products have the same adverse effects when taken with alcohol.

It is important to remember that alcohol itself is a drug, probably one of the oldest drugs known to man. When alcohol is taken by itself, especially in large amounts, it can have a strong depressant effect on the nervous system that can cause drowsiness and difficulty in walking, driving, and thinking. If you are taking prescription or over-the-counter drugs, even small amounts of alcohol (a glass of beer or wine) can doubly affect the slowing down of performance skills, judgment, and alertness.

Alcohol can alter the way drugs do their job. The use of alcohol can speed up the process of drug metabolism. This makes many drugs less effective because they do not stay in the body as long as they should to be of use. In such cases larger doses of the drug may be necessary. Among drugs that respond in this way are anticoagulants such as Coumadin and the antidiabetic drug Orinase.

Mixing alcohol with drugs can also produce the opposite effect, slowing down the metabolism of drugs in the body. Thus, drugs remain in the body longer than they should, and even small amounts of such drugs as antidepressants, tranquilizers (Valium), and aspirin will increase the possibility of side effects.

Knowing when it is safe to have a drink when taking drugs presents some problems. In general, the information on alcohol-drug interactions is provided by

A Sampling of Alcohol-Drug Effects

Drugs that interact with Alcohol	Possible Effects
aspirin Coumadin	Increased risk of bleeding
Valium Dalmane Noctec Elavil Sinequan Librium OTC cold and allergy preparations	Increased risk of excessive drowsiness and dizziness
Lasix HydroDIURIL Dyrenium nitroglycerin	Reduction in blood pressure that may result in dizziness
Orinase	Symptoms of high blood sugar
Insulin	Symptoms of low blood sugar
codeine Darvon	Increased risk of dizziness, drowsiness

Caution: The drugs cited on this list are among the most widely prescribed medicines, but they represent only a few of the hundreds of drugs that involve significant alcohol-drug interactions. Remember: always check with your medical provider or pharmacist about the use of alcohol when taking medications.

drug companies only to a medical provider and pharmacist. Whether you get the message or not depends upon your medical provider and pharmacist giving you this information or your asking about it. Another problem is that labels on over-the-counter drugs do not always warn about alcohol-drug interactions. It should be noted that a number of popular OTC cold medicines contain alcohol.

To be on the safe side, I have included some tips on how you can avoid unpleasant alcohol-drug interactions.

- Always inform your medical provider about your drinking habits when given a drug prescription.
- Always check with your pharmacist if you have any questions about the use of alcohol with either prescription or over-the-counter drugs.
- Read the labels on all over-the-counter drug products for alcohol content.
- When you are taking drugs, always report any changes in your drinking habits to your medical provider.
- When in doubt, do not take a single drink while on medication.

Anticoagulants

Anticoagulants inhibit blood-clotting. They are used to prevent unwanted blood-clotting in people who have had clots form in the lungs, legs, or heart. The major danger involved in taking these drugs is that abnormal bleeding may occur. These medications should be taken only with careful monitoring by a medical provider. Some specific points to be aware of when taking anticoagulants follow.

- Guard against cuts, especially while working in the kitchen and garden or doing similar work. Wear shoes; wear gloves. When shaving, use an electric shaver.
- Do not stop taking the anticoagulant unless so directed by a medical provider. Travelers should carry sufficient amounts of medication with them.
- Fill drug prescriptions at a drugstore that keeps records of all the medications their customers use. This way, the pharmacist can identify drug interactions.
- Ask a medical provider or pharmacist about taking any over-the-counter drug. Aspirin, some cold remedies, mineral oil, vitamin supplements, sleeping pills, laxatives, antacids, and alcoholic beverages may affect the action of anticoagulants.
- Avoid food fads and marked changes in diet. Discuss any dieting plans with a medical provider. Certain foods are high in vitamin K, the vitamin that promotes coagulation. These need not be avoided, but marked change in their consumption will alter the response to oral anticoagulants. Foods high in vitamin K include: alfalfa, cabbage, cauliflower, liver, soybeans, spinach, and fish.
- Inform dentists about anticoagulant medication before having dental work done. Discuss dental work with a medical provider as well.
- Carry identification at all times that indicates you are taking an oral anticoagulant.
- Notify a medical provider about the following symptoms:
  - red urine
  - black bowel movements
  - severe, persistent headaches or stomachaches
  - excessive bleeding after cutting yourself
  - dizziness
  - increased pulse or breathing rate
  - excessive bruising

Taking Medication

People do not always take their medications *exactly* as prescribed by a care giver. In fact, the more medicines necessary, the greater the risk of skipping some doses, eliminating some medications, or making mistakes. Sometimes people get a prescription but fail to fill it because they feel it is too expensive.

Sometimes mistakes are made because people do not understand how and why a drug works. For instance, digoxin is a heart medication that also relieves swollen ankles. I have seen people adjust their dose of digoxin on the basis of their ankle swelling. This can be very dangerous—even fatal.

A third error occurs when people hoard and trade their medications. They wind up taking or giving to friends out-of-date drugs. In general, any drug more than three months old may be out of date. Ask a medical provider if it is still safe. And *never* give or trade medicines.

If you cannot open the newer child-proof bottles, ask your care giver to instruct the pharmacist to give you a screw-cap bottle. Always keep medicines away from places where children can get to them—this is a common source of poisoning in children.

Drugs can be very helpful when used properly. Each of us has the responsibility for our drug treatment by making sure we get the information we need to understand exactly why and how to take the medicine. Remember, it is your health that is at stake. The following medication tips will help you get the information you need to use your medicines safely.

Medication Tips

- Understand the reasons for the medication
- So that medications will be taken on time, understand the drug dosage schedule
- So that therapy will not be interrupted, get medications refilled on time
- To prevent concern over side effects and to prevent unnecessary discontinuance of medication, ask about the side effects caused by drugs and understand the importance of these effects
- To promote safe and effective use of medications, ask if there are any special directions for using them (for example, can they be taken with food?)
- To guard against drug side effects and to know that the drug is doing what it is intended to do, understand how to monitor therapy, including the reporting of any untoward effects
- To prevent misuse of drugs and to prevent serious accidents, understand that prescriptions are individually tailored and should not be shared or offered to friends
- To prevent drug interactions and misuse of medications, understand that pharmacists can give useful advice about prescription and nonprescription medications

Taking Medication

All persons taking medications should understand why, how, and when to take medication that he or she will receive from the doctor or pharmacy. Be aware of the following general medication instructions:

Medication name: The name and strength of all medications should be properly labeled. Know the name and strength of all medications you receive. Keep an up-to-date list of all medicines you are taking. If you go to more than one physician, tell each the name of all medications you are taking.

Medication purpose: The doctor or pharmacist should explain why medications have been prescribed for you and how they work in your body. Ask for written instructions.

How and when to use the medications: If there is a special way to administer your medications, this should be fully explained. Remember: to get the best therapeutic response, some drugs should be taken before meals or after meals, whereas other drugs must be taken alone. If you have trouble remembering when to take your medications, ask your doctor or pharmacist for help. If you have trouble opening medications with child-proof tops, ask your doctor to indicate on the prescription that you are to have a non–child-proof top.

Dosage: Know the maximum amount that may be taken safely in a day. Some medications are taken only "as needed," but this does not mean as often as you want.

Side effects: Certain drugs produce untoward effects, and you should be made aware of these facts. Contact your physician if you:

- develop nausea and vomiting, diarrhea, or lose your appetite
- develop a rash
- have a sore throat for several days
- feel dizzy or faint
- feel weak, tired, or short of breath

Some medicines lose their strength or even become dangerous after several months. If your medicine is over three months old, ask your doctor if it is still safe to take. Because a number of medications may cause temporary drowsiness, be particularly careful when driving a car or operating dangerous machinery. Try to avoid alcoholic beverages when taking any medications.

How long to use the medication: Take the exact number or amount ordered. Do not be lulled into a false sense of security if you start feeling better after a day or two. Stopping your medication too soon may cause a flare-up of the original problem. Do not skip any medication dosages. If you have skipped a dose of your medication, do not try to catch up by doubling the next dose on your own—call your doctor. Do not let your medicine run out. Get prescriptions refilled early. Stop taking medicines only on your physician's instruction. Never take more than has been prescribed; extra medication may be dangerous.

Use of other medications: Your medicine is only for you. Do not give it to anyone else, as it might be dangerous to them. Do not take anyone else's medicine, even if you both have the same illness. Some medicines interfere with actions of other medications. Do not take medicine you can buy without a prescription (aspirin, antacids, vitamins, cold medicines, laxatives, nerve pills, sleeping medicine) until you check with your physician.

Storage and handling: Each time you take a medication, read the label. For some drugs to maintain their full potency, certain storage requirements are necessary (e.g., refrigerate, avoid moisture, etc.). Do not mix medicines together in one bottle or box—keep each one separate. Your name, the name of the medicine, and the directions for taking it should be on each package of medicine. Keep your medicine away from children.

Drugs and special diets: If you are on a low-sodium, low-potassium, diabetic, or peptic ulcer diet, certain foods and drugs must be avoided. These should be explained by your doctor.

• To help in taking medication, know that easy-to-open pill bottle tops are available for the asking from doctors and pharmacists

• Prepare and carry a wallet card on which the following information is printed: name, age, address, the name of a person to notify in an emergency, the name and telephone number of personal physician, allergies, illnesses, and a list of current prescription and non-prescription drugs being taken

• To avoid unexpected drug interactions and to assure the proper action of prescribed drugs, understand that many over-the-counter drug products may interfere with the action of prescription drugs

Medication Record

Drug	Directions	Dose	Physician Prescribing	Drugs to Avoid

Fill out this chart, with the help of your medical provider if necessary.
Keep a copy of this chart with you, in your purse or wallet.
Take it with you when visiting your medical provider, clinic, or emergency room.
Make additional copies to give to family, so they can help in an emergency.

Medication Schedule

Drug	Time	Dosage	Sun.	Mon.	Tue.	Wed.	Thurs.	Fri.	Sat.

1. In the column marked DRUG, put the names of the drugs you are taking.
2. In the column marked TIME, put the time of day you take your medication.
3. In the column marked DOSAGE, put the number of pills or the amount of liquid you are to take at that time.
4. In the remaining columns marked SUN. through SAT., indicate with an X or checkmark that you have taken the drug.

This chart is good for one week. Copy or make photocopies for every week.

Medication Checklist

Before you leave your doctor's office:

_____ Is your medication identified?
_____ Do you know what the medication is for?
_____ Do you have written instructions on the use of your medications?
_____ Are you able to open child-proof bottle tops?
_____ Have you asked about large-print labels for your pill bottles?
_____ Are you certain about the side effects you may encounter? Are the directions for reporting side effects specific?
_____ Are you certain about which over-the-counter medications to avoid while taking medications?

Chapter 25
Common Medications

Hank Pizer, PA-C; and Rein Tideiksaar, PA, PhD

The following tables list medications that are commonly prescribed for or purchased over the counter by people over fifty-five. These listings are not designed to replace the counseling provided by your medical care giver, but are to be used as a resource for additional information about medications. Nor are the data in these tables exhaustive: do not assume that, because your favorite remedy is not listed, it will not interact with other drugs or cause adverse effects. *Always* advise your medical care giver about *any* medication (including OTC) that you are taking before being treated.

The tables are split into listings for prescription and over-the-counter drugs and are divided into six categories. The first category lists the condition to be treated and/or the drug family to which a particular drug belongs. The second column lists the generic name of the drug, plus some (but not all) commonly prescribed or purchased brand names. The third column contains commonly occurring side effects. These are typical, often unavoidable reactions that many people have to a particular drug. Although usually not very dangerous, you should always report these side effects to your medical provider. The fourth column describes adverse effects that appear to be connected to taking that drug. These reactions are abnormal and potentially dangerous. They signal an allergy or a malfunction of the drug in your body. Report them immediately to a medical provider. Again, these listings are not exhaustive—you should report any reaction that you think may possibly be connected with a drug to your medical provider. The fifth column lists those substances that have been found to interact with a particular drug. Your medical provider can advise you about the effects of these interactions and can tell you whether using these substances is prohibited or merely requires an adjustment to your dosage schedule. The final column provides precautions you should keep in mind when using a drug.

Prescription Drugs

Condition/Drug Type	Drug	Side Effects	Adverse Effects	Interactions	Precautions
Angina (vasodilator)	nitroglycerin	flushing, throbbing of head, quickened pulse, light-headedness	skin rash, headache, dizziness, fainting, nausea, vomiting	alcohol, antidepressants, propranolol (Inderal), other antihypertensives, many OTC medications for allergies, colds, and coughs (consult your medical provider before using such medication)	If chest pain is not relieved within 5 minutes, call your medical provider. Keep tablets in their container to preserve potency. Avoid shaking the bottle. Use only fresh tablets.
Anxiety (tranquilizers)	chlordiazepoxide (Librium)	drowsiness, lethargy, unsteadiness	dizziness, fainting, blurred vision, double vision, slurred speech, nausea, vivid dreaming, rashes, jaundice, susceptibility to infection, unusual bleeding or bruising, excitement, rage, parkinsonism, depression, impaired bladder control, constipation	alcohol, sunshine, sedatives, other tranquilizers, antidepressants, antihypertensives, anticonvulsants, Coumadin	Can produce psychological or physical dependence. Do not discontinue dosage abruptly. Can impair mental alertness—avoid driving and hazardous activities.
	diazepam (Valium)	drowsiness, lethargy, unsteadiness	rash, dizziness, fainting, blurred vision, double vision, slurred speech, nausea, jaundice, susceptibility to infection, eye pain, depression, agitation, rage, impaired bladder control, constipation	alcohol, sedatives, other tranquilizers, antidepressants, antihypertensives, anticonvulsants, Coumadin	Can produce psychological or physical dependence. Do not discontinue dosage abruptly. Can impair mental alertness—avoid driving and hazardous activities.
	lorazepam (Ativan)	drowsiness, lethargy, unsteadiness	dizziness, blurred vision, headaches, nausea, indigestion, excessive dreaming, sweating, agitation, depression, impaired bladder control, constipation	alcohol, antihistamines, sedatives, other tranquilizers, antidepressants	Can produce psychological or physical dependence. Do not discontinue dosage abruptly. Can impair mental alertness—avoid driving and hazardous activities

Blood-Clotting Disorders (anticoagulants)	warfarin (Coumadin)	increased tendency to bleed	rash, hives, hair loss, fever, nausea, vomiting, diarrhea, excessive bleeding or bruising	alcohol, aspirin, acetaminophen (e.g., Tylenol), antacids, vitamin C (in large doses), phenylpropanolamine (in OTC antihistamines, e.g., Allerest, Contac, Sinutab, Triaminic), tranquilizers, sedatives, barbiturates, antidepressants, antibiotics, insulin, oral antidiabetics, cortisones, estrogens, digitalis, thyroid preparations, reserpine (e.g., Serpasil), guanethidine (e.g., Ismelin), methyldopa (e.g., Aldomet), furosemide (Lasix), phenytoin (e.g., Dilantin), griseofulvin, cimetidine (Tagamet)	Always carry identification that you take anticoagulant medication. Consult your medical provider before beginning any new prescription or OTC drug. Report any illness that causes fever, vomiting, or diarrhea, as these may affect dosage of anticoagulants. See also Chapter 24, *Drug Guide, Anticoagulants.*
Depression (antidepressants)	amitriptyline (Elavil)	drowsiness, blurred vision, dry mouth, constipation, impaired urination	rash, hives, swelling of face or tongue, nausea, indigestion, mouth irritation, peculiar taste, headache, dizziness, weakness, fainting, unsteadiness, tremors, confusion, heart palpitation, agitation, numbness or tingling in extremities, parkinsonism	alcohol, sunshine, antihistamines, sedatives, tranquilizers, amphetamines, levodopa (e.g., Dopar), Coumadin, clonidine (e.g., Catapres), guanethidine (e.g., Ismelin), thiazide diuretics (e.g., HydroDIURIL), other antihypertensives, phenytoins (e.g., Dilantin), thyroid preparations	Do not discontinue dosage abruptly. Can impair mental alertness—avoid driving and hazardous activities.

(*continued*)

Condition/Drug Type	Drug	Side Effects	Adverse Effects	Interactions	Precautions
Depression (antidepressants) *(continued)*	doxepin (Sinequan)	drowsiness, blurred vision, dry mouth, constipation, impaired urination	rash, hives, swelling of face or tongue, nausea, indigestion, mouth irritation, peculiar taste, headache, dizziness, weakness, fainting, unsteadiness, tremors, confusion, heart palpitations, agitation, numbness or tingling in extremities, parkinsonism	alcohol, sunshine, antihistamines, sedatives, tranquilizers, amphetamines, levodopa (e.g., Dopar), Coumadin, clonidine (e.g., Catapres), thiazide diuretics (e.g., HydroDIURIL), phenytoin (e.g., Dilantin), thyroid preparations	Do not discontinue dosage abruptly. Can impair mental alertness—avoid driving and hazardous activities.
	imipramine (Tofranil)	drowsiness, blurred vision, dry mouth, constipation, impaired urination	rash, hives, swelling of face or tongue, nausea, indigestion, mouth irritation, peculiar taste, headache, dizziness, weakness, fainting, unsteadiness, tremors, confusion, heart palpitations, agitation, numbness or tingling in extremities, parkinsonism	alcohol, sunshine, antihistamines, sedatives, tranquilizers, amphetamines, levodopa (e.g., Dopar), Coumadin, clonidine (e.g., Catapres), guanethidine (e.g., Ismelin), thiazide diuretics (e.g., HydroDIURIL), other antihypertensives, phenytoin (e.g., Dilantin), thyroid preparations	Do not discontinue dosage abruptly. Can impair mental alertness—avoid driving and hazardous activity.
Diabetes (oral antidiabetics)	acetohexamide (Dymelor)	none	rash, headache, ringing in the ears, indigestion, heartburn, nausea, diarrhea, jaundice, fatigue, weakness, confusion	alcohol, sunshine, aspirin, niacin supplements, sedatives, Coumadin, cortisone, estrogen, propranolol (Inderal), furosemide (Lasix), thiazide diuretics (e.g., HydroDIURIL), thyroid preparations	This drug is not a substitute for a properly prescribed diabetic diet. Periodic checkups are necessary to monitor the continued effectiveness of this drug. Use caution when exercising. Be able to recognize symptoms of a hypoglycemic reaction. Report acute infections, injuries,

					and any illness that causes vomiting or diarrhea.
	chlorpropamide (Diabinese)	none	rash, headache, ringing in the ears, indigestion, heartburn, nausea, diarrhea, jaundice, fatigue, weakness, confusion	alcohol, sunshine, aspirin, niacin supplements, sedatives, Coumadin, cortisone, estrogen, propranolol (Inderal), furosemide (Lasix), thiazide diuretics (e.g., HydroDIURIL), thyroid preparations	This drug is not a substitute for a properly prescribed diabetic diet. Periodic checkups are necessary to monitor the continued effectiveness of this drug. Use caution when exercising. Be able to recognize the symptoms of a hypoglycemic reaction. Report acute infections, injuries, and any illness that causes vomiting or diarrhea.
	tolazamide (Tolinase)	none	rash, headache, ringing in the ears, indigestion, heartburn, nausea, diarrhea, jaundice, fatigue, weakness, confusion	alcohol, sunshine, aspirin, niacin supplements, sedatives, Coumadin, cortisone, estrogen, propranolol (Inderal), furosemide (Lasix), thiazide diuretics (e.g., HydroDIURIL), thyroid preparations	This drug is not a substitute for a properly prescribed diabetic diet. Periodic checkups are necessary to monitor the continued effectiveness of this drug. Use caution when exercising. Be able to recognize the symptoms of a hypoglycemic reaction. Report acute infections, injury, and any illness that causes vomiting or diarrhea.

(*continued*)

Condition/Drug Type	Drug	Side Effects	Adverse Effects	Interactions	Precautions
Diabetes (oral antidiabetics) *(continued)*	tolbutamide (Orinase)	none	rash, headache, ringing in the ears, indigestion, heartburn, nausea, diarrhea, jaundice, fatigue, weakness, confusion	alcohol, sunshine, aspirin, niacin supplements, sedatives, Coumadin, cortisone, estrogen, propranolol (Inderal), furosemide (Lasix), thiazide diuretics (e.g., HydroDIURIL), thyroid preparations	This drug is not a substitute for a properly prescribed diabetic diet. Periodic checkups are necessary to monitor the continued effectiveness of this drug. Use caution when exercising. Be able to recognize the symptoms of a hypoglycemic reaction. Report acute illness, injury, and any illness that causes vomiting or diarrhea.
Estrogen Replacement (estrogens)	estrogen (Premarin)	fluid retention, weight gain, susceptibility to yeast (monilia) infection	rash, nausea, vomiting, indigestion, bloating, migraine, speech disturbances, vision difficulties, hearing problems, vertigo, weakness, angina, leg pains, increased blood pressure	nicotine, sunshine, oral antidiabetics, Coumadin	This drug has been linked with uterine cancer; consult your medical provider for advice if you have personal or family history of cancer.
Heart Failure (digitalis)	digoxin, digitoxin	sensitivity in male breast tissue	rash, hives, drowiness, lethargy, vision problems, confusion, disorientation, reduced appetite, nausea, vomiting, diarrhea	nicotine, caffeine, antacids, laxatives, epinephrine (in certain OTC nasal sprays), cortisone, diuretics, reserpine (e.g., Serpasil), guanethidine (e.g., Ismelin), propranolol (Inderal), phenytoin (e.g., Dilantin), thyroid preparations	Always carry identification that you take digitalis medication. Adhere strictly to prescribed dosage; do not discontinue dosage without consulting a medical provider. Report any illness that causes vomiting, diarrhea, dehydration, or jaundice.

Hypertension (antihypertensives, diuretics, thiazide diuretics)	clonidine (Catapres)	drowsiness, dry nose and mouth, constipation, light-headedness	rash, hives, swelling, dizziness, depression, insomnia, nightmares, fainting, nausea, vomiting, dryness and burning in eyes	alcohol, antihistamines, sedatives, tranquilizers, antidepressants, thiazide diuretics (e.g., HydroDIURIL), other antihypertensives	Do not discontinue dosage abruptly—severe or fatal reaction may result. Can cause drowsiness—avoid driving and hazardous activities. Use caution in cold weather. Report any illness that causes vomiting.
	furosemide (Lasix)	light-headedness, muscle weakness and cramping	rash, hives, nausea, vomiting, diarrhea, dizziness, blurred vision, fatigue, fever, sore throat	licorice, alcohol, aspirin, sedatives, antidepressants, oral antidiabetics, insulin, Coumadin, gout medications, thiazide diuretics (e.g., HydroDIURIL), digitalis, other antihypertensives	Avoid activities and climates that cause excessive perspiration. Report any illness that causes vomiting or diarrhea. This drug decreases potassium levels in the body; you may wish to add foods with high potassium content to your diet.
	guanethidine (Ismelin)	light-headedness, dizziness, weakness, fainting, blurred vision, nasal congestion, dry mouth, water retention	rash, hair loss, drowsiness, lethargy, indigestion, nausea, vomiting, diarrhea, muscular ache, impaired ejaculation, ulcer	carbonated beverages, alcohol, nicotine, antihistamines, amphetamines, insulin, Coumadin, Elavil, Tofranil, (not Sinequan), digitalis, reserpine (e.g., Serpasil), thiazide diuretics (e.g., HydroDIURIL), other antihypertensives	Arising suddenly from a sitting or lying position may cause dizziness, light-headedness, and fainting. Can impair mental alertness—use caution when driving or engaging in hazardous activities. Avoid hot weather and overheated environments if possible.

(continued)

Condition/Drug Type	Drug	Side Effects	Adverse Effects	Interactions	Precautions
Hypertension (antihypertensives, diuretics, thiazide diuretics) *(continued)*	hydralazine (Apresoline)	light-headedness, nasal congestion, constipation, difficult urination	rash, hives, fever, headache, dizziness, heart palpitation, flushing, reduced appetite, nausea, vomiting, diarrhea, tremors, muscle cramps, angina, fainting, numbness or tingling of extremities	alcohol, nicotine, amphetamines, antidepressants, diuretics (e.g., Aldactone, Lasix, Dyrenium, HydroDIURIL, etc.)	Use caution in cold weather; cold may cause angina. Heavy exercise may also cause angina.
	hydrochlorothiazide (HydroDIURIL)	muscle weakness, light-headedness, cramps	rash, hives, reduced appetite, indigestion, nausea, vomiting, diarrhea, headache, dizziness, yellow vision, blurred vision, fatigue, weakness, jaundice, abdominal pain, fever	licorice, alcohol, sunshine, barbiturates, antidepressants, oral antidiabetics, insulin, gout medications, cortisone, digitalis, other antihypertensives	Avoid activities and climates that cause excessive perspiration. Report any illness that causes vomiting or diarrhea. This drug decreases potassium levels in the body; you may wish to add foods with high potassium content to your diet.
	methyldopa (Aldomet)	drowsiness, lethargy, weakness, light-headedness, nasal stuffiness, dry mouth	rash, muscle discomfort, headache, dizziness, nausea, vomiting, diarrhea, water retention, weight gain, fever, fainting, parkinsonism, depression	alcohol, amphetamines, antidepressants, levodopa (e.g., Dopar), thiazide diuretics (e.g., HydroDIURIL), other antihypertensives, Coumadin	Can cause drowsiness—avoid driving and hazardous activities. Use caution when exercising.
	prazosin (Minipress)	light-headedness	headache, dizziness, drowsiness, weakness, restlessness, depression, blurred vision, ringing in the ears, nasal congestion, dry mouth, palpitation, shortness of breath, nausea, vomiting, diarrhea,	alcohol, nicotine, amphetamines, nitroglycerin, amitriptyline (e.g., Elavil), other antihypertensives	Follow dosage instructions exactly. Exercise caution in cold weather; cold may cause angina. Use caution when exercising; heavy exertion may cause angina.

			urinary frequency, angina, fluid retention		
	propranolol (Inderal)	lethargy, cold hands and feet, light-headedness	rash, hair loss, fever, reduced appetite, nausea, vomiting, diarrhea, insomnia, vivid dreaming, asthma, depression, fainting	alcohol, nicotine, aspirin, antihistamines, barbiturates, oral antidiabetics, insulin, cortisone, digitalis, reserpine (e.g., Serpasil), phenytoin (e.g., Dilantin), Coumadin, other antihypertensives	Do not discontinue this drug abruptly—severe or fatal reaction may occur. Carry identification that you are taking this drug. Can cause drowsiness—use caution when driving or engaging in hazardous activities. Use caution in cold weather. Report any illness that causes vomiting.
	reserpine (Serpasil)	drowsiness, lethargy, red eye, nasal stuffiness, dry mouth, hunger, indigestion, diarrhea, water retention	rash, bruising, nausea, vomiting, headache, dizziness, nasal congestion, depression, parkinsonism, nosebleeds, ulcers, impaired sex drive	highly spiced foods, carbonated beverages, alcohol, aspirin, antihistamines, sedatives, tranquilizers, Coumadin, levodopa (e.g., Dopar), digitalis, propranolol (Inderal), other antihypertensives, anticonvulsants	This drug has been linked to cancer in laboratory animals—consult your medical provider for advice on its use if you have personal or family history of cancer. Can impair mental alertness—avoid driving and hazardous activities.
	spironolactone (Aldactone)	none	rash, headache, drowsiness, lethargy, confusion, indigestion, nausea, vomiting, diarrhea, ulcers	aspirin, triamterene (e.g., Dyrenium), other antihypertensives, Coumadin	Do not take potassium supplements with this drug.
	triamterene (Dyrenium)	blue urine	rash, nausea, vomiting, diarrhea, dry mouth, headache, weakness, dizziness	sunshine, oral antidiabetics, digitalis, spironolactone (e.g., Aldactone), other antihypertensives	Do not take potassium supplements with this drug. Do not discontinue dosage abruptly.

(continued)

Condition/Drug Type	Drug	Side Effects	Adverse Effects	Interactions	Precautions
Infection (antibiotics)	ampicillin	none	rash, irritation of mouth and tongue, nausea, vomiting, diarrhea, itching in genital and anal regions	antacids, erythromycin, tetracycline	Most effective if taken 1 hour before or 2 hours after eating. Take full dosage as your medical provider prescribes; do not discontinue dosage just because symptoms disappear.
	erythromycin	none	rash, hives, nausea, vomiting, diarrhea, itching in anal and genital regions	bronchodilators, ampicillin	Most effective if taken 1 hour before or 2 hours after eating. Take full dosage as your medical provider prescribes; do not discontinue dosage just because symptoms disappear.
	tetracycline	yeast infections	rash, photosensitivity, loss of appetite, nausea, vomiting, diarrhea, irritation of tongue and mouth, sore throat, asthma, fever, swollen joints, bleeding, itching in anal and genital regions	dairy products, sunshine, antacids, iron and mineral supplements, Coumadin, lithium	Most effective if taken 1 hour before or 2 hours after eating.
Inflammation (cortisone)	prednisone	fluid retention, weight gain, sweating, increased appetite, susceptibility to infection	headache, dizziness, insomnia, indigestion, muscle cramping and weakness, emotional disturbance, ulcer, high blood pressure, bone thinning (osteoporosis), cataracts	nicotine, aspirin, antihistamines, barbiturates, sedatives, stimulants, insulin, oral antidiabetics, Coumadin, digitalis, thiazide diuretics (e.g., HydroDIURIL), propranolol (Inderal), phenytoin (e.g., Dilantin)	Can cause functional dependence (body relies on the drug to perform normally). Do not discontinue dosage abruptly. Report your use of this drug when getting any kind of medical treatment for at least 2 years after you stop taking it.

					Report any infections, acute illnesses, or injury. Carry identification that you take this drug. Vaccination procedures should be used cautiously; you should, with medical provider's advice, discontinue before getting measles, smallpox, rabies, and yellow fever vaccinations.
Insomnia (sedatives)	chloral hydrate (Noctec)	light-headedness, unsteadiness, weakness	rash, indigestion, nausea, heartburn, vomiting, nightmares, dizziness, confusion, loss of bladder control, constipation	alcohol, antihistamines, tranquilizers, other sedatives, Coumadin, cortisone	Can produce psychological or physical dependence. Do not discontinue dosage abruptly. Can impair mental alertness—avoid driving and hazardous activities.
	flurazepam (Dalmane)	drowsiness, lethargy, unsteadiness	rash, burning eyes, dizziness, light-headedness, staggering, blurred vision, slurred speech, headache, nausea, indigestion, confusion, loss of bladder control, constipation	alcohol, anticonvulsants, tranquilizers, other sedatives	May produce psychological or physical dependence if used in large doses over extended periods. Can impair mental alertness—avoid driving and hazardous activities.

(continued)

Condition/Drug Type	Drug	Side Effects	Adverse Effects	Interactions	Precautions
Parkinsonism (anti-Parkinsonism)	amantadine (Symmetrel)	light-headedness, dizziness, weakness, faintness, dry mouth, reddish-blue discoloration of legs and feet	rash, headache, nervousness, irritability, poor concentration, dizziness, insomnia, nightmares, unsteadiness, visual disturbance, slurred speech, loss of appetite, nausea, vomiting, constipation, confusion, depression, impaired urination, urine retention	alcohol, levodopa, amphetamines	Adhere strictly to prescribed dosage; do not discontinue dosage abruptly. Periodic checkups are necessary to monitor the continued effectiveness of this drug. May increase susceptibility to rubella (German measles). Can impair judgment—avoid driving and hazardous activities. Use with caution in cold.
	benztropin (Cogentin)	nervousness, blurred vision, dry mouth, constipation	rash, drowsiness, dizziness, headache, nausea, vomiting, urinary hesitancy, confusion, nightmares	antihistamines, tranquilizers, antidepressants, levodopa (e.g., Dopar), cortisone	Do not discontinue dosage suddenly. Can cause drowsiness—avoid driving and hazardous activities. Use with caution in hot environments, as this drug may reduce sweating and cause heat stroke.
	levodopa (Dopar, Larodopa)	fatigue, lethargy, light-headedness, pink-to-red urine	rash, reduced appetite, nausea, vomiting, headache, dizziness, faintness, unsteadiness, blurred vision, palpitation, body odor, depression, agitation, confusion, ulcer, sore throat, fever, involuntary movement	vitamin B_6, foods containing vitamin B_6, methyldopa (e.g., Aldomet), reserpine (e.g., Serpasil), other anti-Parkinson drugs	Avoid excessive and hurried activity. May cause fainting. See also Chapter 19, *The Nervous System.*
	levodopa/carbidopa (Sinemet)	same as levodopa	same as levodopa	same as levodopa EXCEPT does not react with vitamin B_6	Same as levodopa.

	trihexylphenidyl (Artane)	nervousness, blurred vision, dry mouth, constipation	rash, drowsiness, dizziness, headache, nausea, vomiting, urinary hesitancy, confusion, nightmares	antihistamines, tranquilizers, antidepressants, levodopa (e.g., Dopar), cortisone	Do not discontinue dosage suddenly. Can cause drowsiness—avoid driving and hazardous activities. Use with caution in hot environments as this drug may reduce sweating and cause heat stroke.
Respiratory Conditions (bronchodilators)	theophyllines (Quibron, Theodar, Elixophyllin, Slo-phyllin, Theolair)	nervousness, insomnia	rash, stomach irritation, nausea, vomiting, diarrhea, headache, dizziness, palpitations, fluid retention	epinephrine (in some OTC nasal sprays), gout medication, lithium, propranolol (Inderal), furosemide (Lasix), reserpine (e.g., Serpasil), erythromycin, chlordiazepoxide (e.g., Librium), antiasthma preparations	None beyond standard precautions for any drug.

Over-the-Counter Drugs

Drug Type	Drug	Side Effects	Adverse Effects	Interactions	Precautions
Analgesics (painkillers)	acetaminophen (Datril, Tylenol, Nyquil, Bromo-Seltzer, many others)	none	rash, hives, impaired concentration, swelling of vocal cords, abnormal bruising or bleeding	oral anticoagulants (Coumadin)	Use with caution if you have bronchial asthma and are allergic to aspirin, or if you have impaired liver or kidney function.

(continued)

Drug Type	Drug	Side Effects	Adverse Effects	Interactions	Precautions
Analgesics (painkillers) *(continued)*	aspirin (Anacin, Ascriptin, Arthritis Pain Formula, Alka-Seltzer, Bayer, Bufferin, Dristan, Empirin, Excedrin, Vanquish, numerous other OTC drugs for many ailments)	none	rash, hives, nasal discharge, stomach irritation, heartburn, nausea, vomiting, asthma, unusual bruising, ulcer, fatigue, weakness, sore throat, jaundice, irritability, ringing in the ears, deafness, loss of appetite, gray-to-black stools	alcohol, antacids, vitamin C (in large doses), penicillins (e.g., ampicillin), insulin, oral antidiabetics, cortisone, spironolactone (e.g., Aldactone), furosemide (Lasix), propranolol (Inderal), reserpine (e.g., Serpasil), phenytoin (e.g., Dilantin), Coumadin	Can cause excessive, "silent" bleeding in stomach lining; drink a full glass of water with dose to reduce irritation. May cause psychological dependence. Discontinue use at least 1 week prior to surgery. Do not use if you have an active peptic ulcer. Use with caution if you have gout. Remember, aspirin is a drug. See also Chapter 24, *Drug Guide, Aspirin.*
Antacids	sodium bicarbonate (Alka-Seltzer, Brioschi, Bromo-Seltzer, Rolaids)	belching, weight gain	high blood pressure, fluid retention, urinary tract infections, constipation, diarrhea	vitamin A and C, iron supplements, Coumadin, digitalis, penicillins (e.g., ampicillin), tetracycline	These antacids have a high sodium content and so should be limited to occasional use by healthy individuals. They should not be taken by those with hypertension.
	aluminum hydroxide (Amphojel, Di-Gel, Maalox, Mylanta, Gelusil, Rolaids, Camalox, Ducon)	constipation	nausea, vomiting, intestinal obstruction	vitamin A and C, iron supplements, Coumadin, digitalis, penicillins (e.g., ampicillin), tetracycline, pseudoephedrine (e.g., Sudafed and other OTC cold remedies)	May cause osteomalacia. Do not use regularly for more than 2 weeks without advice from medical provider. Use with caution if you have hypertension, any disorder that causes fluid retention, chronic constipation or diarrhea, or a history of kidney disease or congestive heart failure.

	calcium carbonate (Titralac, Tums, Camalox, Ducon)	belching, constipation	none	vitamin A and C, iron supplements, Coumadin, digitalis, penicillins (e.g., ampicillin), tetracycline.	In large doses, can cause excessive calcium levels in the body. Can also cause kidney stones. Do not use regularly for more than 2 weeks without advice from medical provider. Use with caution if you have hypertension, any disorder that causes fluid retention, chronic constipation or diarrhea, or a history of kidney disease or congestive heart failure.
	magnesium hydroxide (milk of magnesia, Di-Gel, Maalox, Mylanta, Camalox, Ducon)	diarrhea	none	vitamin A and C, iron supplements, Coumadin, digitalis, penicillins (e.g., ampicillin), tetracycline	May cause toxic effect on nervous system in those with decreased kidney function. Do not use regularly for more than 2 weeks without advice from medical provider. Use with caution if you have hypertension, any disorder that causes fluid retention, chronic constipation or diarrhea, or a history of kidney disease or congestive heart failure.
Bronchodilators	pseudoephedrine (Co-Tylenol, Novahistine, Sudafed)	nervousness, insomnia	rash, headache, dizziness, palpitation, tremors, angina	epinephrine, antidepressants, digitalis, guanethidine (e.g., Ismelin), other antihypertensives	Use with caution if you have hypertension, heart disease, or hyperthyroidism.

(continued)

Drug Type	Drug	Side Effects	Adverse Effects	Interactions	Precautions
Bronchodilators *(continued)*	ephedrine (Bronkaid tablets, Nyquil)	nervousness, insomnia	headache, dizziness, chest discomfort, sweating, nausea, vomiting, difficult urination, angina	epinephrine, antidepressants, digitalis, guanethidine (e.g., Ismelin), other antihypertensives	Use with caution if you have hypertension, heart disease, hyperthyroidism, diabetes. You can develop a tolerance for this drug, requiring more frequent use.
	epinephrine (Bronkaid mist, Primatene tablets and mist)	restlessness, anxiety, headache, tremor, palpitation, cold hands and feet, dry mouth and throat	rash, weakness, dizziness, pallor, angina, impaired urination in men	alcohol, cocaine, ephedrine, antidepressants, oral antidiabetics, insulin, digitalis, guanethidine (e.g., Ismelin), reserpine (e.g., Serpasil), propranolol (Inderal), thyroid preparations	Do not use if you have glaucoma or have recently suffered a stroke or heart attack. Use with extreme caution if you have hypertension, heart disease, diabetes, hyperthyroidism, enlarged prostate, Parkinson's disease, or a history of stroke. Do not increase size or frequency of dosage if drug does not provide relief. Discard all preparations that are discolored (pink, red, brown) or cloudy.
Cold and Allergy Medications (antihistamines and decongestants)	chlorpheniramine (antihistamine—A.R.M., Alka-Seltzer Plus, Allerest, Chlor-Trimeton, Comtrex, Contac, Coricidin, Co-Tylenol, Dristan, Novahistine, Sinarest, Sine-Off, Sinutab, Triaminic	drowsiness; weakness; dry nose, mouth, and throat	rash, headache, nervousness, dizziness, double vision, blurred vision, ringing in the ears, tremor, reduced appetite, heartburn, nausea, vomiting, diarrhea, impaired urination in men	alcohol, sedatives, tranquilizers, Coumadin	Can impair mental alertness—avoid driving and hazardous activities. Avoid prolonged, continuous use. Use with caution if you have glaucoma.

	phenylpropanolamine (decongestant—Allerest, Contac, Sinutab, Triaminic, A.R.M., Comtrex, Coricidin Cough Syrup, Novahistine, Sinarest, Sine-Aid, Sine-Off, Sucrets, Formula 44-D)	nervousness, insomnia	headache, dizziness, nausea, vomiting, high blood pressure, disturbed heart rhythm, angina	epinephrine, antidepressants, digitalis, guanethidine (e.g., Ismelin), other antihypertensives	Do not exceed recommended dosage. Use with caution if you have hypertension, heart disease, or hyperthyroidism.
Cough Medications (expectorants and suppressants)	dextromethorphan (suppressant—Romilar, Robitussin, St. Joseph Cough Formula, Cheracol-D, Dristan Cough Formula, Formula 44-D, Hold Cough Suppressant, Nyquil, Vicks Cough Syrup, Chloraseptic Lozenges, Comtrex, Coricidin, Sucrets)	drowsiness	rash, dizziness, nausea, indigestion, constipation, unsteadiness	none—but see note under Precautions	Use with caution if you have bronchial asthma. May cause psychological dependence. Many of these drugs also contain alcohol—do not use if taking a medication that interacts with alcohol.
	guaifenisin (expectorant—Robitussin, Cheracol, Chlor-Trimeton, Dristan Cough Formula, Formula 44-D, Vicks Cough Syrup, Novahistine Cough Formula, Triaminic Expectorant)	none	rash, drowsiness, nausea, indigestion	Coumadin	Drink 3 to 4 pints (1½ to 2 l) of fluid per day to ensure drug's effectiveness. Many of these drugs have high sugar contents—use with caution if you are diabetic.

The Contributors

Donald Abrams, RPA: Albany Hudson Valley Physician Assistant Program; Field Aidman, U.S. Army; Vietnam veteran; Staff Sergent, Massachusetts Army National Guard; Registered Physician Assistant.

Blair Ardman, MD: MD, Thomas Jefferson University, College of Medicine, Philadelphia; Fellowship, Department of Hematology and Oncology, Tufts College of Medicine, New England Medical Center.

Betty Barry: B.S., Salem State College, Salem, MA; Chief Photographer, Boston Seniority, a 35,000-circulation newspaper for seniors, published by the mayor's office, Boston; Free lance; exhibits: *Seniors in the City; Shades of Grey in Black and White.*

Marcia Bowling, MD: MD, University of Massachusetts, Worcester; Residency, University of Massachusetts, Department of Obstetrics and Gynecology; Assistant in Gynecology, Massachusetts General Hospital, Boston; Clinical Fellow in Gynecologic Oncology, Harvard Medical School, Cambridge, MA; Junior Fellow, American College of Obstetrics and Gynecology.

Peggy Clark: BA, Smith College, Northampton, MA; MS, Art Education, Massachusetts College of Art, Boston; Art Specialist, Newton Public Schools; Free-lance medical illustrator.

John Coblyn, MD: MD, Johns Hopkins University, Baltimore; Residency, Stanford University Hospital, Stanford, CA; Research Fellow in Rheumatology, Robert Breck Brigham Hospital, Boston; Assistant Professor of Medicine, Harvard Medical School, Cambridge, MA; Associate Physician, Department of Rheumatology and Immunology, Brigham and Women's Hospital, Boston.

Christopher H. Fanta, MD: MD, Harvard University School of Medicine, Cambridge, MA; Medical Residency, Peter Bent Brigham Hospital, Boston; Fellowship in Pulmonary Medicine, Peter Bent Brigham Hospital; Instructor in Medicine, Harvard Medical School; Junior Associate in Medicine, Brigham and Women's Hospital, Boston; Head of Pulmonary Consultation Service, Brigham and Women's Hospital.

Michael L. Glenn, MD: MD, Columbia College of Physicians and Surgeons, New York; Internship, Bronx Municipal Hospital, New York; Residency, New York State Psychiatric Institute; Instructor of Social Medical Sciences, Boston University, School of Medicine, Boston; Board of Directors, Kantor Family Institute, Cambridge, MA; Private practice, Everett, MA.

Jerilou Hammett: BA, MS, Hofstra University, Hempstead, NY; Director of Consumer Education, State of New Mexico, Office of the Attorney General; Serves on: New Mexico Bar Committee on Senior Citizens and the Law, Lt. Governor's Task Force on Medigap Insurance, New Mexico Advisory Committee for Energy Training Grants to Senior Citizens.

Mark Huberman, MD: MD, Tufts School of Medicine, Medford, MA; Clinical Associate in Oncology, National Cancer Institute; Fellowship in Hematology, Boston University, Boston; Member American Boards of Internal Medicine, American Society of Clinical Oncology; Instructor in Medicine, Harvard Medical School, Cambridge, MA; Staff Oncologist, New England Deaconess Hospital, Boston.

Amy Jacobsen, PA-C: BS cum laude, University of Massachusetts, Amherst; George Washington University, Physician Assistant Program, Washington, DC; Health Professionals for Social Responsibility; Vice-President, Massachusetts Association of Physician Assistants; Member Gray Panthers; Private practice, Greenfield, MA; Certified Physician Assistant.

C. William Kaiser, MD: MD, Tufts School of Medicine, Medford, MA; Internship, Charity Hospital, New Orleans; Residency, Boston City Hospital, Boston; Chief of Surgery, Veterans Administration Hospital, Manchester, NH; Member American College of Surgeons; Fellow, Royal College of Physicians and Surgeons, Canada.

Peter Lockhart, DDS: DDS, University of North Carolina, School of Dentistry; Postdoctoral Residency, University of Vermont College of Medicine; Assistant Professor of Oral Medicine and Oral Pathology, Harvard School of Dental Medicine, Cambridge, MA; Junior Associate in Surgery (Dentistry), Department of Surgery, Brigham and Women's Hospital, Boston.

Gerry Marcus, RD: BS, University of Maine; MS, Nutrition, Framingham State College, Framingham, MA; Nutrition Project Director, Council of Elders, Boston; Registered Dietician.

Patti Marcus, RPT: BS, Physical Therapy, Sargent College of Allied Health Professions, Boston University, Boston; MEd, Rehabilitation Administration, Northeastern University, Boston; Coordinator of Rehabilitation Services and Director of Physical Therapy, Jewish Memorial Hospital, Boston; Registered Physical Therapist.

Paula McBrine, MD: MD, Loyola University, Chicago; Residency and Fellowship in Hematology and Oncology, Boston Veterans Administration Hospital, Boston; American Boards of Internal Medicine; Board Certified Subspecialty Hematology; Medical Director, Hospice Collaborative, Pondville Hospital, Walpole, MA.

Hank Pizer, PA-C: BA, University of Wisconsin; Albany Hudson Valley Physician Assistant Program; Fenway Community Health Center; Member, American Medical Writer's Association; Author of *The New Birth Control Program, The Post-Partum Book, Coping with a Miscarriage, Guide to the New Medicine;* Past President, Massachusetts Association of Physician Assistants; Certified Physician Assistant.

Stella Young Pizer: BA, MA, Brooklyn College, New York; Postgraduate studies, guidance and counseling, Teacher's College, Columbia University, New York; Guidance counselor, New York City Public Schools; Instructor, Women's Studies Program, Great Neck Public Schools, Long Island, NY.

Neil Robertson, PA-C: Emergency Medical Technician, Mount Auburn Hospital, Boston; Northeastern University Physician Assistant Program, Boston; Project Place Emergency Services; President, Massachusetts

Association of Physician Assistants; Member, Massachusetts Public Health Association, American Public Health Association; Internal and Emergency Medicine, Fallon Clinic, Worcester, MA; Certified Physician Assistant.

Alice Rothchild, MD: MD, Boston University School of Medicine, Boston; Medical internship, Lincoln Hospital, Bronx, NY; Residency, Beth Israel Hospital, Department of Obstetrics and Gynecology, Boston; Urban Woman and Child Health; Clinical Instructor, Department of Obstetrics and Gynecology, Harvard Medical School, Cambridge, MA; American College of Obstetrics and Gynecology; Women's Health Network.

Rhona Selkowitz, RPT: BS, Physical Therapy, University of Pennsylvania; Senior Physical Therapist and Coordinator of Student Education, Jewish Memorial Hospital, Boston; Registered Physical Therapist.

Ann Stewart, RN, NP: BS, MS in Nursing, Boston College, Boston; Nurse Consultant in Internal Medicine, Harvard Community Health Plan, Cambridge, MA; Nursing Education Committee, American Heart Association, Boston Chapter. Registered Nurse, Nurse Practitioner.

Rein Tideiksaar, PA-C, PhD: BA, Hofstra University, Hempstead, NY; BS, SUNY Stony Brook, Stony Brook, NY; Physician Assistant Program, SUNY Stony Brook; PhD, Columbia Pacific University; Coordinator of Geriatric Education, Jewish Institute for Geriatric Care, Representative to White House Conference on Aging; Clinical Assistant Professor of Allied Health, Department of Family Medicine, Health Science Center, SUNY Stony Brook.

Barbara Maloney Turner, RN, NP: BSN, Lowell State College, Lowell, MA; MSN, University of Lowell; Certified Adult Nurse Practitioner with the Urban Medical Group, Boston; Adjunct Clinical Instructor in Gerontological Nursing, University of Lowell.

Lynn Zashin, MD: MD, New York Medical College; Residency, Family Practice, University of Massachusetts Medical Center, Worcester; American Academy of Family Physicians; Board Certification American Academy of Family Physicians; Physicians for Social Responsibility; Clinical Faculty, University of Massachusetts Medical School; Private practice, Greenfield, MA.

Index

Index

About the Author

Hank Pizer works as a physician associate in community health in Boston. He is a graduate of the University of Wisconsin, Madison, and has done postgraduate work at the University of California, Berkeley, and the City University of New York. He has also served as president of the Massachusetts Association for Physician Assistants. A medical writer as well as practitioner, Mr. Pizer is the author of the recently published *Guide to the New Medicine: What Works, What Doesn't*, and coauthor of *The New Birth Control Book, The Post Partum Book,* and *Coping with Miscarriage,* the last of which won an Honorable Mention award from the American Medical Writers' Association in 1981. He firmly believes in making medical information in nontechnical terms easily available to laypeople, so that we can all learn to take better care of our bodies and be more knowledgeable when we use professional medical services.